Intensity Modulated Radiation Therapy

A clinical overview

IPEM–IOP Series in Physics and Engineering in Medicine and Biology

About the Series

Series in Physics and Engineering in Medicine and Biology will allow IPEM to enhance its mission to 'advance physics and engineering applied to medicine and biology for the public good.'

Focusing on key areas including, but not limited to:

- clinical engineering
- diagnostic radiology
- informatics and computing
- magnetic resonance imaging
- nuclear medicine
- physiological measurement
- radiation protection
- radiotherapy
- rehabilitation engineering
- ultrasound and non-ionising radiation.

A number of IPEM–IOP titles are published as part of the EUTEMPE Network Series for Medical Physics Experts.

Intensity Modulated Radiation Therapy

A clinical overview

Indra J Das
Department of Radiation Oncology, Northwestern University Feinberg School of Medicine, Chicago, USA

Nicholas J Sanfilippo
Department of Radiation Oncology, Weill Cornell Medical College, New York, USA

Antonella Fogliata
Department of Radiotherapy, Humanitas Clinical and Research Center IRCCS, Milan-Rozzano, Italy

Luca Cozzi
Department of Radiotherapy, Humanitas Clinical and Research Center IRCCS, Milan-Rozzano, Italy
and
Humanitas University, Milan-Rozzano, Italy

IOP Publishing, Bristol, UK

Multimedia content is available for this book from http://iopscience.iop.org/book/978-0-7503-1335-3.

ISBN 978-0-7503-1335-3 (ebook)
ISBN 978-0-7503-1336-0 (print)
ISBN 978-0-7503-1769-6 (myPrint)
ISBN 978-0-7503-1337-7 (mobi)

DOI 10.1088/978-0-7503-1335-3

Version: 20201201

IOP ebooks

British Library Cataloguing-in-Publication Data: A catalogue record for this book is available from the British Library.

Published by IOP Publishing, wholly owned by The Institute of Physics, London

IOP Publishing, Temple Circus, Temple Way, Bristol, BS1 6HG, UK

US Office: IOP Publishing, Inc., 190 North Independence Mall West, Suite 601, Philadelphia, PA 19106, USA

Dedicated to my late grandfather Jagdev Das, who guided me to learning and education early in my childhood.

&

My love and gratitude to my wife Sununta C Das, son Avanindra C Das, and daughter Anita C Das for their constant support of my pursuits.

—Indra J Das

I dedicate this book to my father, Louis J Sanfilippo, MD, who inspired me to pursue a career in radiation oncology and always gave me the best advice. It has been an honor to follow in his footsteps. Also, to my mother, Ismene Sanfilippo, who has been a constant source of strength in my life. I owe both of them everything.

—Nicholas J Sanfilippo

Dedicated to my parents, who instilled in me the joy of finding the beauty in working for the care of the human beings, and thanks to Professor Jacques Bernier, who I worked with and who encouraged me to approach IMRT in the late 90s. Thanks to my daughters and sons who supported me, and to my husband, who encouraged me on this long journey.

—Antonella Fogliata

Thanks to Antonella who assisted my transformation from particle to medical physics! Without her brilliant brain nothing would have been possible! Thanks to our kids. They had to learn how to manage with their parents too frequently at the hospital (we even breast-fed the first during a linac commissioning in the console room!) or travelling around the world. I hope they will develop some of the passion we put in to our jobs and will gain the same satisfaction from their professional lives as we did.

—Luca Cozzi

Contents

Preface

Nearly two-thirds of all radiation treatments currently being delivered use modulated beam therapies due to the overwhelming acceptance of this unique technology that has matured over time. These treatments have provided significant positive clinical responses in every disease site as indicated by the outcomes data. The phrase intensity modulated radiation therapy (IMRT) is used in a generic way applied to all forms of modulated beam delivery, and in a broader sense it applies to both IMRT and volumetric modulated arc therapy (VMAT).

The genesis of this book started in late 2016 through a discussion with Jessica Fricchione (the book editor of IOP at that time) in New York. We realized that there was a need for a comprehensive book on IMRT that could be used with therapy students, dosimetrists, physicists, medical residents and radiation professionals. There have been many edited books on IMRT that have focused on how to conduct IMRT and clinical approaches, but in all these books, fundamental aspects have been missing. We chose the name *Intensity Modulated Radiation Therapy: A clinical overview* for this book. Over several years, the book took shape, but our transitions to different institutions posed challenges in solidifying the book.

In February 2019, Antonella Fogliata and Luca Cozzi were contacted to be co-authors. Both of them have vast amounts of expertise in IMRT, especially of the European perspectives and approaches. Graciously, they agreed to participate in this endeavor. During the COVID-19 pandemic, the process slowed down as our efficiency and productivity dropped significantly, even though we had plenty of time at home to write. Finally, we made significant progress to complete this book, and we hope you will enjoy the fruits of our hard work. We have attempted to provide animations to understand the concepts, a lot of figures, and up-to-date references for reading. Nonetheless, we should say that this is not the ultimate book because there are so many aspects of modulation that need further elaboration. There will be many other issues that will arise in the future that may require additional books.

This book is a compilation of the essential concepts of the physics of modulated techniques and processes along with clinical applications. It provides the cumulative knowledge of 30 years of the evolution of this technology and has relevant references for further reading. It is the result of our labor of love to provide the essentials of modulated treatment. We are thankful to Jessica Fricchione who was instrumental in making this book possible by getting it approved at IOP. We are also grateful to IOP for bearing with us and for waiting such a long time for the completion of this book. Thanks also to Sarah Armstrong, Michael Slaughter, and David McDade at IOP who supported us in the journey of writing this book.

Indra J Das, PhD

Nicholas J Sanfilippo, MD

Antonella Fogliata, MSc

Luca Cozzi, PhD

Author biographies

Indra J Das

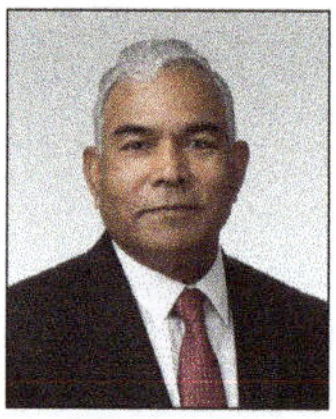

Indra J Das, an Indian born medical physicist, received his initial education (BSc and MSc) from Gorakhpur University and Dip Radiological Physics from Bombay University in India and MS and PhD degrees from USA. He has worked at many academic institutions: University of Massachusetts Medical Center; Fox Chase Cancer Center; University of Pennsylvania; Indiana University School of Medicine; and NYU Langone Medical Center. He is currently Vice Chair, Professor and Director of Medical Physics at Northwestern University Feinberg School of Medicine in Chicago. Dr Das is internationally known in clinical innovations and research contributions in the field of radiation dosimetry, treatment planning, nanoparticles, proton beam, small field, radiochromic film and MR-linac. He is serving or has served on several journal editorial boards including, *International Journal of Radiation Oncology • Biology • Physics*, *Medical Physics*, *British Journal of Radiology*, and *Journal of Radiation Research*.

Nicholas J Sanfilippo

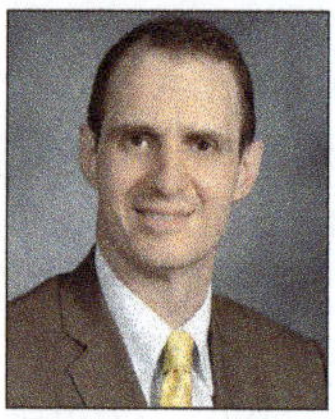

Dr Sanfilippo is a radiation oncologist with special interest in treatment of head and neck, thoracic, cutaneous, and genitourinary malignancies. He received his undergraduate and medical degrees from the University of Virginia and completed his residency training in radiation oncology at the University of Pennsylvania. He then spent an additional year of training in brachytherapy at the Gustave-Roussy Institute in Villejuif, France. Following a short time in private practice, Dr Sanfilippo joined the faculty at New York University School of Medicine where he was a member of the disease management groups in head and neck, genitourinary, and melanoma services. He also served as Clinical Medical Director and later Vice Chairman for Clinical Operations in the Department of Radiation Oncology. He was promoted to Associate Professor of Radiation Oncology in 2014.

Dr Sanfilippo has authored numerous original reports, reviews, and textbook chapters. He has received numerous research grants from both private and public entities including the National Institutes of Health. Dr Sanfilippo joined Weill Cornell Medicine in 2018 as Vice Chairman of the Department of Radiation Oncology, Residency Program Director, and Director of Quality Assurance.

Antonella Fogliata

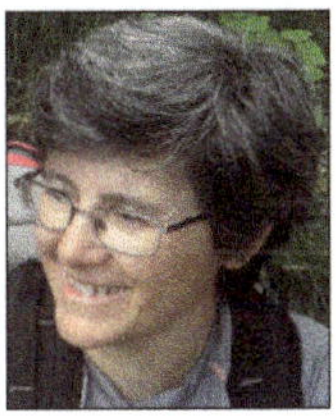

Antonella Fogliata, Italian, graduated at the University of Milan, Italy, in medical physics and specialized at the SSRPM in Switzerland. She spent almost 25 years at the Oncology Institute of Southern Switzerland in Bellinzona as medical physicist, working in the team pivotal for the clinical introduction of IMRT in 1999 and VMAT in 2008; then she moved to the Humanitas Research Hospital in Milan-Rozzano, where she is a research scientist. The main interests in her career have been mostly focused in the pre-clinical investigation of novel treatment technologies and treatment planning modalities for photons and protons, as well as the dose calculation algorithms and all the aspects of treatment quality. Ms Fogliata teaches many courses dedicated to medical physicists and clinicians on the radiotherapy advanced technologies. She serves as associate editor of some journals, including *Physica Medica*.

Luca Cozzi

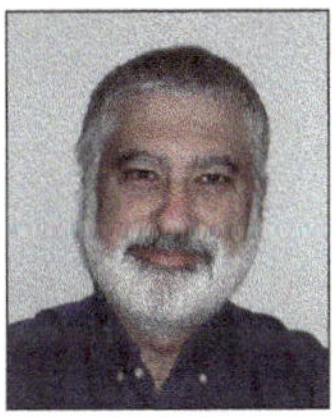

Luca Cozzi, Italian, graduated at the University of Milan in particle physics and did his PhD at CERN on the early simulations for the LHC collider. He moved into the field of Medical Physics and spent his clinical time at the Oncology Institute of Southern Switzerland in Bellinzona (as the head of the physics unit) and at the Humanitas Research Hospital in Rozzano-Milan (as a research scientist). He has acted also as a Privat Docent at the University of Lausanne and as an Adjunct Professor at the Humanitas University. The main interests of Dr Cozzi are focused in the pre-clinical investigation of novel treatment technologies and treatment planning modalities for photons and protons. Dr Cozzi was president of the Swiss Society of Radiobiology and Medical Physics and editorial board member or section editor of several journals including *Radiotherapy and Oncology*, *Radiation Oncology*, *Journal of Applied Medical Physics* and others.

Acronyms

2D	Two-Dimensional
3D	Three-Dimensional
3DCRT	Three-Dimensional Conformal Radiation Therapy
4DCT	Four-Dimensional Computed Tomography
AAA	Anisotropic Analytical Algorithm
AAPM	American Association of Physicists in Medicine
AIP	Average Intensity Projection
ASTRO	American Society of Radiation Oncology
CBCT	Cone-Beam Computed Tomography
CI	Conformity Index
CNN	Convolution Neural Network
CT	Computed Tomography
CTV	Clinical Target Volume
DAO	Direct Aperture Optimization
DNN	Deep Neural Network
DRR	Digitally Reconstructed Radiograph
DSC	Dice Similarity Coefficient
DTA	Distance to Agreement
DVH	Dose Volume Histogram
EPID	Electronic Portal Imaging Device
EPL	Equivalent Path Length
ESTRO	European Society for Radiotherapy and Oncology
EUD	Equivalent Uniform Dose
FFF	Flattening Filter Free
FFT	Fast Fourier Transform
gEUD	Generalized Equivalent Uniform Dose
GPU	Graphics Processing Unit
GTV	Gross Target Volume
HI	Homogeneity Index
HU	Hounsfield Unit
IAEA	International Atomic Energy Agency
ICRU	International Commission on Radiation Units and Measurement
IGRT	Image-Guided Radiation Therapy
IM	Internal Margin
IMAT	Intensity modulated Arc Therapy
IMPT	Intensity Modulated Proton Therapy
IMRT	Intensity Modulated Radiation Therapy
IROC	Imaging and Radiation Oncology Core, Houston
ITV	Internal Target Volume
LBTE	Linear Boltzmann Transport Equation
Linac	Linear Accelerator
MAR	Metal Artifact Reduction
MI	Modulation Index
MIMiC	Multileaf Intensity Modulating Collimator
MIP	Maximum Intensity Projection
MLC	Multi-Leaf Collimator
MR	Magnetic Resonance

MRI	Magnetic Resonance Imaging
MU	Monitor Unit
NSCLC	Non-Small Cell Lung Cancer
NTCP	Normal Tissue Complication Probability
OAR	Organs At Risk
OF	Output Factor
PDD	Percentage Depth Dose
PET	Positron Emission Tomography
PRV	Planning organ at Risk Volume
PSQA	Patient Specific Quality Assurance
PTV	Planning Target Volume
QA	Quality Assurance
QUANTEC	Quantitative Analyses of Normal Tissue Effects in the Clinic
RTOG	Radiation Therapy Oncology Group
SBRT	Stereotactic Body Radiation Therapy
SD	Standard Deviation
SE	Standard error of the mean
SM	Set-up Margin
TAR	Tissue-Air Ratio
TERMA	Total Energy Released per Mass
TPR	Tissue-Phantom Ratio
TPS	Treatment Planning System
TCP	Tumor Control Probability
VMAT	Volumetric Modulated Arc Therapy
WF	Wedge Factor

Chapter 1

Introduction

Radiation oncology has evolved from a traditional two-dimentional (2D) approach to more complex modern treatments. Traditionally, radiation treatment has been performed with radiographic visualization of the anatomical structures. The 2D option started with a simple radiographic approach that used imaging to localize a tumor on a plane. A radiograph in a beam angle is taken to show the projection of the tumor and its location with respect to critical structures, such as organs that would be damaged by the radiation dose for the tumors. The physician chooses the angle for the radiograph that may provide separation between target and normal structures. This has been an iterative process: when an optimum radiograph is visualized, it provides the beam angle for treatment. Figure 1.1 provides a historical view of 2D approaches for treatment planning and indicates corner blocks. These images were rudimentary by today's standard. Figure 1.1 depicts the treatment approach showing anterior/posterior (AP) and lateral view of head and neck patients. A physician with radiographic knowledge blocks the normal structures by using a wax pencil on the radiograph. The original shielding of normal structures was by lead (Pb) blocks. Later the development of more conformal blocks was realized; the blocks required a low melting point high atomic number (Z) alloy. Lipowitz's metal commonly known as Cerrobend is an alloy with a composition of Bi (50%), Pb (26.7%), Sn (13.3%) and Cd (10%). This alloy is unique with a melting point of 70 °C and a density of 9.4 g cm^{-3}, and it provides nearly the same attenuation as Pb. Cerrobend became the choice for custom block making and is still used today.

For 2D treatments, radiographs were acquired using x-ray machines. Physicists realized that an x-ray machine that mimicked treatment was needed to reduce multiple exposures of patients during treatment planning and was termed a 'simulator' [1]. A detailed description of a simulator was published in 1975 by British Institute of Radiology in Special Report 10 [2]. Simulators provided radiographs in any possible angle that a patient could be treated on the treatment unit,

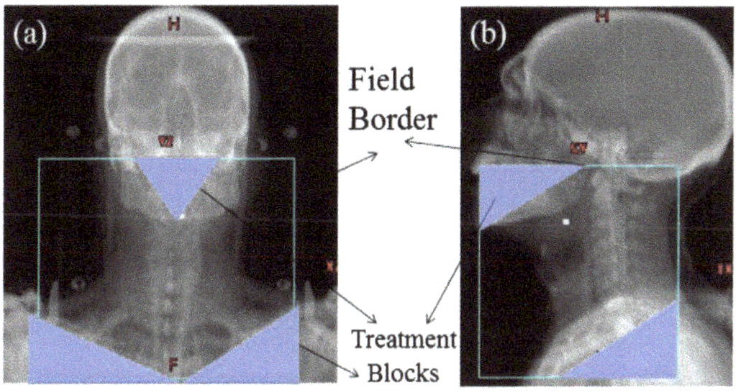

Figure 1.1. Two-dimensional (2D) treatment approach shows; (a) AP and (b) left lateral radiographs. The outer line indicates the field border and blue triangles are conventional Pb blocks placed to block normal structures.

and these revolutionary ideas, which were adopted in the last century, still are used in many parts of the world. Understanding and visualization of tumors from radiographs remained a rudimentary idea, as the depth information was still needed. Since the invention of computed tomography (CT) [3] in 1972, our field has totally changed as we can now see structures on the axial view slice by slice. The application of CT was immediately realized for providing three-dimensional (3D) information. The structures in the body can be further refined and visualized in 3D. By 1980, CT had became an integral part of medicine and the backbone of radiology. For radiation treatment, CT provided many critical aspects of imaging for planning and gave birth to 3D conformal radiation therapy (3DCRT). Within 10 years, *International Journal of Radiation Oncology Biology and Physics* published a special issue that described the innovations in 3D and 3DCRT [4] and contained seminal work with innovative approaches in visualization, 3D rendering, dose volume histograms (DVH), and treatment techniques for many disease sites.

In the same time frame and context, ICRU-50 [5] provided the volume nomenclatures of gross target volume (GTV), clinical target volume (CTV), and planning target volume (PTV). Additionally it provided recommendations for dose specifications such that clinical data could be compared throughout the world. The GTV, CTV, PTV concepts have now become well-established in the alphabet of radiation oncology.

Similar to the original simulator, the idea of a CT-simulator became a reality in 1993 with advances in virtual simulation [6–9]. The CT-simulator has three components: a CT-scanner (hardware), a laser aligning system (hardware) and a virtual simulator (software), and it became an icon of patient care. Details of these innovations can be found in the textbook *A Practical Guide To CT Simulation* [10]. The CT-simulator provided a unique opportunity to use CT data and draw target volumes along with normal structures that could be excluded from treatment fields. Digitally reconstructed radiographs (DRR) [11] became synonymous with traditional radiographs. Such images could be made without exposing patients to radiation again. The DRR could be made from a CT data set from any possible angle, and thus avoiding unnecessary radiation exposure.

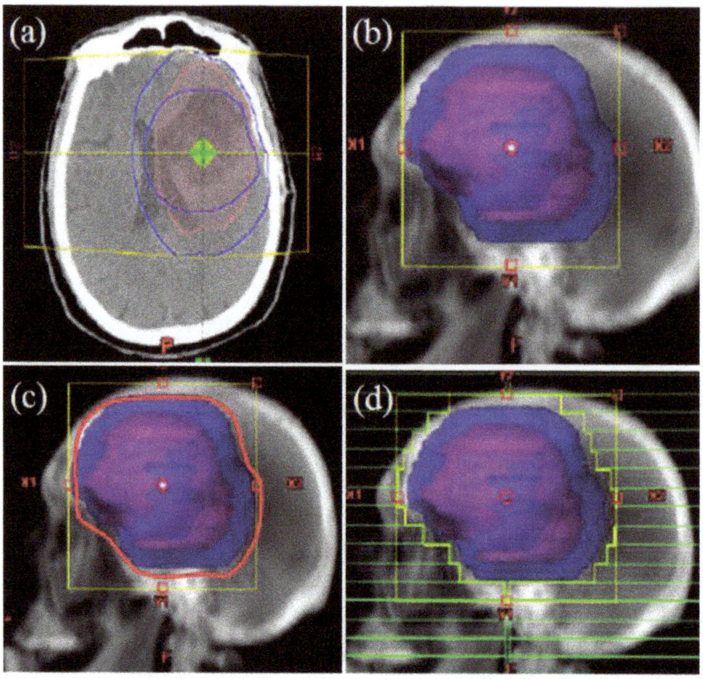

Figure 1.2. Concept of 3DCRT, (a) indicating contours GTV, CTV, PTV on a CT axial slice and treatment fields for a brain tumor, (b) color wash of the structures, (c) conformal block for desired coverage to the tumor and (d) blocks with MLC.

3DCRT relies on DRR to calculate the treatment parameters for conforming the radiation treatment to an irregular-shaped tumor. Figure 1.2 shows the concept of 3DCRT indicating axial as well as lateral views from the reconstructed image mainly known as DRR. Such a rendering has enabled physicians to visualize tumors in any special coordinates and block the normal structures. Additional innovations came with the introduction of multi-leaf collimators which allowed us to shape radiation fields dynamically, as previously Cerrobend blocks had been static and unable to provide beam shaping flexibility. The multi-leaf collimator (MLC) provided a new dimension in the radiation treatment for shaping the treatment fields. Based on the CT datasets, MLC provided ease in designing blocks that can be managed dynamically, which is shown in figure 1.2(c,d) that provides an example of such an approach. Details of MLC can also be found in many references by many vendors [12–25]. The designs of MLCs have been clearly thought through from the process from curved leaves to double focus leaves with each providing unique capabilities and functionality for shipping the fields.

The goal in radiation oncology is to deliver the desired dose to the tumor and spare the normal tissues, also known as organs at risk (OAR), as much as possible. This mantra needs to be followed for every successful therapy. Takahashi [26] in 1965 before the computer era provided an innovative approach to achieve this goal by rotational therapy using pre-MLC blocks. He showed that critical structures

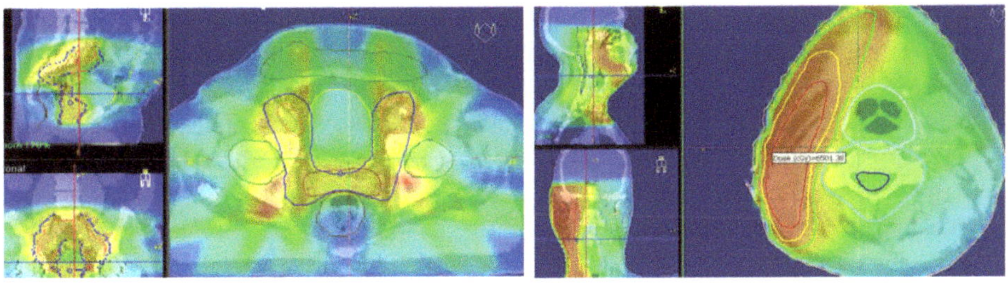

Figure 1.3. IMRT plan of (a) prostate and lymph nodes and (b) head and neck nodes.

could be spared by using this rotational technique. Similar efforts were also given by Proimos *et al* [27] at Memorial Sloan–Kettering Cancer Center in New York who provided a gravity oriented block in arc therapy for Co-60 treatment to block normal structures. This technique was successfully employed for selectively sparing normal tissues and only irradiating lymph nodes [28].

Unfortunately, 3DCRT cannot provide an optimum balance with even complex and very innovative ideas as proposed by various investigators [26–28]. Joint Center of Radiation Therapy (JCRT) in Boston attempted to spare normal tissues and provide a uniform dose to the tumor using a computer controlled approach by changing the collimator gantry and table orientation and even making a wedge beam [29, 30]. This was a unique approach used way before the current concept of volumetric modulated arc therapy (VMAT), which will be discussed later.

Maximizing the dose to a tumor and minimizing the dose to OAR then became a mathematic issue, which is solved through an iterative process in many walks of life: business (trading), aviation (optimum route) and other industrial use. Intensity modulated radiation therapy (IMRT) was introduced in the early 1980s and did not succeed because of the limited computational powers at that time. Figure 1.3 shows a prostate cancer being treated indicating dose painting to prostate lymph nodes and the bladder. Similarly figure 1.3(b) shows the symmetric capabilities of IMRT indicating sequential dose painting of three structures: GTV CTV and PTV. Such selections on the dose painting are only possible with IMRT.

References

[1] Kramer S, Kusner D and Gunn W G 1966 Clinical experience with the Jefferson Hospital Radiotherapy Simulator *Radiology* **87** 134–6

[2] Bomford C K, Craig L M and Hanna F A *et al* 1975 *Treatment Simulators.* (London: British Institute of Radiology)

[3] Hounsfield G N 1973 Computerized transverse axial scanning (tomography): part I. Description of system *Br. J. Radiol.* **46** 1016–22

[4] Smith A R and Purdy J A 1991 Three-dimensional photon treatment planning: report of the collaborative working group on the evaluation of treatment planning for external photon beam radiotherapy *Int. J. Radiat. Oncol. Biol. Phys.* **21** 1–265

[5] ICRU Report 50 1993 *Prescribing, Recording, and Reporting Photon Beam Therapy* (Bethesda, MD: International Commission on Radiation Units and Measurements)

[6] Sherouse G W, Novins K and Chaney E 1990 Computation of digitally reconstructed radiography for use in radiotherapy treatment design *Int. J. Radiat. Oncol. Biol. Phys.* **18** 651–8

[7] Sherouse G W, Bourland J D and Reynolds K *et al* 1990 Virtual simulation in the clinical setting: some practical considerations *Int. J. Radiat. Oncol. Biol. Phys.* **19** 1059–65

[8] Rosenman J, Chaney E L and Sailer S *et al* 1991 Recent advances in radiotherapy treatment planning *Cancer Investig.* **9** 465–81

[9] Rosenman J, Sailer S L and Sherouse G W *et al* 1991 Virtual simulation: initial clinical results *Int. J. Radiat. Oncol. Biol. Phys.* **20** 843–51

[10] Coia L R, Schultheiss T E and Hanks G E 1995 *A Practical Guide to CT Simulation* (Madison, WI: Advanced Medical Publishing)

[11] Das I J, McGee K P and Desobrey G E 1995 The digitally reconstructed radiograph *A Practical Guide to CT Simulation* ed L R Coia, T E Schultheiss and G E Hanks (Madison, WI: Advanced Medical Publishing) 39–50

[12] Budgell G J, Mott J H and Williams P C *et al* 2000 Requirements for leaf position accuracy for dynamic multileaf collimation *Phys. Med. Biol.* **45** 1211–27

[13] Kallman P, Lind B and Brahme A 1988 Shaping of arbitrary dose distributions by dynamic multileaf collimator *Phys. Med. Biol.* **33** 1291–300

[14] Boyer A L, Ochran T G and Nyerick C E *et al* 1992 Clinical dosimetry for implementation of a multileaf collimator *Med. Phys.* **19** 1255–61

[15] Galvin J M, Smith A R and Moeller R D *et al* 1992 Evaluation of multileaf collimator design for a photon beam [published erratum *Int. J. Radiat. Oncol. Biol. Phys. 1992 24(3) 579*]. *Int. J. Radiat. Oncol. Biol. Phys.* **23** 789–801

[16] Galvin J M, Smith A R and Lilly B 1993 Characterization of a multi-leaf collimator system *Int. J. Radiat. Onol. Biol. Phys.* **25** 181–92

[17] LoSasso T, Chui C S and Kutcher G J *et al* 1993 The use of a multi-leaf collimator for conformal radiotherapy of carcinomas of the prostate and nasopharynx *Int. J. Radiat. Oncol. Biol. Phys.* **25** 161–70

[18] Jordan T J and Williams P C 1994 The design and performance characteristics of a multileaf collimator *Phys. Med. Biol.* **39** 231–51

[19] Brewster L, Mohan R and Mageras G *et al* 1995 Three dimensional conformal treatment planning with multileaf collimators *Int. J. Radiat. Oncol. Biol. Phys.* **33** 1081–9

[20] Helyer S J and Heisig S 1995 Multileaf collimation versus conventional shielding blocks: a time and motion study of beam shaping in radiotherapy *Radiother. Oncol.* **37** 61–4

[21] Huq M S, Yu Y and Chen Z P *et al* 1995 Dosimetric characteristics of a commercial multileaf collimator *Med. Phys.* **22** 241–7

[22] LoSasso T and Kutcher G J 1995 Multileaf collimation versus alloy blocks: analysis of geometric accuracy *Int. J. Radiat. Oncol. Biol. Phys.* **32** 499–506

[23] Palta J R, Yeung D K and Frouhar V 1996 Dosimetric considerations for a multileaf collimator system *Med. Phys.* **23** 1219–24

[24] Boyer A L and Li S 1997 Geometric analysis of light-field position of a multileaf collimator with curved ends *Med. Phys.* **24** 757–62

[25] Das I J, Desobry G E and McNeeley S W *et al* 1998 Beam characteristics of a retrofitted double-focused multileaf collimator *Med. Phys.* **25** 1676–84

[26] Takahashi S 1965 Conformation radiotherapy: rotation techniques as applied to radiography and radiotherapy of cancer *Acta Radiol. Suppl.* **242** 1–142

[27] Proimos B S, Tsialas S P and Coutroubas S C 1966 Gravity-oriented filters in arc cobalt therapy *Radiology* **87** 933–7

[28] Proimos B S and Goldson A L 1981 Dynamic dose-shaping by gravity-oriented absorbers for total lymph node irradiation *Int. J. Radiat. Oncol. Biol. Phys.* **7** 973–7

[29] Levene B M, Kijewski P K and Chin L M *et al* 1978 Computer controlled radiation therapy *Radiology* **129** 769–75

[30] Cheng C W and Chin L M 1987 A computer-aided treatment planning technique for universal wedge *Int. J. Radiat. Oncol. Biol. Phys.* **13** 1927–35

Chapter 2

Beam modulation

Traditionally, radiation beams are made uniform by inserting a flattening filter in the beam that is specific to a particular beam energy. The design of a flattening filter is such that it produces a flat beam (±2%) at a depth of 10 cm for the central 80% of the beam width. Due to such selection, the beam is usually non-uniform at shallower depths say d_{max} (depth of maximum dose) with a pronounced horn, e.g., a higher dose towards periphery compared to the dose at the central axis. The flat beam profile at depth thus produces uniform dose distributions that cover the target volume uniformly.

Frequently a non-uniform dose is needed due to the sloping surfaces of the chest wall, pelvis and breast. Such changes are required and achieved by inserting a metallic wedge-shaped device known as a 'wedge'. Initially, wedges were made for a specific energy and field size in a limited increment of dose angle from the central angle. These were 15°, 30°, 45°, and 60° wedges. These wedges could produce tilted isodose lines defined by their wedge angle. Figure 2.1 shows a metallic device and associated isodose lines tilted in one plane characterized by the wedge angle. Hence in the past, dose distributions were modulated in a single plane. With the combination of two wedges, specific isodoses suitable for patient treatment were created. Wedge factor (WF) for each beam and device is measured as dose with wedge to dose without wedge and is generally < 1.0. As expected WF (E, d, F, W) is a function of beam energy (E), treatment depth (d), field size (F) and wedge angle (W) and has been studied extensively as shown in references [1–6].

There are a lot of problems with wedges for handling, quality assurance, and limitation in dose modulations; thus, electronic or soft wedges were introduced. Each linear accelerator vendor opted to design a unique soft wedge with a proprietary name, e.g., Varian called it the dynamic wedge; Siemens, the virtual wedge; and Elekta, the Universal or Omni wedge [7–13]. The genesis of these soft wedges came from work performed in Boston [14, 15]. Petti *et al* [15] showed that if a 60° wedge is created, then with the combination of an open (unwedged) beam and a 60° wedge, any

doi:10.1088/978-0-7503-1335-3ch2

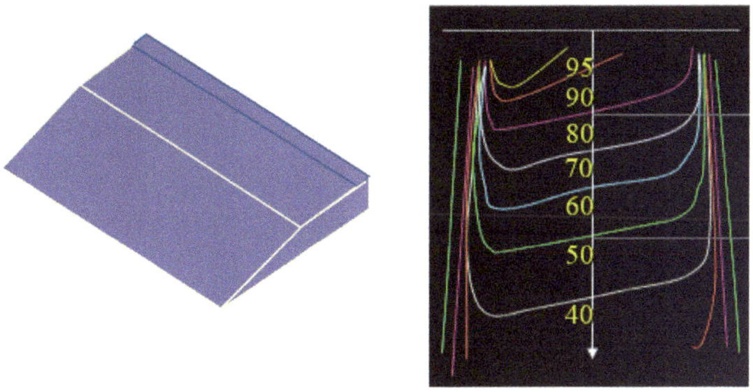

Figure 2.1. Wedge and associated 2D modulated isodose lines.

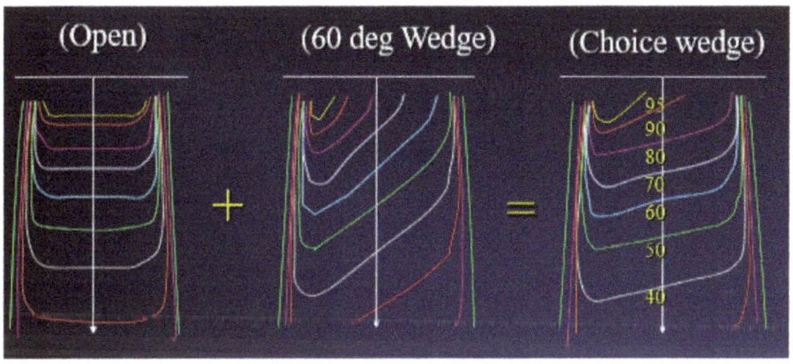

Figure 2.2. Concept of soft wedge based on combination of open and 60° wedge combination as described by Petti *et al* [15].

angled wedge can be created. This paved the way for the creation of an advanced soft wedge from most vendors and hence the ability to modulate the beam in one plane uniformly. Figure 2.2 shows the concept of creating the wedge beam.

2.1 Forward planning

The target receives the dose based on percent depth dose (PDD) or tissue maximum ratio (TMR). Since the target dose is always < 100%, normalization is used. To give a uniform dose to the volume, multiple beams are used based on beam angles to avoid the normal structures. Forward planning requires inputting a beam profile either flat or modulated by the wedge. The forward planning process requires a lot of trial and error in repeating beam angles, weights, and then dose calculation. With open and wedged beams, a uniform dose distribution is possible which has been practiced for nearly 100 years in radiation oncology. Multiple beams can be added at a given beam angle with proper beam weights. Figure 2.3 shows the concept of forward planning.

2.2 Paradigm shift

With development of computers and fast processing time, beam eye view (BEV) visualization was possible. Thus, target and normal structures can be seen in the

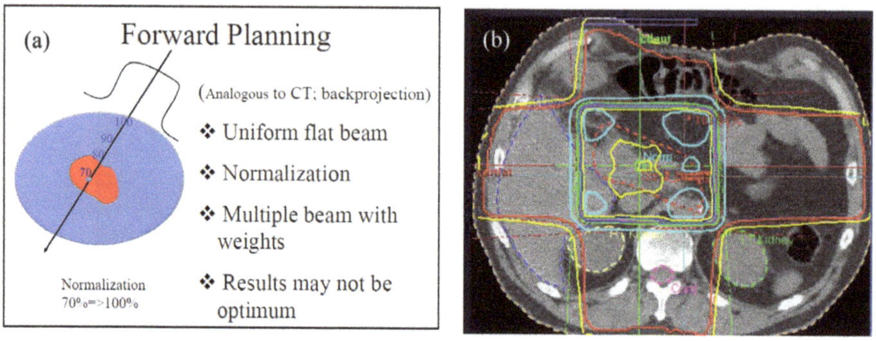

Figure 2.3. (a) Concept of forward planning where a uniform beam is shown in the entrance of the surface. (b) A four field plan properly weighted provides uniform dose. To give 100% dose to the target volume, isodose is normalized.

beam. A planner can then avoid normal structures by choosing a suitable beam angle. It was realized that with traditional analog treatments, the manipulation of isodose was always difficult. A digital innovation was needed where each target volume element could be painted with a different dose based on the clinical need. This certainly was a bold idea moving away from the uniform beam to a non-uniform beam and paint dose in subsection of the target that may be deterministic. This would also allow for no trial and error in the treatment planning thus saving countless hours.

This revolutionary idea was first proposed by Brahme [16] with a conceptual view of sparing normal structures as shown in figure 2.4. The term 'reverse approach' was used to provide the desired dose distribution to the target volume without the trial and error of the forward planning. The animation in figure 2.4 shows that a beam based on BEV is chosen. A pencil beam is cast that passes through the target volume. Depending on the desired dose and body contour, a fluence based on the forward plan can be assigned. Such a process is repeated for each ray in each beam, thus giving an uneven fluence. Depending on the normal structure and location of the target, conformation-convergent beam irradiation was possible. The resultant fluence is shown in each beam arrangement. So if the incident fluence could be created, as shown by Brahme [16], then an ideal solution of the problem is achieved. This idea was further implemented with the help of simulated annealing and then the term 'inverse planning' was introduced.

Brahme [16] detailed the discussion and the mathematical approach to the solution of inverse planning that was later picked up by Steve Webb [17–21], who expanded this field, which is now known as intensity modulated radiation therapy (IMRT).

2.3 Simulated annealing

Simulated annealing (SA) is a highly advanced mathematical tool using a probabilistic approach to find the global optimum (maximum or minimum) solution in one dimension or multi-dimensions. It applies to every walk of life when an optimum choice among multiple iterative variables is sought, such as finding places

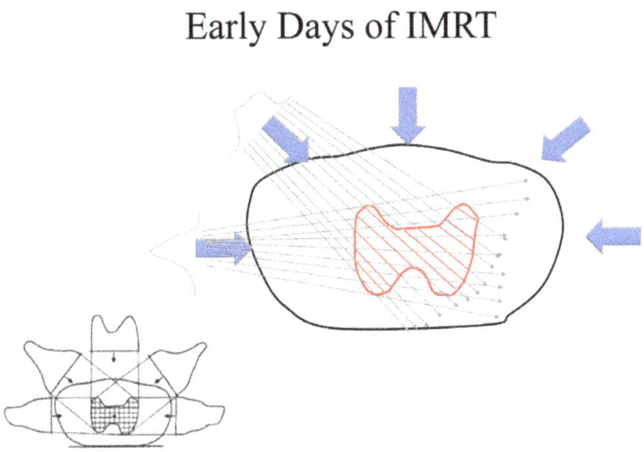

Figure 2.4. Concept of inverse planning as introduced by Brahme [16], reprinted with permission of Elsevier. The animation on the left provides the ray tracing concept and dividing the beam in smaller beam called beamlet. The composition of these provides beam fluence. A typical beam fluence to cover a hatched target from various beams is shown on the right. Such an approach eliminates the trial and error approach of the forward planning. Animation available at https://iopscience.iop.org/book/978-0-7503-1335-3.

to visit for a tourist, the return of money in the stock exchange, airline routing, the procurement of products, etc. If a function $f(x)$ is analytical, the optimum can be found by the gradient such that

$$\frac{df(x)}{dx} = 0 \in \text{max or min} \tag{2.1}$$

$$\frac{d^2f(x)}{dx^2} = \begin{cases} - \text{ for maximum} \\ + \text{ for minimum} \end{cases} \tag{2.2}$$

The criterion can be simple if it has functional and limited dimensions. SA is a term used in chemistry for processing metallurgical components to refine and find a product by iteratively heating and cooling. SA considers a state x^* of a current position x based on probabilistic approach. The differences (x^*-x) are compared and continuously modified such that $(x^*-x = 0)$ in all dimensions. The function is iteratively searched for the global maximum or minimum in multi-dimensions. The SA field has evolved from a simple application in the middle of the 19th century to a highly sophisticated, computationally challenging approach from gradient search, heuristics to Monte Carlo simulation. A simple outline of SA can be found in this review article by Fleischer [22]. Finding the global max or min is very difficult, as shown in figure 2.5, depending on the nature of the function. In a Newtonian approach where the function is well defined without uncertainty, the global minimum is easily reached (figure 2.5(a)). However, when it is stochastic, there is a probability associated with the function and it may have a hard time finding the global minimum (figure 2.5(b)).

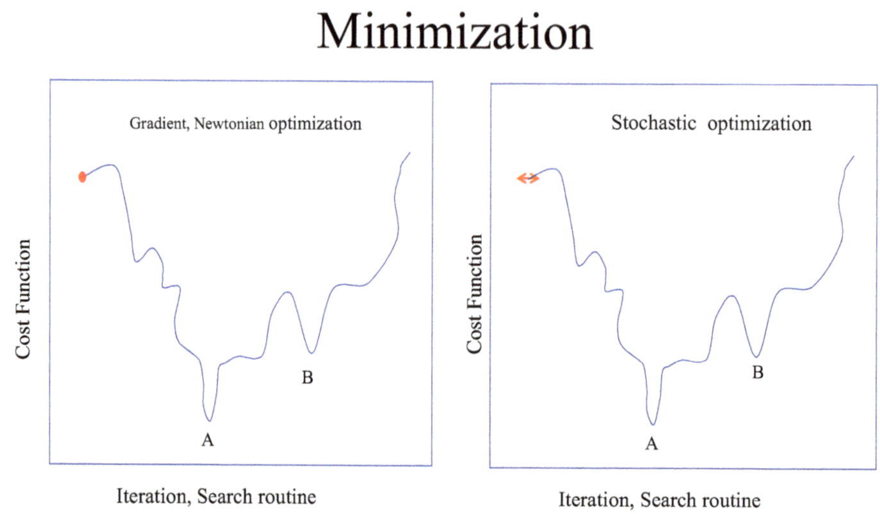

Figure 2.5. Concept of Newtonian and stochastic approaches for finding global minimum. Play simulation and see the difference between the figure on the left and then the figure on the right. Animation available at https://iopscience.iop.org/book/978-0-7503-1335-3.

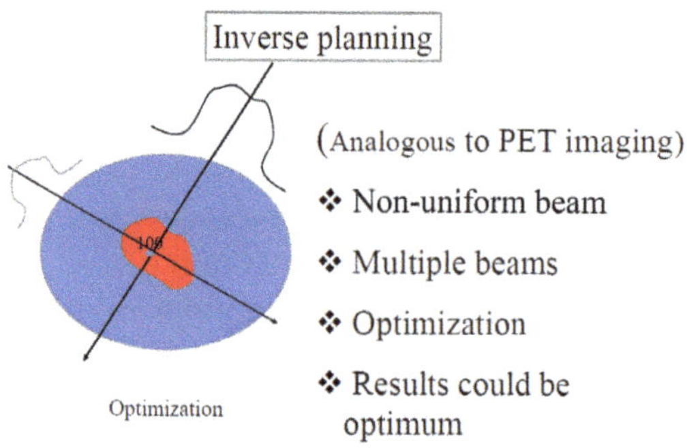

Figure 2.6. Conceptual analogy of inverse planning in terms of positron emission tomography, where a known source produces non-uniform fluence at surface based on attenuation property of the tissue.

In radiation therapy, it was Steve Webb who introduced the concept of SA for the optimization of beams in 3DCRT and later in IMRT [17–19, 21, 23, 24]. He wrote many seminal works on IMRT. The SA process in radiation treatment is also known as inverse planning as indicated in figure 2.6, where the input parameter is not known but rather searched iteratively. One can think of this process like positron emission tomography where the source in the center is known, but on the surface, it is traced. A descriptive process of inverse planning is shown in figure 2.4. A ray line from uniform fluence is traced back depending upon the attenuation of the beam. Additional details can be found in chapter 6. The same process is repeated in each ray line, thus providing a non-uniform beam at the surface. This process is then repeated in each field orientation giving a non-uniform fluence at the surface. The details of the complex IMRT processes will be elaborated in further chapters.

References

[1] McCullough E C, Gortney J and Blackwell C R 1988 A depth dependence determination of the wedge transmission factor for 4-10 MV photon beams *Med. Phys.* **15** 621–3

[2] Palta J R, Daftari I and Suntharlingam N 1988 Field size dependence of wedge factors *Med. Phys.* **15** 624–6

[3] Thomas S J 1990 The variation of wedge factors with field size on a linear accelerator *Br. J. Radiol.* **63** 355–6

[4] Heukelom S, Lanson J H and Mijnheer B J 1994 Wedge factor constituents of high energy photon beams: head and phantom scatter components *Radiother. Oncol.* **32** 73–83

[5] Sharma S C and Johnson M W 1994 Recommendations for measurement of tray and wedge factors for high energy photons *Med. Phys.* **21** 573–5

[6] Myler U and Szabo J J 2002 Dose calculation along the nonwedged direction *Med. Phys.* **29** 746–54

[7] Klein E E, Low D A and Meigooni A S *et al* 1995 Dosimetry and clinical implementation of dynamic wedge *Int. J. Radiat. Oncol. Biol. Phys.* **31** 583–92

[8] Klein E E, Gerber R and Zhu X R *et al* 1998 Multiple machine implementation of enhanced dynamic wedge *Int. J. Radiat. Oncol. Biol. Phys.* **40** 977–85

[9] Leavitt D D and Klein E 1997 Dosimetry measurement tools for commissioning enhanced dynamic wedge *Med. Dosim.* **22** 171–6

[10] van Santvoort J 1998 Dosimetric evaluation of the Siemens virtual wedge *Phys. Med. Biol.* **43** 2651–63

[11] Verhaegen F and Das I J 1999 Monte Carlo modelling of a virtual wedge *Phys. Med. Biol.* **44** N251–9

[12] Shackford H, Bjarngard B E and Vadash P 1995 Dynamic universal wedge *Med. Phys.* **22** 1735–41

[13] Phillips M H, Parsaei H and Cho P S 2000 Dynamic and omni wedge implementation on an Elekta SL linac *Med. Phys.* **27** 1623–34

[14] Kijewski P K, Chin L N and Bjärngard B E 1978 Wedged-shaped dose distribution by computer controlled collimator motion *Med. Phys.* **5** 426–9

[15] Petti P L and Siddon R L 1985 Effective wedge angles with universal wedge *Phys. Med. Biol.* **30** 985–91

[16] Brahme A 1988 Optimization of stationary and moving beam radiation therapy techniques *Radiother. Oncol.* **12** 129–40

[17] Webb S 1989 Optimisation of conformal radiotherapy dose distributions by simulated annealing *Phys. Med. Biol.* **34** 1349–70

[18] Webb S 1994 Optimizing the planning of intensity-modulated radiotherapy *Phys. Med. Biol.* **39** 2229–46

[19] Webb S 1998 Configuration options for intensity-modulated radiation therapy using multiple static fields shaped by a multileaf collimator. II: constraints and limitations on 2D modulation *Phys. Med. Biol.* **43** 1481–95

[20] Webb S 1998 Intensity-modulated radiation therapy: dynamic MLC (DMLC) therapy, multisegment therapy and tomotherapy. An example of QA in DMLC therapy *Strahlenther. Onkol.* **174** 8–12

[21] Webb S 2000 *Intensity-Modulated Radiation Therapy* (Bristol: Institute of Physics Publishing)

[22] Fleischer M 1995 Simulated annealing: past, present and future *Proccedings of the 1995 Winter Simulation Conf.* ed K Alexopolus, K Kang and W R Lilegdon *et al* pp 155–61

[23] Webb S 2003 The physical basis of IMRT and inverse planning *Br. J. Radiol.* **76** 678–89

[24] Webb S, Convery D J and Evans P M 1998 Inverse planning with constraints to generate smoothed intensity-modulated beams *Phys. Med. Biol.* **43** 2785–94

Indra J Das, Nicholas J Sanfilippo, Antonella Fogliata and Luca Cozzi

Chapter 3

Definitions and terminology

The IMRT process is very complex and has many terminologies. The intent of this chapter is primarily to educate students, trainees, and novices about the concept of IMRT and its terminologies before we move to higher level discussion of the process. The following concepts that appear in IMRT literature are explained in this chapter:

- Pixel
- Voxel
- Bixel/Beamlet
- Level (intensity)
- Segment
- Concept of dose painting

Additionally, IMRT is a digital concept as compared to 2D and 3DCRT, where dose distributions are mainly analog. So to understand IMRT, we need to think of every aspect in digital form including the dose at every point in space. This is due to the fact that IMRT dose planning is performed from CT or MRI data, which is digital in nature and made out of small building blocks. So the concepts critical for IMRT are explored in the following sections.

3.1 Pixel

The genesis of IMRT started in the late 1980s and has picked up rapid momentum since then. So before we move to the details, the fundaments of IMRT need to be explored. All images created in the modern day are digital, i.e., they are composed of small elements called pixels which stands for Picture Element as the smallest building block. Figure 3.1 shows such a concept. When imaging a patient using CT, images are acquired sequentially slice by slice. A slice is a 2D image. This image is further divided by the smallest element, which is called a pixel. Hence, a collection of pixels makes a 2D CT slice. This can be generalized to any image, e.g., CT,

doi:10.1088/978-0-7503-1335-3ch3

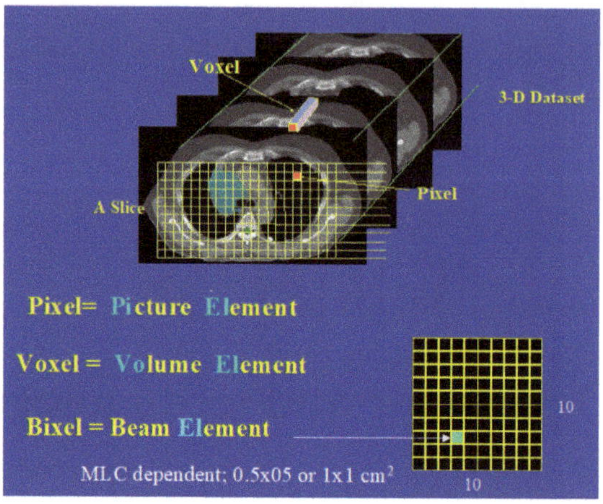

Figure 3.1. Schematic of the 3D data set that represents a patient. This 3D data is divided by a planar slice that represents the slice thickness. The smallest element that makes up a slice is known as a pixel. Please note that all the picture elements; pixel, voxel and bixel are shown.

magnetic resonance imaging (MRI), PET, or ultrasound (US). In the context of radiation therapy, CT images are mainly used as they contain information about tissue attenuation that is correlated with the electron density, ρ_e (#e cm^{-3}). In general, each pixel is vital with unique characteristics of the tissue in terms of the attenuation coefficient, μ, that relates to ρ_e for a given beam energy. The CT number or Hounsfield number (HU) is related to μ associated with each pixel.

The picture of a plane or slice that we see is the collection of the content of pixels, which is represented by μ, which represents the gray value on the screen. The correlation of HU and ρ_e is typical in treatment planning that provides dosimetric information based on the composition of the tissue [1]. Every pixel in an image has an identical square dimension. The smaller the pixel size, the higher the resolution of the image or better information of dose. In a CT data set, the typical pixel values are 1×1 mm^2. When we decrease the pixel size, it requires more memory to store the information. Therefore, pixel size is directly related to the square of the amount of memory needed for the data.

For example, if an image is 10×10 cm^2, it is 100×100 mm^2. Thus, this image would contain 10 000 pixels with a dimension of 1×1 mm^2, 2500 pixels with a dimension of 2×2 mm^2, 400 pixels at 5×5 mm^2 and 100 pixels at 10×10 mm^2. It should be clear now that as the pixel size gets smaller, the memory requirement increases exponentially. In the beginning of the computer age, memory was very expensive and so was computation. Hence, early implementation of IMRT in the 1990s and 2000s took weeks to process for dose calculations. Currently with faster computers and cheaper memory, an IMRT calculation can be performed in less than a minute, but the entire IMRT process can still take hours; in chapter 4 it will be seen that the IMRT process is very complex and time consuming.

3.2 Voxel

The CT images of a patient contain many slices (planar images). The entire 3D data is a collection of slices. However, a slice has finite thickness called the 'slice thickness' and usually it is in millimeters. The spacing between slices is called the slice width, which is between 5–10 mm. So two parameters, slice thickness and slice width, need to be considered when making 3D data set for the entire body. The pixels connecting two adjacent slices are called voxels, which stands for Volume Elements. As described earlier, pixels have square dimensions, but voxels are usually a rectangular box as shown in figure 3.1. So the voxel dimension is pixel × slice width. There has been a lot of discussion on the dosimetry and slice thickness. In general, a smaller thickness (smaller voxels) provides better dose distribution [2].

In reality, a voxel is always a rectangular cube, as it is not possible to make the slices thin enough to match the pixel size. Dose calculations are performed in individual voxels, and then distributions are plotted. To visualize in high resolution and to appreciate dose gradient, one should try to reduce the size of the voxel.

3.3 Bixel (beamlet)

Radiation treatment field sizes were traditionally square or rectangular fields that were then shaped with blocks to spare the normal structures. Imagine that the treatment field can be made up of small elements to form the fields, similar to pixels creating an image. The smallest entity is called a bixel (beam element). It was introduced for a finite size of the treatment field and named bixel to make it phonetically similar to pixel for a treatment field [3]. As will be seen later, the IMRT treatment field is divided into small fields called beamlets. In the old days, a term fixel (field element) was also introduced but did not become popular. At the present time, the terms bixel and beamlet are used interchangeably.

The size of the bixel, or the minimum achievable field size by definition, is determined by the MLC of the treatment machine that creates these beamlets. In older machines, the MLC width was 1 cm wide, later it became 0.5 cm, and for high definition MLC it is now 0.25 cm. Making the size of the beamlet small is a challenging process as the MLC blades cannot be made too thin due to safety reasons and accommodating a large number of motor drives is not possible in the limited space in the treatment head. It should be clear by now that bixels can have any rectangular size whose width is governed by the MLC width and length is controlled by the other jaw. Figure 3.1 shows the beamlets/bixels. It should be intuitive that a smaller size of bixel can provide a higher dose gradient, which is a hallmark of IMRT; but due to optimization and multiple fields, the MLC size does not directly impact the quality of IMRT dose distribution [4–7]. However, for small structures in the brain or for small field SBRT, the MLC size does make a small but visible difference in dose distribution [8–11].

3.4 Intensity level

Another parameter for IMRT is level or intensity level. It is an integer number of intensity that can be delivered to a bixel. So for a linear accelerator, the intensity is synonymous with the monitor unit (MU). It is possible to deliver any integer number of the MU to a bixel. However, machine characteristics at low MUs are not as reliable as large MUs [12, 13]. For this reason, a minimum MU is administratively selected for IMRT in treatment planning. This is typically 2–5 MU. However, with the advent of newer technology, machines are more reliable and fractional MUs can be delivered safely and accurately which occurs in the case for the sliding window treatment in VMAT. Figure 3.2 shows the concept of levels using color representation. In other words, since IMRT is digital in nature, we can add levels in a bixel.

In the beginning of the IMRT era, the level was a selectable entity and typically 1, 3, 5, 7, ... 20 were chosen. The selection of intensity in a bixel is governed by the

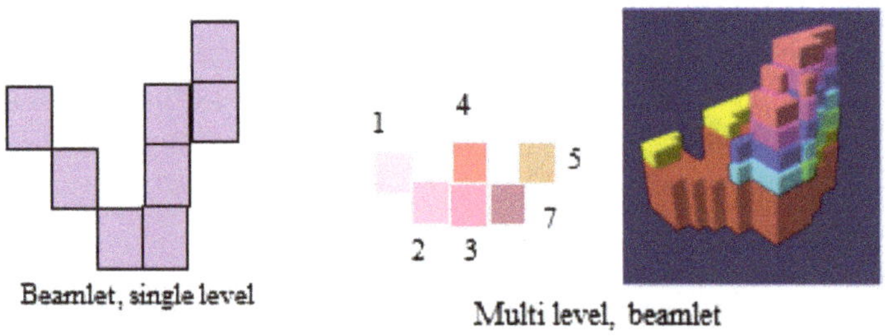

Figure 3.2. Showing level (intensity, dose) is a bixel. One can have different levels in different bixels which is shown in multilevel bixels. A combined level for a beam is also shown with different colors indicating different intensity levels.

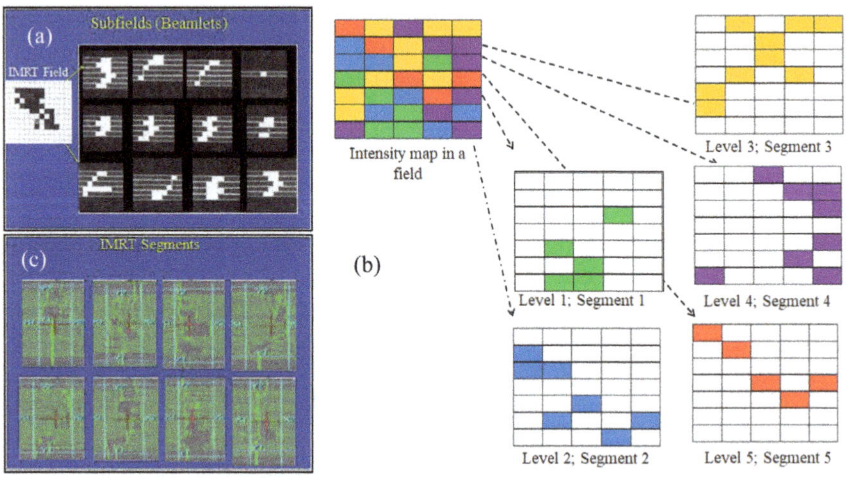

Figure 3.3. (a) An IMRT field is composed of beamlets (segments). (b) An example of how a fluence (intensity) map of a field is composed based on intensity level. A collection of the same intensity pixels makes a segment. So in this diagram, a treatment field is composed of five segments whose pixels have the same intensity level (MU) represented by different colors. (c) Actual IMRT segments are generated by the planning system. Animation available at https://iopscience.iop.org/book/978-0-7503-1335-3.

treatment planning system which is derived for a given prescribed dose and depth of a target. Sun *et al* [14] showed that increasing level does not improve the quality of the plan, rather it increases the treatment time.

3.5 Segment

A collection of bixels for the same MU (level as discussed in the previous section) is called a segment. An IMRT field is composed of many segments that are delivered based on intensity (MU) level needed. Figure 3.3 shows a treatment field, which is created with many segments.

3.6 Concept of dose painting

IMRT allows us to selectively provide the desired dose in specific voxels or structures such as the target and organs at risk (OAR). As the goal of radiation therapy is to give the highest dose in the target and the minimum dose to OAR, this is much easier to achieve in IMRT with the concept of dose painting. Figure 3.4 provides a pictorial view as to how dose painting is achieved using intensity levels in a voxel. In a beam's

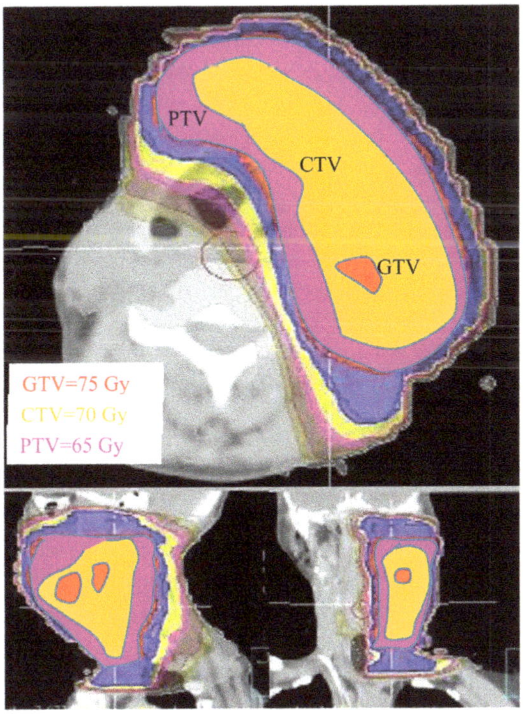

Figure 3.4. Concept of dose painting, e.g., variable dose to GTV, CTV and PTV in this head and neck cancer. Animation available at https://iopscience.iop.org/book/978-0-7503-1335-3.

eye view, structures are represented by the voxel based on its size. The computer optimization selectively chooses the desired dose in each voxel.

This process will be discussed in later sections. Dose painting is a hallmark of IMRT where one can deliver selectively high dose and reduce dose to normal structures. This process is generally beneficial where cone down are used to deliver higher dose to GTV (figure 3.4). In IMRT, this can be done sequential thus treatment time can be saved. This is a common practice now in most head and neck cancers.

References

[1] Das I J, Cheng C W and Cao M *et al* 2016 CT imaging parameters for inhomogeneity correction in radiation treatment planning *J. Med. Phys.* **41** 1–11

[2] Srivastava S P, Cheng C W and Das I J 2016 The effect of slice thickness on target and organs at risk volumes, dosimetric coverage and radiobiological impact in IMRT planning *Clin. Transl. Oncol.* **18** 469–79

[3] Markman J, Low D A and Beavis A W *et al* 2002 Beyond bixels: generalizing the optimization parameters for intensity modulated radiation therapy *Med. Phys.* **29** 2298–304

[4] Wu V W 2007 Effects of multileaf collimator parameters on treatment planning of intensity-modulated radiotherapy *Med. Dosim.* **32** 38–43

[5] Leal A, Sanchez-Doblado F and Arrans R *et al* 2004 MLC leaf width impact on the clinical dose distribution: a Monte Carlo approach *Int. J. Radiat. Oncol. Biol. Phys.* **59** 1548–59

[6] Burmeister J, McDermott P N and Bossenberger T *et al* 2004 Effect of MLC leaf width on the planning and delivery of SMLC IMRT using the CORVUS inverse treatment planning system *Med. Phys.* **31** 3187–93

[7] Hong C S, Ju S G and Kim M *et al* 2014 Dosimetric effects of multileaf collimator leaf width on intensity-modulated radiotherapy for head and neck cancer *Med. Phys.* **41** 021712

[8] Fiveash J B, Murshed H and Duan J *et al* 2002 Effect of multileaf collimator leaf width on physical dose distributions in the treatment of CNS and head and neck neoplasms with intensity modulated radiation therapy *Med. Phys.* **29** 1116–9

[9] Wu Q J, Wang Z and Kirkpatrick J P *et al* 2009 Impact of collimator leaf width and treatment technique on stereotactic radiosurgery and radiotherapy plans for intra- and extracranial lesions *Radiat. Oncol.* **4** 3

[10] Jin J Y, Yin F F and Ryu S *et al* 2005 Dosimetric study using different leaf-width MLCs for treatment planning of dynamic conformal arcs and intensity-modulated radiosurgery *Med. Phys.* **32** 405–11

[11] Dvorak P, Georg D and Bogner J *et al* 2005 Impact of IMRT and leaf width on stereotactic body radiotherapy of liver and lung lesions *Int. J. Radiat. Oncol. Biol. Phys.* **61** 1572–81

[12] Cheng C W and Das I J 2002 Comparison of beam characteristics in intensity modulated radiation therapy (IMRT) and those under normal treatment condition *Med. Phys.* **29** 226–30

[13] Das I J, Kase K R and Tello V M 1991 Dosimetric accuracy at low monitor unit settings *Br. J. Radiol.* **64** 808–11

[14] Sun X, Xia P and Yu N 2004 Effects of the intensity levels and beam map resolutions on static IMRT plans *Med. Phys.* **31** 2402–11

Chapter 4

IMRT devices

Beam modulations require particular methods to change photon fluence. The simplest method is to use a wedge to change fluence uniformly in one dimension; however, for IMRT, 2D fluence modifications are needed. In the late 1980s, it was realized that a true conformal dose distribution including irregular contours and inhomogeneities could be delivered by multiple beams with varied intensity rather than the presumed notion of uniform intensity beams. This was proposed by many investigators, building the notion for non-uniform beam profiles, which is also called intensity modulation [1–3]. To execute IMRT plans, various devices must be used; these are mainly dynamic jaws, masks and filters, and MLC based.

The concept of intensity modulation was first proposed by Brahme [2] in 1988. He proposed that, rather than iteratively planning dose distribution, it is possible to find a deterministic dose by beam modulation. He provided a theoretical model where the tumor dose could be optimized based on a modulated (non-uniform) beam, depending on the beam angle of the tumor, from the beam's eye view (BEV). Input photon fluence can be shaped based on the ray line passing the tumor and the depth of the underlying tissue. With the combination of many non-uniform beams, a uniform dose in the tumor can be achieved as shown in figure 4.1. The same approach was suggested for sparing the organs at risk by avoiding radiation fluence [2].

These 2D intensity profiles can be pictorially represented in 3D, as shown in figure 4.2, indicating smooth, wire frame, and digitized profiles. For the treatment, these theoretically generated intensity profiles require specific methods to generate devices. Before the development of MLC, there were two options: filters and jaws. One could imagine that this is easy to achieve by filter. So the inverse of profiles was created by metallic filters that can be placed in the respective beam as we used to make compensators. Another approach could be to digitize the fluence, and then use dynamic jaws, i.e., jaws that can be moved independently. With independent jaws that can move in x and y direction, one can create a fluence suitable for IMRT. Such ideas have been attempted and used successfully for IMRT.

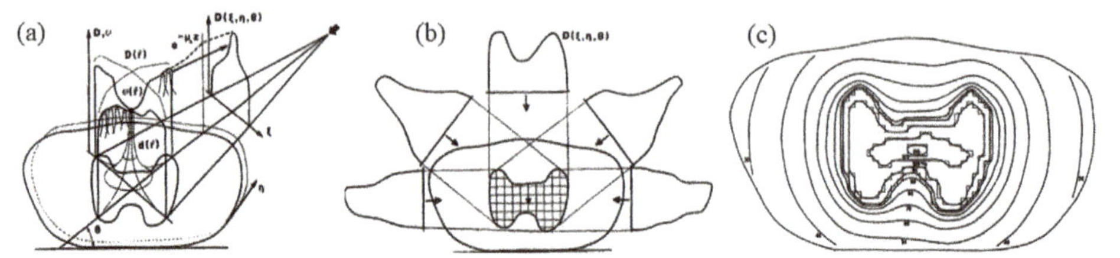

Figure 4.1. (a) Concept of beam's eye view (BEV) and making of the intensity profile by the decomposition of the point dose by the inverse back projection based on the target shape and depth of each ray line, (b) Intensity profile as derived from (a) in each BEV, and (c) Resultant dose distribution to provide the uniform dose in the target volume. Adapted from Brahme [2] with permission from Elsevier.

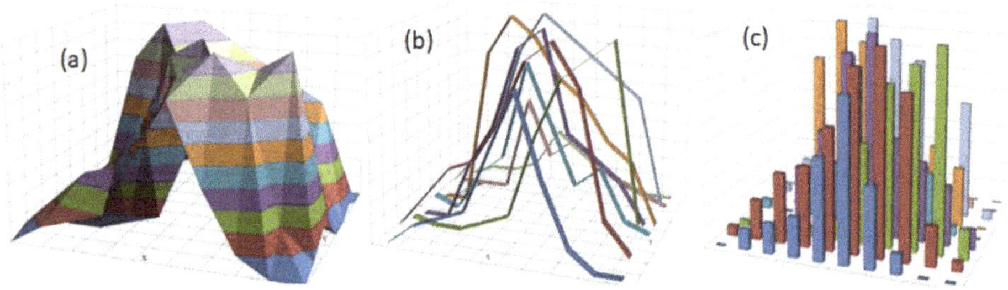

Figure 4.2. Schematic diagram of the intensity profile of one of the BEV for target coverage (a) smooth profile, (b) wire frame and (c) digitized profile that can be executed by one of the available methods described in the text.

4.1 Intensity modulation filter/compensator

Metallic filters/compensators can be made to modulate the fluence as desired as long as the primary attenuation and scatter is accurately modeled in the treatment planning system [4, 5]. These devices offer the opportunity for IMRT on machines that are old and for institutions that do not have resources to retrofit MLC. They also provide increased reliability, less downtime and repair, reduced requirements of quality assurance (QA) procedures, and shorter treatment times leading to less influence of patient motion during treatment. The filter process for IMRT is extremely economical as older machines can be used. The filter fabrication is easy to accomplish either in house or through third party vendors who specialize in fabricating filters. One such company is dot decimal (decimal® Sanford, FL 32771) and they have contracted hospitals all over the USA to make 3DCRT blocks. IMRT filter making is an extension of their business, providing field-shaping blocks and electron cutouts. Users can upload the encrypted files containing *x*, *y*, and the height of filter (figure 4.2(c)) for each gantry angle and send it to the vendor. The vendor then mills the filter using a specialized milling machine with a very high degree of accuracy (<0.1 mm). These filters are made out of brass for durability for a given energy. The typical shielding block material, Cerrobend, is not used due to the need for stability, durability, and transportability. Usually most IMRT is performed with 6 MV beams since high-energy beams do not provide much advantage if the number of fields is ⩾5 as indicated by Pirzkall *et al* [6]. Additionally, high-energy photon beams for IMRT should be avoided due to additional weight of the filter and an increased risk of neutron contamination and total body burden [7–9]. The manufactured filters contain the patient name and identification number as well as the orientation inscribed on the metal. These are then shipped to the site for QA and treatment.

To extend the filter concept, Van Schelt *et al* [10] proposed a ring-based device for poor and developing countries to be able to use IMRT where MLC is not available. This ring holds the physical compensators for the IMRT for a patient that has been calculated. So the physical device can be loaded before the treatment in each planned gantry angle. Obviously such an invasive process with a heavy load of metallic filters requires extra QA for error and to reduce the chance of a filter falling on a patient. The costs associated with the fabrication of filters can be exhaustive in some countries as well, as it can include the costs of transporting it from the place of manufacture to the hospital for treatment. Disposal of these devices after treatment is another issue; thus the storage of these devices in a crowded department should be carefully evaluated.

Another difficulty with using a filter is its resolution, as shown in figure 4.3, indicating planned fluence and truncated fluence due to discretization of the intensity level. There are several articles that have provided methodology pros and cons of filters that should be clearly evaluated if one is attempting to use the filter/compensator concept for IMRT [11–13].

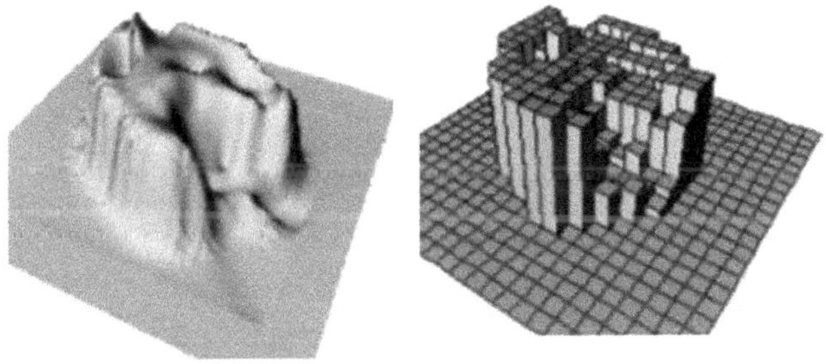

Figure 4.3. IMRT using filter/compensator. Filter of a fluence map for a specific field and corresponding digitized filter as described in figure 4.2(c). Adapted from open source, Chang *et al* [13] CC BY 3.0.

4.2 Dynamic Jaw

In principal, the modulation of the beam can also be accomplished with the movement of the jaws, which was proposed in Boston in the 1980s [14, 15]. Before the evolution of MLCs, manufacturers made the upper and lower jaws of the machines dynamic, and called them independent jaws. This provided flexibility in moving the jaws independently of each other, allowing for the creation of asymmetrical fields, and later became the backbone of soft wedges [14, 16–19]. However, since the jaws are heavy and have a limited range of motion and speed, the fluence modulation needed for delivery may not be feasible. Webb *et al* provided a theoretical solution to such challenges in a series of papers [20–25]. However, simply using jaws is a theoretical concept and cannot provide

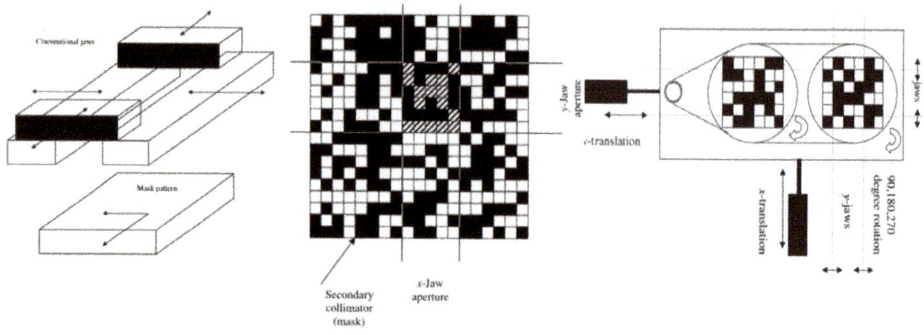

Figure 4.4. Intensity modulation in a beam's eye view can be achieved by moving the jaws. A binary pattern of jaw position is shown in the central figure. To refine the fluence, a mask was introduced. The schematic execution of these patterns using X and Y motors is seen in the right-most image. Adapted from Webb [26] with permission. Copyright IOP Publishing Ltd. All rights reserved.

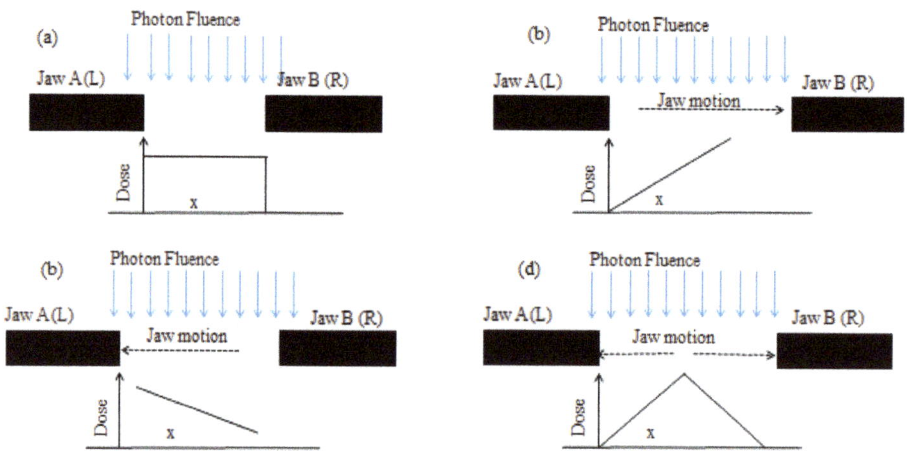

Figure 4.5. With the position of the left and right banks of jaws or MLC, in principle, any shape of dose can be created. (a) A box dose profile, (b) linearly increasing dose, (c) linearly decreasing dose, and (d) a wedge shaped dose profile can be generated by the motion of the leaves as indicated by the arrow.

the smooth function of beam modulation. Figure 4.4 provides a conceptual view of Webb's ideas where the jaws are moved to create an exposure pattern. Later, he designed a mask to fine-tune the details of implementation [26], as shown in figure 4.4.

4.3 MLC based

Modern linear accelerators are equipped with MLC that can be used for dose modulation. The concept of fluence based on target dose has been described in figure 4.2. The implementation is shown in figure 4.5 in a very simplistic form. Assuming constant fluence, a constant speed of the MLC/jaw speeds, and unlimited positions of leaves, the four patterns of dose are shown depending on the motion of the left, right, or both jaws.

In a much more rigorous and mathematical way, the combination of all leaves can be programmed to produce any fluence map as shown by several investigators [3, 27–32]. The clinical implementation in many disease sites also has been shown using the motions of the leaves with proper constraints on the leaf motion, which is the case for most vendors [33–35]. At the present time, the majority of IMRT patients are treated with linear accelerators using the concept described above.

4.4 Direct aperture optimization (DAO)

There are many hurdles with the above concepts, e.g., logistics, QA, beam time, and accuracy in beam delivery. With the development of MLC, it was possible to create an intensity fluence much more discretely than with the jaws. However, these fluences needed to be executed using constraints imposed by vendors and the design of the MLC. So there is a two-step process: First, generating an intensity map and then using a leaf-sequencing algorithm to create beams that can be delivered. Many alternatives were implemented for IMRT that relied on some forms of MLC as an automated process for the beam delivery. The DAO concept was introduced by Shepard *et al* [36–39] and led to the intensity modulated arc therapy, which was later introduced by Yu *et al* [37, 38]. In the DAO concept, the traditional optimization is eliminated; instead try to directly optimize the shape and weight of the aperture to achieve the desired dose.

4.5 Systems for IMRT

Before the days of modern IMRT that is exclusively delivered with a linear accelerator, various innovative devices were introduced, such as the NOMOS Peacock system. In the beginning, the clinical IMRT treatments were mainly performed on the NOMOS system. Later, helical tomotherapy was introduced, both of which are described below.

4.5.1 Peacock-MIMiC

The Peacock three-dimensional (3D) conformal system developed primarily for radiosurgery was a sequential rotational therapy (tomotherapy) developed by NOMOS Corp (Swickley, PA, USA). Mark Carol, a neurosurgeon, was interested in radiotherapy during his medical training, and he introduced a prototype delivery system in 1992. Under the investigational device exemption (IDE), his prototype was installed in Methodist-Baylor College of Medicine in Houston, TX. Mainly skull-based patients were treated on this system for three years before the FDA approved its use for other sites. The Peacock system incorporated a binary multi-leaf collimator called the Multileaf Intensity Modulating Collimator (MIMiC), which was a specialized device developed by the NOMOS corporation [40]. This device could create a peacock feather-like dose pattern with the MIMiC system, which used an electropneumatic device that could be attached to a wedge/tray holder of a linear accelerator for rotational therapy. The first device was attached to a Siemens Mevatron unit as shown in figure 4.6 [41].

Another component of the Peacock system is CORVOUS, an inverse treatment planning system that produced the output file for delivery of the desired beamlets via floppy disk. The MIMiC system has 20 leaf pairs of 1×1 cm^2 at the isocenter that could cover 20 cm length and 2 cm width with 40 binary (on/off) leaves as shown in

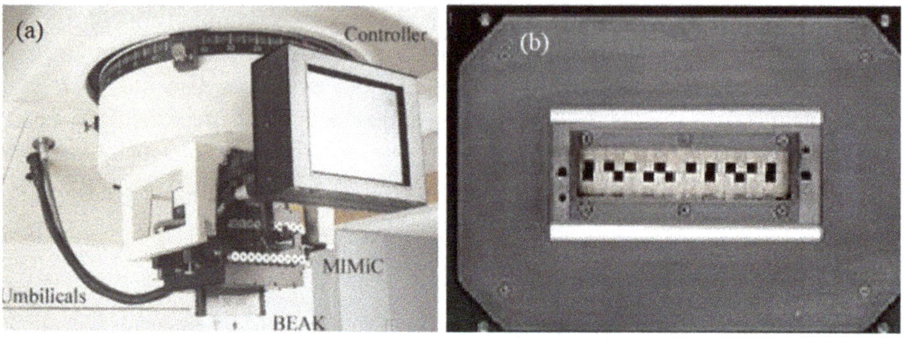

Figure 4.6. (a) Gantry mounted NOMOS Peacock serial tomotherapy system on a linear accelerator and (b) on-face view of MIMiC system showing 2-rows of leaves. A combination of 40 independent openings of 1 × 1 cm^2 is possible. Axial coverage of 2 cm width in one sweep is performed followed by table motion by a specialized system called Beak. Courtesy of Best Nomos, PA, USA, a Team Best Global company http://www.teambest.com.

figure 4.6. The leaves are divergent 8 cm long tungsten rods with transmission <0.4%. The motion is powered by miniature pneumatic pistons controlled by electrical solenoid valves with a lot of safety interlocks. The switch rate is very fast and takes a mere 40–60 milliseconds to turn on/off. The device rotates on an axial basis as the machine is rotated.

Details of the MIMiC system, including the electronic safety, lock feature, sensors, etc are described in many publications [40–43]. In the MIMiC system, the gantry rotates axially around the patient. At every 5 degrees of angle rotation, the treatment is called a port. Therefore, for complete rotation, there are 72 ports. It requires 2–7 arcs for each table position before it is manually indexed to a new position. The manual table movement was imprecise and time tasking. This was later overcome by a device called a crane that has an accuracy of table motion to 0.1 mm at increments of 0.5 mm with a special high precision to avoid junction dosimetry [44]. Due to the high precision and delivery of high gradient dose, this device was initially implemented in neurological treatment and prostate cancer [45–48]. The imaging was rudimentary, with a slice width of 2 × 20 cm^2, and hence the planner would need to provide feedback for anatomical landmarks that may not be in the vicinity of the tumor and a shift was always needed between imaging and treatment.

4.5.2 Tomotherapy

The MIMiC system delivery was slice-by-slice, relatively noisy, and slow. It also did not provide imaging information, which is needed for modern and complex treatment. The genesis of tomotherapy has its roots in three facts (a) the limitation of target volume coverage due to the vicinity of critical structures, (b) the verification of beam and structure through imaging, and (c) the safety aspect of the machines due to collision in a dynamic therapy. For target volume coverage in the vicinity of normal structures, solutions have been found using multiple fields with dynamic conformal techniques with variable shapes to change the intensity of the beam as described in the beginning of this chapter and by various investigators [20, 32, 49, 50]. This is a mature field. The second component of imaging remained a big obstacle since megavoltage portal imaging was not satisfactory and image quality was relatively poor. The solution was to introduce low energy x-ray beams, such as CT scans, for imaging. The third component was collisions, which is still not resolved but can be eliminated if we limit the radiation to a co-planar treatment. All of this led Rock Mackie to design the tomotherapy concept in 1993 [51]. Many influences were taken from radiosurgery that used gantry rotation with a fixed head frame. The first prototype was built with many early decisions that were dropped such as CT (figure 4.7), and new ones (slit MLC) were later adopted as described by Mackie [52].

The helical tomotherapy unit differed from that of NOMOS in many ways, but most importantly, the treatment was delivered in a spiral fashion. This was a significant improvement from NOMOS manually moving the patients between arcs. It also eliminated the hot and cold junction that required the feathering between arcs. The tomotherapy device is mounted upon a CT ring gantry and combines MLC to create a dedicated IMRT delivery methodology (figure 4.7).

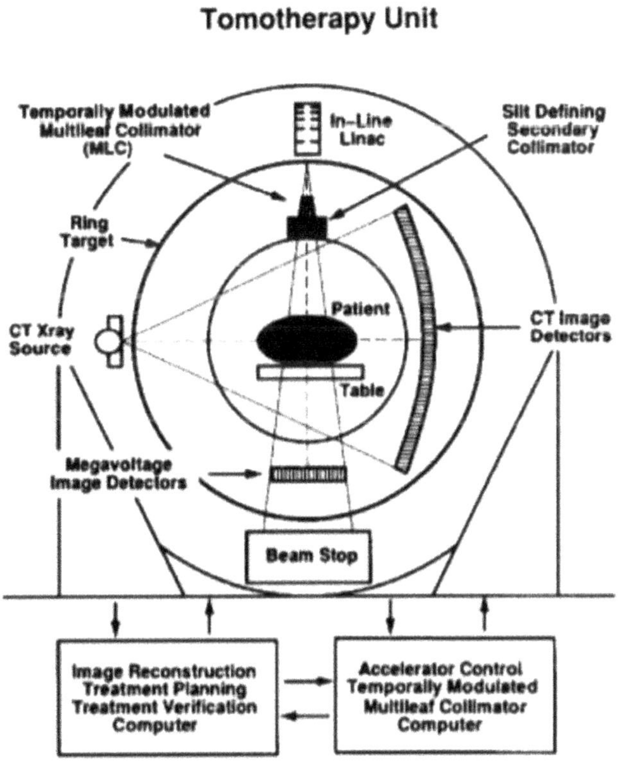

Figure 4.7. Early concept of tomotherapy to include beam modulation, imaging, and collision avoidance. Various components are shown: linac, MLC, CT, and detectors. However, the CT scanning part was dropped from the tomotherapy unit in the first prototype. Adapted from Mackie *et al* [51] John Wiley & Sons. Copyright 1993 American Association of Physicists in Medicine.

The concept of the ring gantry was a radical decision to accomplish all three factors. The gantry ring originally was designed to house a mega-voltage linear accelerator for treatment, as well as imaging. It included a CT-x-ray tube perpendicular to the accelerator with an image panel; hence, it was a CT scanner fitted with a treatment option. Originally, it was thought that the tomotherapy unit could be used as a stand-alone CT scanner for image acquisition for treatment planning and also for treatment verification. The unit has a conical secondary collimator followed by MLC for beam modulation. Since MIMiC was proven to be successful, tomotherapy adopted this technology with slight modifications. The new device was called tomotherapy [51] and could deliver the dose based on helical motion of the table and the CT-like motion of the linear accelerator. It used slip-ring technology, which is used in modern CT scanners.

The MLC design was borrowed from MIMiC as a binary MLC with significant improvements in terms of speed and width. The jaws could be continuously moved and completely opened or closed to form the maximum fan beam width of 5 cm. The MLC leaves were very fast, which was achieved by a compressed air system enabling them to close or open in approximately 20 milliseconds. Unlike MIMiC, tomotherapy uses 64 interleaved leaves with a nominal width of 6.25 mm at the isocenter, providing a maximum field size of 5 cm × 40 cm at isocenter. To limit the leakage and transmission to a minimum ($\leqslant 0.5\%$), the leaves are 10 cm thick and have a tongue and groove design.

Unlike NOMOS, the couch translation allows unrestricted treatment volume lengths for the large majority of deliveries. The maximum treatment length is 160 cm for a single spiral with the couch at the isocenter height. Additionally, due to the helical motion, the issue of feathering is eliminated. The helical tomotherapy deliveries provided another parameter pitch as in spiral CT. This resulted in the table translation longitudinally by the amount of pitch times the width of the beam for each full rotation. This latter effect can be thought of in the same way as the step size or spatial discretization of intensity profiles in leaf sequencing for fixed field IMRT beams.

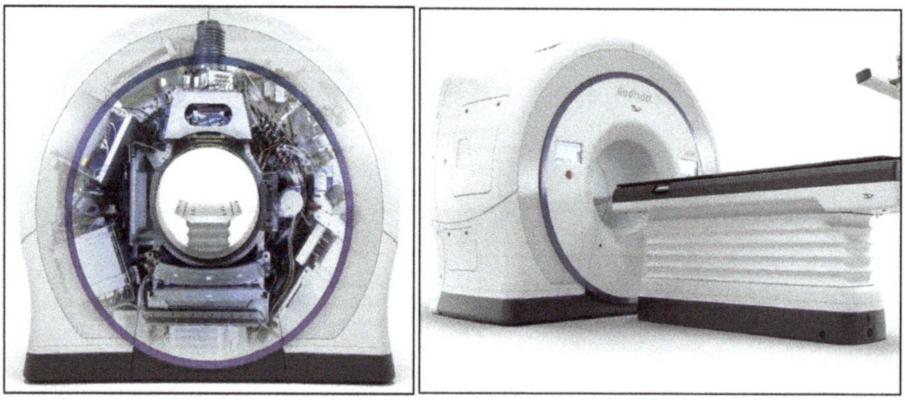

Figure 4.8. Tomotherapy unit marketed now as Radixact by Accuray. Please note that there is no x-ray unit in the system that was originally proposed, instead an MV imaging is used. Left panel internal view and right panel tomotherapy, Radixact unit. Images used with permission from Accuray Incorporated, https://www.accuray.com/radixact/.

Tomotherapy used all the features of CT along with a 6 MV linear accelerator mounted in the head. Imaging was easily accomplished using the MV portal. In the final phases, the diagnostic imaging (CT) was eliminated from the system (figure 4.8) and only mega-voltage images were allowed with 3.5 MV beam. At this point, the imaging of the tomotherapy machine is not intended to be used for diagnostic purposes or its role in the treatment planning of radiotherapy patients. The final tomotherapy unit had a bore size of 85 cm to include most patients with an immobilization device. The unit is a single energy x-ray machine without a flattening filter since it was meant for intensity modulation and a dedicated unit for IMRT. It provided high dose rate treatment.

References

[1] Convery D J and Rosenbloom M E 1995 Treatment delivery accuracy in intensity-modulated conformal radiotherapy *Phys. Med. Biol.* **40** 979–99

[2] Brahme A 1988 Optimization of stationary and moving beam radiation therapy techniques *Radiother. Oncol.* **12** 129–40

[3] Bortfeld T R, Kahler D L and Waldron T J *et al* 1994 X-ray field compensation with multileaf collimators *Int. J. Radiat. Oncol. Biol. Phys.* **28** 723–30

[4] du Plessis F C and Willemse C A 2006 Inclusion of compensator-induced scatter and beam filtration in pencil beam dose calculations *Med. Phys.* **33** 2896–904

[5] Opp D, Forster K and Feygelman V 2011 Commissioning compensator-based IMRT on the Pinnacle treatment planning system *J. Appl. Clin. Med. Phys.* **12** 310–25

[6] Pirzkall A, Carol M P and Pickett B *et al* 2002 The effect of beam energy and number of fields on photon-based IMRT for deep-seated targets *Int. J. Radiat. Oncol. Biol. Phys.* **53** 434–42

[7] Kry S F, Salehpour M and Followill D S *et al* 2005 Out-of-field photon and neutron dose equivalents from step-and-shoot intensity-modulated radiation therapy *Int. J. Radiat. Oncol. Biol. Phys.* **62** 1204–16

[8] Kry S F, Salehpour M and Followill D S *et al* 2005 The calculated risk of fatal secondary malignancies from intensity-modulated radiation therapy *Int. J. Radiat. Oncol. Biol. Phys.* **62** 1195–203

[9] Kry S F, Howell R M and Titt U *et al* 2008 Energy spectra, sources, and shielding considerations for neutrons generated by a flattening filter-free Clinac *Med. Phys.* **35** 1906–11

[10] Van Schelt J, Smith D L and Fong N *et al* 2018 A ring-based compensator IMRT system optimized for low- and middle-income countries: design and treatment planning study *Med. Phys.* **45** 3275–86

[11] Dai J R and Hu Y M 1999 Intensity-modulation radiotherapy using independent collimators: an algorithm study *Med. Phys.* **26** 2562–70

[12] Yoda K and Aoki Y 2003 A multiportal compensator system for IMRT delivery *Med. Phys.* **30** 880–6

[13] Chang S X, Cullip T J and Deschesne K M *et al* 2004 Compensators: an alternative IMRT delivery technique *J. Appl. Clin. Med. Phys.* **5** 15–36

[14] Cheng C W and Chin L M 1987 A computer-aided treatment planning technique for universal wedge *Int. J. Radiat. Oncol. Biol. Phys.* **13** 1927–35

[15] Cheng C W, Chin L M and Kijewski P K 1987 A coordinate transfer of anatomical information from CT to treatment simulation *Int. J. Radiat. Oncol. Biol. Phys.* **13** 1559–69

[16] Leavitt D D, Martin M and Moeller J H *et al* 1990 Dynamic wedge field techniques through computer-controlled collimator motion and dose delivery *Med. Phys.* **17** 87–91
[17] Petti P L and Siddon R L 1985 Effective wedge angles with universal wedge *Phys. Med. Biol.* **30** 985–91
[18] van Santvoort J 1998 Dosimetric evaluation of the Siemens virtual wedge *Phys. Med. Biol.* **43** 2651–63
[19] Klein E E, Low D A and Meigooni A S *et al* 1995 Dosimetry and clinical implementation of dynamic wedge *Int. J. Radiat. Onol. Biol. Phys.* **31** 583–92
[20] Webb S 1994 Optimizing the planning of intensity-modulated radiotherapy *Phys. Med. Biol.* **39** 2229–46
[21] Webb S and Oldham M 1996 A method to study the characteristics of 3D dose distributions created by superposition of many intensity-modulated beams delivered via a slit aperture with multiple absorbing vanes *Phys. Med. Biol.* **41** 2135–53
[22] Webb S, Bortfeld T and Stein J *et al* 1997 The effect of stair-step leaf transmission on the 'tongue-and-groove problem' in dynamic radiotherapy with a multileaf collimator *Phys. Med. Biol.* **42** 595–602
[23] Webb S 1998 Configuration options for intensity-modulated radiation therapy using multiple static fields shaped by a multileaf collimator *Phys. Med. Biol.* **43** 241–60
[24] Webb S 1999 Conformal intensity-modulated radiotherapy (IMRT) delivered by robotic linac-testing IMRT to the limit? *Phys. Med. Biol.* **44** 1639–54
[25] Webb S 2000 *Intensity-modulated Radiation Therapy.* (Bristol: Institute of Physics Publishing)
[26] Webb S 2002 Intensity-modulated radiation therapy using only jaws and a mask *Phys. Med. Biol.* **47** 257–75
[27] Spirou S V and Chui C S 1994 Generation of arbitrary intensity profiles by dynamic jaws or multileaf collimators *Med. Phys.* **21** 1031–41
[28] Chui C S, Chan M F and Yorke E *et al* 2001 Delivery of intensity-modulated radiation therapy with a conventional multileaf collimator: comparison of dynamic and segmental methods *Med. Phys.* **28** 2441–9
[29] Chui C S, Spirou S and LoSasso T 1996 Testing of dynamic multileaf collimation *Med. Phys.* **23** 635–41
[30] LoSasso T, Chui C S and Ling C C 1998 Physical and dosimetric aspects of a multileaf collimation system used in the dynamic mode for implementing intensity modulated radiotherapy *Med. Phys.* **25** 1919–27
[31] Chui C-S, Spriou S and LoSasso T 1996 Testing of dynamic multifleaf collimation *Med. Phys.* **23** 635–41
[32] Källman P, Lind B and Eklöf A *et al* 1988 Shaping of arbitrary dose distributions by dynamic multileaf collimation *Phys. Med. Biol.* **33** 1291–300
[33] LoSasso T, Chui C S and Kutcher G J *et al* 1993 The use of a multi-leaf collimator for conformal radiotherapy of carcinomas of the prostate and nasopharynx *Int. J. Radiat. Oncol. Biol. Phys.* **25** 161–70
[34] Chui C S, LoSasso T and Spirou S 1994 Dose calculation for photon beams with intensity modulation generated by dynamic jaw or multileaf collimations *Med. Phys.* **21** 1237–44
[35] Ling C C, Burman C and Chui C S *et al* 1996 Conformal radiation treatment of prostate cancer using inversely-planned intensity-modulated photon beams produced with dynamic multileaf collimation *Int. J. Radiat. Oncol. Biol. Phys.* **35** 721–30

[36] Shepard D M, Earl M A and Li X A *et al* 2002 Direct aperture optimization: a turnkey solution for step-and-shoot IMRT *Med. Phys.* **29** 1007–18

[37] Yu C, Li A and Ma L *et al* 2002 Clinical implementation of intensity-modulated arc therapy *Int. J. Radiat. Oncol. Biol. Phys.* **53** 453–63

[38] Yu C X, Li X A and Ma L *et al* 2002 Clinical implementation of intensity-modulated arc therapy *Int. J. Radiat. Oncol. Biol. Phys.* **53** 453–63

[39] Earl M A, Shepard D M and Naqvi S *et al* 2003 Inverse planning for intensity-modulated arc therapy using direct aperture optimization *Phys. Med. Biol.* **48** 1075–89

[40] Carol M P 1995 Peacock: a system for planning and rotational delivery of intensity-modulated fields *Int. J. Imag. Sys. Tecnol.* **6** 56–61

[41] Curran B 2001 Where goest the Peacock? *Med. Dosim.* **26** 3–9

[42] Tsai J S, Rivard M J and Engler M J 2000 Dependence of linac output on the switch rate of an intensity-modulated tomotherapy collimator *Med. Phys.* **27** 2215–25

[43] Salter B J 2001 NOMOS Peacock IMRT utilizing the Beak post collimation device *Med. Dosim.* **26** 37–45

[44] Carol M, Grant W H III and Bleier A R *et al* 1996 The field-matching problem as it applies to the Peacock three dimensional conformal system for intensity modulation *Int. J. Radiat. Oncol. Biol. Phys.* **34** 183–7

[45] Carol M, Grant W H 3rd and Pavord D *et al* 1996 Initial clinical experience with the Peacock intensity modulation of a 3-D conformal radiation therapy system *Stereotact. Funct. Neurosurg.* **66** 30–4

[46] Woo S Y, Grant W H 3rd and Bellezza D *et al* 1996 A comparison of intensity modulated conformal therapy with a conventional external beam stereotactic radiosurgery system for the treatment of single and multiple intracranial lesions *Int. J. Radiat. Oncol. Biol. Phys.* **35** 593–7

[47] Uy N W, Woo S Y and Teh B S *et al* 2002 Intensity-modulated radiation therapy (IMRT) for meningioma *Int. J. Radiat. Oncol. Biol. Phys.* **53** 1265–70

[48] Salter B J, Fuss M and Sarkar V *et al* 2009 Optimization of isocenter location for intensity modulated stereotactic treatment of small intracranial targets *Int. J. Radiat. Oncol. Biol. Phys.* **73** 546–55

[49] Webb S 1989 Optimisation of conformal radiotherapy dose distributions by simulated annealing *Phys. Med. Biol.* **34** 1349–70

[50] Convery D J and Webb S 1998 Generation of discrete beam-intensity modulation by dynamic multileaf collimation under minimum leaf separation constraints *Phys. Med. Biol.* **43** 2521–38

[51] Mackie T R, Holmes T and Swerdloff S *et al* 1993 Tomotherapy: a new concept for the delivery of dynamic conformal radiotherapy *Med. Phys.* **20** 1709–19

[52] Mackie T R 2006 History of tomotherapy *Phys. Med. Biol.* **51** R427–53

IOP Publishing

Intensity Modulated Radiation Therapy
A clinical overview
Indra J Das, Nicholas J Sanfilippo, Antonella Fogliata and Luca Cozzi

Chapter 5

IMRT, IMAT and VMAT

The implementation of modulated treatment has been approached with various modalities such as static (step and shoot) IMRT, dynamic (sliding window), IMAT, helical (tomotherapy), and rotational (VMAT). A brief outline of some of the approaches was discussed in chapter 4. In this chapter IMRT, IMAT and VMAT will be discussed.

For over 30 years, IMRT has been used for patient treatment. A large number of developments, due to advances in MLC technology, have provided improved patient care with IMRT. Static IMRT became dynamic, and then in 2008 it became rotational [1] as VMAT. The rise of these technologies is shown in figure 5.1 indicating significant clinical interest and advances in most disease sites. These modulated beam delivery approaches have nearly the same outline and end-results but the implementation is different. Features of these different methodologies will be presented in this chapter.

5.1 IMRT

Historically, IMRT evolved with inverse planning using simulated annealing as described in the previous chapters of this book. However, IMRT has two main components, static and dynamic depending upon the delivery techniques as described below.

5.1.1 Step and shoot IMRT

A schematic diagram of an IMRT process is shown in figure 5.2. It represents the treatment of prostate cancer. The prostate as PTV and rectum as OAR are seen in an anterior–posterior beam. After the beam optimization and dose calculation, as discussed later in chapters 9 and 10, the treatment plan produces a deliverable fluence (figure 5.2(b)). This fluence is digitized based on the machine's MLC for delivery. This fluence is divided into fields (figure 5.2(c)) and then split into segments (figure 5.2(d)) that have different intensities. Each segment is composed of small beamlets defined by the MLC. These segments are static while the beam is on

doi:10.1088/978-0-7503-1335-3ch5

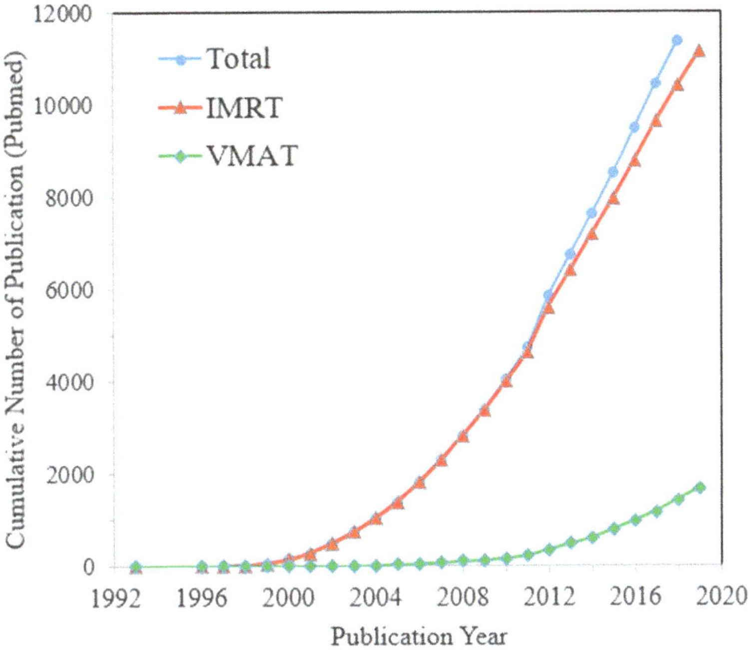

Figure 5.1. Growth of IMRT and VMAT reflected by the number of publications. Data derived from search in PubMed (https://pubmed.ncbi.nlm.nih.gov/).

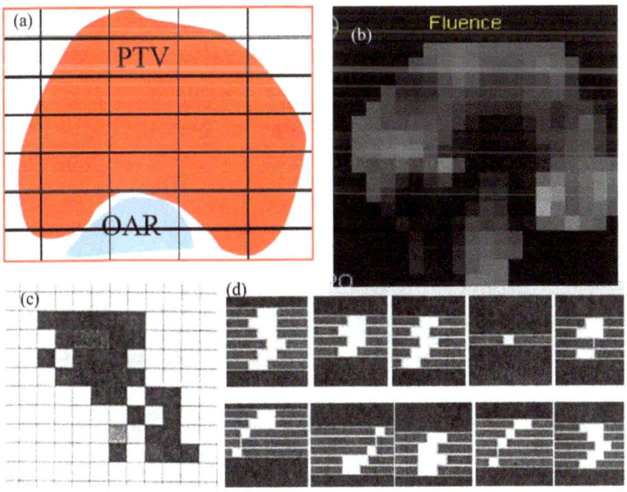

Figure 5.2. (a) Beam's eye view of structures (PTV, OAR) representing prostate and rectum, (b) intensity fluence map generated after optimization and dose calculation, (c) one of the IMRT fields, which is (d) decomposed in segments of same intentity level. In static IMRT, the MLC jaws are static while the beam is on. Animation available at https://iopscience.iop.org/book/978-0-7503-1335-3.

for a given MU, and the MLC only moves when the beam is off. Depending on the beam design and delivery, the machine may be off between the segments, but the waveguide is still active and may produce a small amount of radiation. This is due to the active pulse-forming network of the waveguide, which is known as dark current, and was discussed by Cheng *et al* [2] for the Siemens Primus machine. Thus, it is important to know if the machine is actually not delivering any radiation when the MLC is moving, as this radiation is not modeled and not accounted for in the planning phase of static IMRT. This issue may be critical in older machines and machines of a certain vintage.

The static IMRT process is similar to 3DCRT, where the user chooses the beam angle. In IMRT, it is imperative that the beam angles are not parallel-opposed as may be in 3DCRT. The beam angles should be chosen selectively to provide the maximum sparing of the normal tissues. Typically 5, 7, or 9 beams are chosen in static IMRT. The number of beams is critical, but it is shown that the conformity index does not improve beyond 5–7 fields for most beam energies [3]. Some vendors have provided software for this proccess known as 'beam angle optimizer'. There are some advantages in using a beam angle optimization routine, but a good planner with experience can create a similar selection that provides identical dose distribution; this is shown by various investigators [4, 5]. In many cases, the manual process is better as the user can avoid the table or other metallic objects in a particular beam angle.

Another question often asked in beam angle optimization is if non-co-planar IMRT plans are better than co-planar? The answer is not simple and may depend on the disease site. Chang *et al* [6] showed that there is no disecernable advantage in a non-co-planar beam arrangement in liver cases. However, this is not a universally accepted view.

The static IMRT field delivery scheme is shown in figure 5.3, where a given isodose is composed in many static fields defined by the MLC with a given monitor unit. So in a beam angle, the MLC could change shape with a given MU to provide a suitable iosodose.

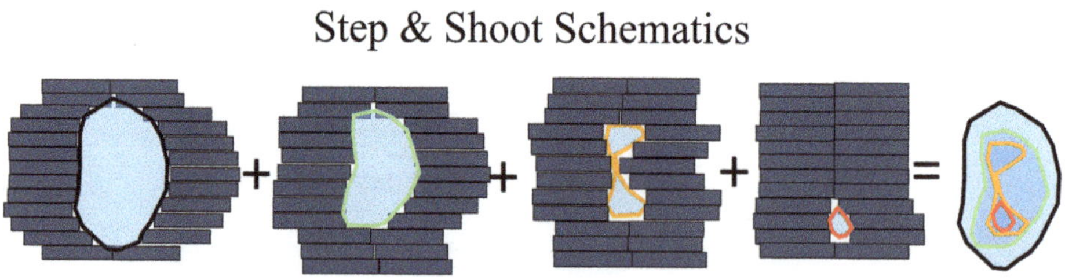

Figure 5.3. Schematic of the step and shoot IMRT with static MLC beamlets providing a desired dose distribution. Animation available at https://iopscience.iop.org/book/978-0-7503-1335-3.

5.1.2 Dynamic delivery IMRT

As discussed previously, in static IMRT, the MLC is static; hence, it usually takes a longer time to deliver the desired dose. As such, dynamic delivery could save time, bringing about the concept of dynamic IMRT. Chapter 4 has provided the basics of fluence modulation with the movement of the leaves based on this concept, as proposed by Bortfeld [7], that led us to the dynamic IMRT. The concept of fluence modulation through the movement of the leaves provides spatial and temporal variation, as shown in figure 5.4, due to the temporal response to a fixed dose rate. Imagine a unidirectional jaw movement at position x and time t, which produces the $t(x)$ profile from the fixed dose rate (fluence of the machine) to create a desired fluence profile $\Phi(x)$. Depending on the movement, e.g., trailing (A) leaf creates positive slopes and the leading (B) leaf creates negative slopes that can be tailored for a desired profile. This concept is also shown in figure 4.5. The difference $t\mathrm{A}(x) - t\mathrm{B}(x)$ provides the desired treatment time translated into MU based on constant dose rate. The temporal profile $t(x)$ provide the positional profile $x(t)$ by inversion as shown in figure 5.4 on the right panel; this can be used to drive the leaves as a function of time for treatment.

The implementation of figure 5.4 in real life is shown pictorially in figure 5.5, where the modulation of the leaves provides the variable intensity profile. When

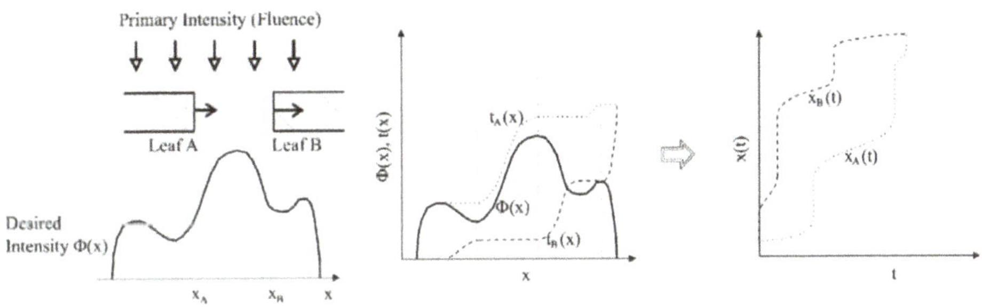

Figure 5.4. Schematic of the MLC motion creating fluence modulation for a fixed dose rate. Adapted from Bortfeld [7] with permission. Copyright IOP Publishing Ltd. All rights reserved.

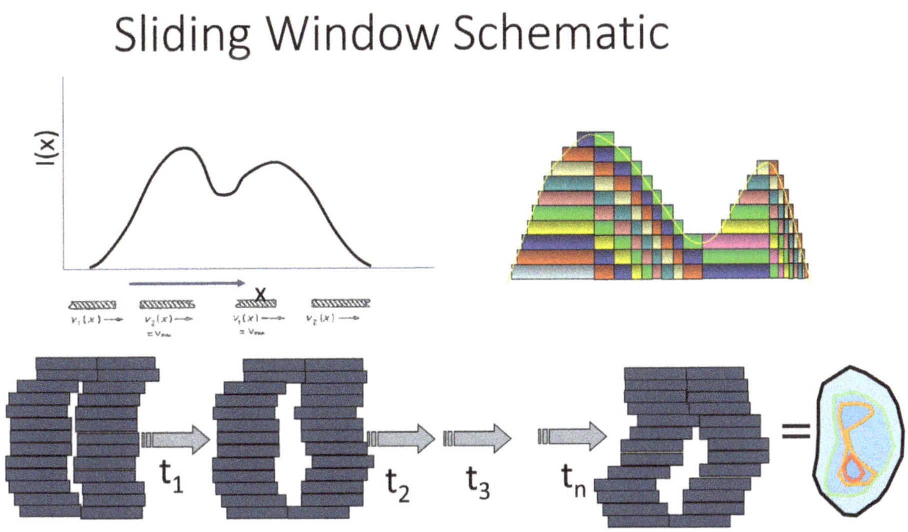

Figure 5.5. Concept of dynamic IMRT of continuous motion of the MLC while the beam is on. The shape changes over time as indicated by t_1, t_2, t_3 etc. The final dose distribution is the sum of all MLC-shaped dose delivery beams in a gantry angle. Animation available at https://iopscience.iop.org/book/978-0-7503-1335-3.

combining, the combination of both sets of jaws modulated by time can provide a digitized intensity level. Similar to the summation of the isodose in figure 5.4, dynamic leaves can provide the desired dose distribution as shown in the bottom panel. Dynamic delivery has many advantages including the treatment of moving targets and reduction in the treatment time. Dynamic IMRT is more susceptible to MLC leaf gap at dynamic speeds as reported in many publications [8–14]. For precise treatment, periodic MLC QA is an essential component in dynamic IMRT. Additionally, wear and tear could put an extra burden on machine maintenance, which should be evaluated.

5.2 IMAT

Soon after the development of cobalt teletherapy machines in 1950, arc therapy became a possibility with isocentric machines. The seed of rotation and conformal therapy was also started in Japan by Takahashi in 1965 [15] who proposed dynamic rotational therapy using MLC. He showed that with rotation and choice of the MLC, conformal dose distribution was achievable. During the 70s and 80s, arc therapy was an important tool for radiation therapy in treating centrally located tumors such as esophagus, prostate, bladder, and mid-line brain tumors. In general, arc therapy provided a cylindrical shaped isodose and could be treated with minimum effort. Arc therapy could be full rotation (360°) or partial rotation to tailor the isodose distributions. However, there was no mechanism to shield normal tissues, and arc therapy faded away with the emergence of 3DCRT in the 90s, which made it possible to provide conformal dose distribution and spare normal tissues.

During this time, a lot of progress was made on modulated treatments, as explained in more detail in previous chapters. It was realized that the number of beams was directly proportional to the conformity index, leading to conformal arc therapy as proposed by Cedric Yu in his two papers [16, 17]. He introduced a method of arc therapy to shield the normal tissue with the help of the MLC and called it intensity modulated arc therapy (IMAT). This was a concept similar to tomotherapy, but IMAT used a totally different approach by performing beam shaping in each beam angle with the MLC. Yu showed that it was possible to create a C-shaped dose distribution; this could be used with the spine to spare the spinal cord, as shown in figure 5.6. It was a revolutionary idea to shape the fields in arc therapy as the gantry moved. The MLC shape could be adjusted in a gantry angle based on the beam's eye view of the PTV and normal structure. Imagine a larger number of static fields that have MLC-shaped fields to provide desired dose distribution.

The methodology improved over time and the clinical applications of IMAT were reported for spine and head, and neck, both of which are very complex treatments [18], along with a large amount of interest reflected by the number of publications [17, 19–24]. The adaptability of IMAT on different MLCs was challenging due to the MLC characteristics that made it harder to adapt [25]. Various attempts took place over 10 years, but because of lack of interest and suitable vendors to create a planning system, IMAT was not a success. Due to lack of interest in suitable vendors to create a planning system, the development of

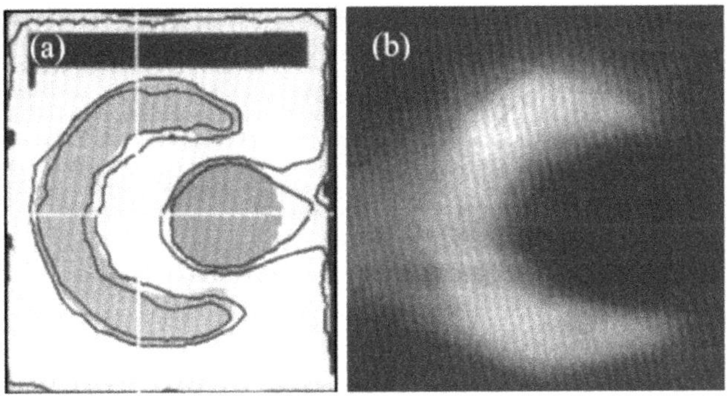

Figure 5.6. (a) Treatment plan on a phantom using IMAT and (b) IMAT delivered dose distribution. Adapted from Yu [16] with permission. Copyright IOP Publishing Ltd. All rights reserved.

IMAT did not take place and ultimately IMRT took over during this time. However, the dynamic approach did not stop there. Rather, it flourished using gantry and MLC movements simultaneously in a new technique called VMAT, which will be discussed in the following section.

5.3 Volumetric, modulated arc therapy, VMAT

The IMAT proposed by Yu in 1995 [16, 17] aimed at increasing flexibility in delivering highly conformal plans by using a large number of beam directions at the limits of the arc approaches. However, the efficiency of that technique was limited by the MLC leaf motion constraints, since leaf position changes between consecutive gantry positions have to be restricted. To overcome this limitation, multiple arc settings were investigated to allow for a clinical approach, but this increased the treatment time [26]. Another limitation was the coarse sampling of the gantry and MLC leaf positions, resulting in unacceptable dosimetric errors.

Volumetric modulated arc therapy, VMAT, was born as the solution to overcome the limitations encountered with IMAT. By efficiently optimizing in a single arc, VMAT provided high dose conformality and high-resolution sampling for MLC and gantry positions. The fundamental concept was published by Otto in 2008 [1], when the approach was going to be clinically implemented as RapidArc in Varian systems. In his work, Otto described an alternative approach to IMRT and IMAT. The differences between IMAT and RapidArc (subsequently VMAT) were very subtle and became the subject of copyright and patent litigation, which was settled out of court between Elekta and Varian. The word VMAT is now a generic and universally used term irrespective of the vendor.

VMAT dose optimization was based on a method similar to an aperture-based optimization process, incorporating the MLC leaf positions (MLC aperture) and the MU weights [27]. During the optimization, these two parameters are also constrained so that only aperture shapes and MU values physically achievable in practice are allowed to be used, thus preserving continuous delivery. In practice, considering the maximum gantry speed ($(d\theta/dt)_{max}$) of 6 deg s^{-1}, and the maximum leaf motion speed ($(dx/dt)_{max}$) of 3.0 cm s^{-1} (achievable on a Varian Linac), the two constraints are summarized in equations (5.1) and (5.2), as:

$$\left(\frac{dx}{d\theta}\right)_{max} = \left(\frac{dx}{dt}\right)_{max} \Big/ \left(\frac{d\theta}{dt}\right)_{max} = 0.5 \text{ cm/deg} \tag{5.1}$$

$$\left(\frac{dMU}{d\theta}\right)_{max} = \left(\frac{dMU}{dt}\right)_{max} \Big/ \left(\frac{d\theta}{dt}\right)_{max} \tag{5.2}$$

An MU weight that exceeds the maximum allowed dose rate $(dMU/dt)_{max}$ can be delivered by reducing the gantry rotation speed $(d\theta/dt)$. The constraints also aim to ensure that the maximum dose rate is rarely exceeded, as gantry deceleration is undesirable (because it leads to longer treatment times).

The VMAT optimization process proposed by Otto involved a progressive mechanism to sample a dynamic arc by a finite number of static beams that had to be high enough to achieve acceptable accuracy. The progressive concept is reported in figure 5.7. At the beginning of VMAT optimization, a rather coarse sampling of the gantry positions is used, including the start and stop angles of rotation, with evenly distributed samples. After a number of iterations, an additional sample is added at the midway between two existing samples. The leaf positions for the new sample are interpolated from the adjacent gantry angles and the MU is a function of the neighboring beams. The number of samples is increased until adequate dosimetric accuracy is achieved. The coarse sampling at the beginning of the progressive process provides more optimization flexibility, relatively poor accuracy, and fast optimization. Increasing the number of samples decreases the flexibility and, improves the dosimetric accuracy. The addition of any new sample causes a temporary increase in the cost function, which is then lowered during the optimization of the next steps.

The number of samples (control points, CP, in the common terminology) is in relation to the plan accuracy. In figure 5.8, the percentage of volume exceeding 10%, 5%, and 3% dose error is presented as a function of the gantry and spacing, showing that a gantry angle spacing larger than maximum 2 degrees would yield an unacceptably high dosimetric error.

The evaluations in Otto's paper characterizing the relationships between sampling, dose modeling accuracy, and optimization times resulted in:

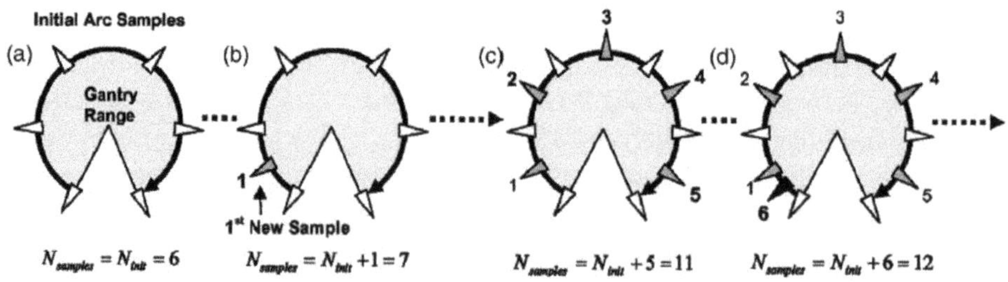

Figure 5.7. Progressive resolution VMAT optimization concept. Adapted from Otto [1] with permission John Wiley & Sons. Copyright 1993 American Association of Physicists in Medicine.

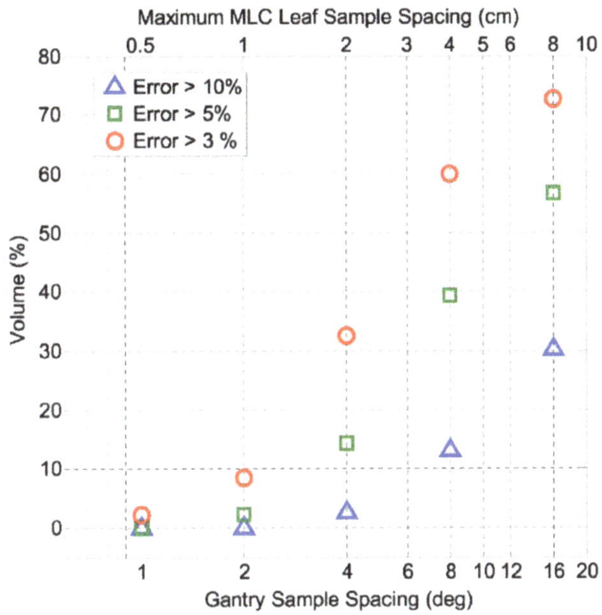

Figure 5.8. Volume exceeding fixed dose errors as a function of the gantry (and MLC leaf) sample spacing. Adapted from Otto [1] with permission John Wiley & Sons. Copyright 1993 American Association of Physicists in Medicine.

- Adequate dosimetric accuracy requires a high sampling frequency of gantry and MLC positions
- Greater sampling of MLC leaf positions exponentially increases optimization time

The progressive introduction of samples during the optimization allows VMAT to rapidly approach a solution without compromising the dosimetric accuracy. The key points of VMAT, pointing to its implementation in the Varian Eclipse system as RapidArc, have been subsequently clarified by Otto [28], describing the VMAT solution of a problem similar to that proposed by Brahme *et al* [29] and elaborated in figure 5.9.

A VMAT (RapidArc) solution very close to the ideal solution is shown by Otto [28] and depicted in figure 5.10. However, to achieve such a result, the whole capabilities of the system, including not only a theoretical optimization approach but also the linac and MLC characteristics, have to be included in the process. In particular, there are three points, which have to be properly adapted to fully utilize the degree of freedom:

- the speed and range of the dynamic MLC motion;
- the dose rate variation (through dose rate or gantry speed variation) during the arc;
- the use of any collimator angle, giving the possibility to use multiple MLC leaf pairs for intensity modulation in a given plane; the choice of the collimator angle equal to zero is the worst possible solution, since in this case only a single leaf pair can be used to modulate the intensity, providing an inferior dose distribution.

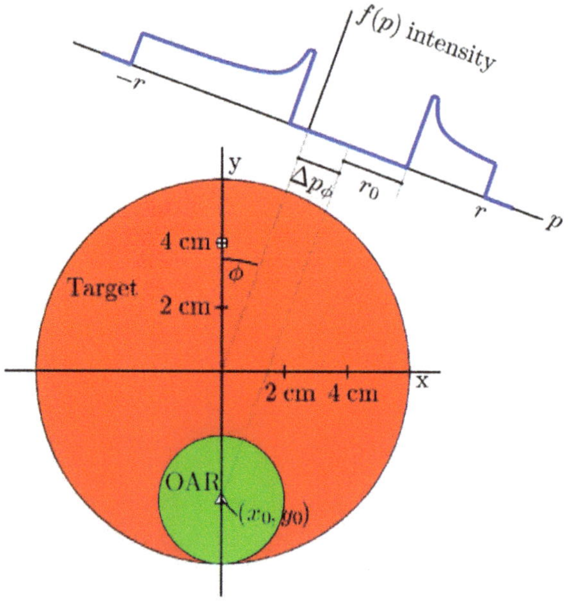

Figure 5.9. Modification of the Brahme's rotational radiation therapy problem [29], with the green OAR (excentric) to be spared inside the red target to treat. The exemplified ideal intensity profile is shown for the gantry angle of 20 degrees. Adapted from Bortfeld and Webb [30] with permission. Copyright 2009 Institute of Physics and Engineering in Medicine. All rights reserved.

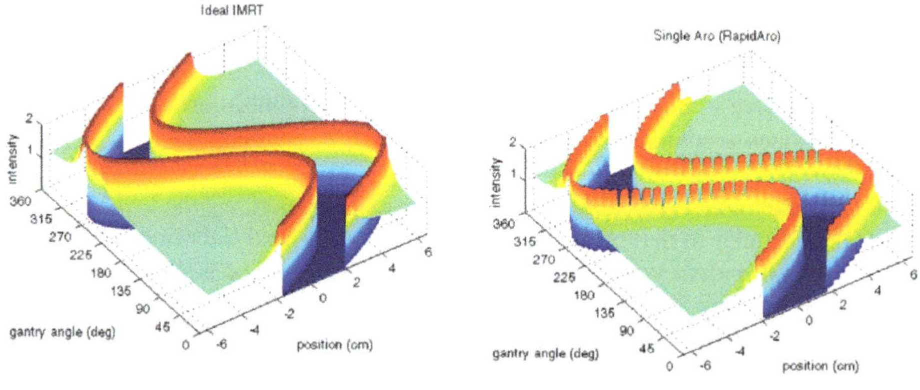

Figure 5.10. On the left: ideal sinogram of the theoretical, ideal, solution of the Brahme problem [29] in figure 5.9. On the right: sinogram of the same, according to the VMAT, RapidArc (single-arc IMRT) solution. Adapted from Otto [28] with permission. Copyright 2009 Institute of Physics and Engineering in Medicine. All rights reserved.

Regarding the collimator angle, Otto also suggested that the potential exists to change the collimator angle during arc rotation to further improve the ability to achieve the desired dose conformality due to the MLC design. This option is not yet available today in clinical commercial systems. The VMAT technique was born as a single full arc IMRT providing the desired dose distribution. However, it is already noted by Otto [1] about the reduced arc ranges that may be applied, as well as the possibility of multiple arc setting for a desired goal.

As soon as VMAT technology was made available for clinical practice (initially by Varian with the RapidArc solution, then by Elekta with the Elekta-VMAT solution), an increasing number of papers started to be published, showing great interest in this new step forward in the intensity modulated era. Most of the studies compared plans obtained with IMRT and VMAT for various anatomical sites. The general message showed VMAT plans having shorter treatment times, similar target coverage and dose homogeneity as IMRT, and improved OAR sparing, even in the cases of the initial VMAT versions available, which, as expected, improved their performances over the subsequent years, as shown in figure 5.1.

In most of the cases, an increased plan complexity (e.g., an increased number of arcs) presented better plan quality. Papers presenting patient-specific QA proved the accurate deliverability of VMAT plans. Practically all anatomical sites have been explored for VMAT planning, for a wide variety of treatments with no limitations of treatment location and target volumes. Here a limited number of the pioneering or seminal studies are reported for further reading in various disease sites with the use of VMAT and its implications [31–45].

5.4 Outlook

IMRT, IMAT, RapidArc, and VMAT have progressively provided better treatment techniques. However, the implementation of VMAT has significantly reduced treatment time as the gantry and MLC both move while delivering the beam [34]. VMAT also provides reduced MU and thus reduces the whole body radiation as compared to similar cases with IMRT. The reduction in MU is nearly 3–5 fold with VMAT. This reduction is associated with a similar possible reduction in long-term complications, mainly secondary cancer, as shown in this long list of publications [33, 36, 46–60].

References

[1] Otto K 2008 Volumetric modulated arc therapy: IMRT in a single gantry arc *Med. Phys.* **35** 310–7

[2] Cheng C W, Das I J and Ndlovu A M 2002 Suppression of dark current radiation in step-and-shoot intensity modulated radiation therapy by the initial pulse-forming network *Med. Phys.* **29** 1974–9

[3] Pirzkall A, Carol M P and Pickett B *et al* 2002 The effect of beam energy and number of fields on photon-based IMRT for deep-seated targets *Int. J. Radiat. Oncol. Biol. Phys.* **53** 434–42

[4] Srivastava S P, Das I J and Kumar A *et al* 2011 Dosimetric comparison of manual and beam angle optimization of gantry angles in IMRT *Med. Dosim.* **36** 313–6
[5] Zhang H H, Gao S and Chen W *et al* 2013 A surrogate-based metaheuristic global search method for beam angle selection in radiation treatment planning *Phys. Med. Biol.* **58** 1933–46
[6] Chang D S, Bartlett G K and Das I J *et al* 2013 Beam angle selection for intensity-modulated radiotherapy (IMRT) treatment of unresectable pancreatic cancer: are noncoplanar beam angles necessary? *Clin. Transl. Oncol.* **15** 720–4
[7] Bortfeld T 2006 IMRT: a review and preview *Phys. Med. Biol.* **51** R363–79
[8] Xu Z, Wang I Z and Kumaraswamy L K *et al* 2016 Evaluation of dosimetric effect caused by slowing with multi-leaf collimator (MLC) leaves for volumetric modulated arc therapy (VMAT) *Radiol. Oncol.* **50** 121–8
[9] LoSasso T, Chui C S and Ling C C 1998 Physical and dosimetric aspects of a multileaf collimation system used in the dynamic mode for implementing intensity modulated radiotherapy *Med. Phys.* **25** 1919–27
[10] LoSasso T, Chui C and Ling C 2001 Comprehensive quality assurance for the delivery of intensity modulated radiotherapy with a multileaf collimator used in the dynamic mode *Med. Phys.* **28** 2209–19
[11] Kumaraswamy L K, Schmitt J D and Bailey D W *et al* 2014 Spatial variation of dosimetric leaf gap and its impact on dose delivery *Med. Phys.* **41** 111711
[12] Chui C-S, Spriou S and LoSasso T 1996 Testing of dynamic multifleaf collimation *Med. Phys.* **23** 635–41
[13] Chui C S, LoSasso T and Spirou S 1994 Dose calculation for photon beams with intensity modulation generated by dynamic jaw or multileaf collimations *Med. Phys.* **21** 1237–44
[14] Kim J, Han J S and Hsia A T *et al* 2018 Relationship between dosimetric leaf gap and dose calculation errors for high definition multi-leaf collimators in radiotherapy *Phys. Imag. Radiat. Oncol.* **5** 31–6
[15] Takahashi S 1965 Conformation radiotherapy: rotation techniques as applied to radiography and radiotherapy of cancer *Acta Radiol. Suppl.* **242** 1–142
[16] Yu C X 1995 Intensity-modulated arc therapy with dynamic multileaf collimation: an alternative to tomotherapy *Phys. Med. Biol.* **40** 1435–49
[17] Yu C X, Symons M J and Du M N *et al* 1995 A method for implementing dynamic photon beam intensity modulation using independent jaws and a multileaf collimator *Phys. Med. Biol.* **40** 769–87
[18] Yu C X, Li X A and Ma L *et al* 2002 Clinical implementation of intensity-modulated arc therapy *Int. J. Radiat. Oncol. Biol. Phys.* **53** 453–63
[19] Yu C, Shepard D and Earl M *et al* 2006 New developments in intensity modulated radiation therapy *Technol. Cancer Res. Treat.* **5** 451–64
[20] Yu C X, Amies C J and Svatos M 2008 Planning and delivery of intensity-modulated radiation therapy *Med. Phys.* **35** 5233–41
[21] Yu C X, Li X A and Ma L *et al* 2002 Clinical implementation of intensity-modulated arc therapy *Int. J. Radiat. Oncol. Biol. Phys.* **53** 453–63
[22] Yu C X, Shao X and Zhang J *et al* 2013 GammaPod-a new device dedicated for stereotactic radiotherapy of breast cancer *Med. Phys.* **40** 051701–11
[23] Yu C X and Wong J W 1993 Implementation of the ETAR method for 3D inhomogeneity correction using FFT *Med. Phys.* **20** 627–31

[24] Yu C X, Yan D and Du M N *et al* 1995 Optimization of leaf positions when shaping a radiation field with a multileaf collimator *Phys. Med. Biol.* **40** 305–8

[25] Huq M S, Das I J and Steinberg T *et al* 2002 A dosimetric comparison of various multileaf collimators *Phys. Med. Biol.* **47** N159–70

[26] Cao D, Afghan M K and Ye J *et al* 2009 A generalized inverse planning tool for volumetric-modulated arc therapy *Phys. Med. Biol.* **54** 6725–38

[27] Earl M A, Shepard D M and Naqvi S *et al* 2003 Inverse planning for intensity-modulated arc therapy using direct aperture optimization *Phys. Med. Biol.* **48** 1075–89

[28] Otto K 2009 Letter to the Editor on 'Single-Arc IMRT?' *Phys. Med. Biol.* **54** L37–41 (author reply L43-34)

[29] Brahme A, Roos J E and Lax I 1982 Solution of an integral equation encountered in rotation therapy *Phys. Med. Biol.* **27** 1221–9

[30] Bortfeld T and Webb S 2009 Single-arc IMRT? *Phys. Med. Biol.* **54** N9–20

[31] Fogliata A, Cozzi L and Clivio A *et al* 2011 Preclinical assessment of volumetric modulated arc therapy for total marrow irradiation *Int. J. Radiat. Oncol. Biol. Phys.* **80** 628–36

[32] Fogliata A, Bergström S and Cafaro I *et al* 2011 Cranio-spinal irradiation with volumetric modulated arc therapy: a multi-institutional treatment experience *Radiother. Oncol.* **99** 79–85

[33] Fogliata A, De Rose F and Franceschini D *et al* 2018 Critical appraisal of the risk of secondary cancer induction from breast radiation therapy with volumetric modulated arc therapy relative to 3D conformal therapy *Int. J. Radiat. Oncol. Biol. Phys.* **100** 785–93

[34] Popescu C C, Olivotto I A and Beckham W A *et al* 2010 Volumetric modulated arc therapy improves dosimetry and reduces treatment time compared to conventional intensity-modulated radiotherapy for locoregional radiotherapy of left-sided breast cancer and internal mammary nodes *Int. J. Radiat. Oncol. Biol. Phys.* **76** 287–95

[35] Nicolini G, Clivio A and Fogliata A *et al* 2009 Simultaneous integrated boost radiotherapy for bilateral breast: a treatment planning and dosimetric comparison for volumetric modulated arc and fixed field intensity modulated therapy *Radiat. Oncol.* **4** 27

[36] Johansen S, Cozzi L and Olsen D R 2009 A planning comparison of dose patterns in organs at risk and predicted risk for radiation induced malignancy in the contralateral breast following radiation therapy of primary breast using conventional, IMRT and volumetric modulated arc treatment techniques *Acta Oncol.* **48** 495–503

[37] Lagerwaard F J, Meijer O W and van der Hoorn E A *et al* 2009 Volumetric modulated arc radiotherapy for vestibular schwannomas *Int. J. Radiat. Oncol. Biol. Phys.* **74** 610–5

[38] Scorsetti M, Bignardi M and Clivio A *et al* 2010 Volumetric modulation arc radiotherapy compared with static gantry intensity-modulated radiotherapy for malignant pleural mesothelioma tumor: a feasibility study *Int. J. Radiat. Oncol. Biol. Phys.* **77** 942–9

[39] Rao M, Yang W and Chen F *et al* 2010 Comparison of Elekta VMAT with helical tomotherapy and fixed field IMRT: plan quality, delivery efficiency and accuracy *Med. Phys.* **37** 1350–9

[40] McGrath S D, Matuszak M M and Yan D *et al* 2010 Volumetric modulated arc therapy for delivery of hypofractionated stereotactic lung radiotherapy: a dosimetric and treatment efficiency analysis *Radiother. Oncol.* **95** 153–57

[41] Clivio A, Fogliata A and Franzetti-Pellanda A *et al* 2009 Volumetric-modulated arc radiotherapy for carcinomas of the anal canal: a treatment planning comparison with fixed field IMRT *Radiother. Oncol.* **92** 118–24

[42] Cozzi L, Dinshaw K A and Shrivastava S K *et al* 2008 A treatment planning study comparing volumetric arc modulation with RapidArc and fixed field IMRT for cervix uteri radiotherapy *Radiother. Oncol.* **89** 180–91

[43] Shaffer R, Morris W J and Moiseenko V *et al* 2009 Volumetric modulated arc therapy and conventional intensity-modulated radiotherapy for simultaneous maximal intraprostatic boost: a planning comparison study *Clin. Oncol. (R Coll. Radiol.)* **21** 401–7

[44] Vanetti E, Clivio A and Nicolini G *et al* 2009 Volumetric modulated arc radiotherapy for carcinomas of the oro-pharynx, hypo-pharynx and larynx: a treatment planning comparison with fixed field IMRT *Radiother. Oncol.* **92** 111–7

[45] Nicolini G, Ghosh-Laskar S and Shrivastava S K *et al* 2012 Volumetric modulation arc radiotherapy with flattening filter-free beams compared with static gantry IMRT and 3D conformal radiotherapy for advanced esophageal cancer: a feasibility study *Int. J. Radiat. Oncol. Biol. Phys.* **84** 553–60

[46] Kry S F, Titt U and Ponisch F *et al* 2007 Reduced neutron production through use of a flattening-filter-free accelerator *Int. J. Radiat. Oncol. Biol. Phys.* **68** 1260–4

[47] Athar B S and Paganetti H 2011 Comparison of second cancer risk due to out-of-field doses from 6-MV IMRT and proton therapy based on 6 pediatric patient treatment plans *Radiother. Oncol.* **98** 87–92

[48] Wang B and Xu X G 2008 Measurements of non-target organ doses using MOSFET dosemeters for selected IMRT and 3D CRT radiation treatment procedures *Radiat. Prot. Dosim.* **128** 336–42

[49] Fontenot J D, Lee A K and Newhauser W D 2009 Risk of secondary malignant neoplasms from proton therapy and intensity-modulated x-ray therapy for early-stage prostate cancer *Int. J. Radiat. Oncol. Biol. Phys.* **74** 616–22

[50] Abo-Madyan Y, Aziz M H and Aly M M *et al* 2014 Second cancer risk after 3D-CRT, IMRT and VMAT for breast cancer *Radiother. Oncol.* **110** 471–6

[51] Ruben J D, Smith R and Lancaster C M *et al* 2014 Constituent components of out-of-field scatter dose for 18-MV intensity modulated radiation therapy versus 3-dimensional conformal radiation therapy: a comparison with 6-MV and implications for carcinogenesis *Int. J. Radiat. Oncol. Biol. Phys.* **90** 645–53

[52] Ruben J D, Lancaster C M and Jones P *et al* 2011 A comparison of out-of-field dose and its constituent components for intensity-modulated radiation therapy versus conformal radiation therapy: implications for carcinogenesis *Int. J. Radiat. Oncol. Biol. Phys.* **81** 1458–64

[53] Murray L J, Thompson C M and Lilley J *et al* 2015 Radiation-induced second primary cancer risks from modern external beam radiotherapy for early prostate cancer: impact of stereotactic ablative radiotherapy (SABR), volumetric modulated arc therapy (VMAT) and flattening filter free (FFF) radiotherapy *Phys. Med. Biol.* **60** 1237–57

[54] Chargari C, Goodman K A and Diallo I *et al* 2016 Risk of second cancers in the era of modern radiation therapy: does the risk/benefit analysis overcome theoretical models? *Cancer Metastasis Rev.* **35** 277–88

[55] Bednarz B, Hancox C and Xu X G 2009 Calculated organ doses from selected prostate treatment plans using Monte Carlo simulations and an anatomically realistic computational phantom *Phys. Med. Biol.* **54** 5271–86

[56] Filippi A R, Vanoni V and Meduri B *et al* 2018 Intensity modulated radiation therapy and second cancer risk in adults *Int. J. Radiat. Oncol. Biol. Phys.* **100** 17–20

[57] Kry S F, Salehpour M and Followill D S *et al* 2005 The calculated risk of fatal secondary malignancies from intensity-modulated radiation therapy *Int. J. Radiat. Oncol. Biol. Phys.* **62** 1195–03

[58] Kry S F, Howell R M and Titt U *et al* 2008 Energy spectra, sources, and shielding considerations for neutrons generated by a flattening filter-free clinac *Med. Phys.* **35** 1906–11

[59] Kry S F, Followill D and White R A *et al* 2007 Uncertainty of calculated risk estimates for secondary malignancies after radiotherapy *Int. J. Radiat. Oncol. Biol. Phys.* **68** 1265–71

[60] Kry S F, Salehpour M and Followill D S *et al* 2005 Out-of-field photon and neutron dose equivalents from step-and-shoot intensity-modulated radiation therapy *Int. J. Radiat. Oncol. Biol. Phys.* **62** 1204–16

Chapter 6

Intensity modulated planning process

6.1 IMRT planning process

The beam modulated treatments IMRT/VMAT, as described in chapter 5, provide the desired dose distribution in the target volume and spare dose to normal tissues. This is truly a beautiful dose distribution similar to the natural beauty of a flower, as shown in figure 6.1. IMRT represents the creativity of the planner like an artist who paints on a canvas. However, to appreciate the IMRT results, one needs to understand all of the processes involved that cannot be negated or ignored. In this chapter, all these processes are described.

6.2 Imaging

As described in chapter 1, historically, radiation treatment in general did not require images. However, in the 3DCRT era [1], imaging became an integral part of the process as GTV, CTV, PTV, and OARs were required based on IRCU-50 and 62 definitions [2, 3]. The dose-volume concept was developed during 3DCRT and has become a pillar for the IMRT process [4]. Without volume, IMRT cannot be implemented, and the volume information comes from imaging. CT has become the standard in radiation oncology after the acquisition of CT-simulators [5, 6]. Even though MRI and PET images are used in radiation treatment, these imaging modalities are used in conjunction with CT. The literature is full of data in terms of the suitability of different imaging types for volume delineation with variable values [7–14]. In general, CT provides a larger volume compared to MRI and PET; however, this is debatable depending upon the MRI sequence and site used [15, 16]. Depending upon the tumor site, selective use of imaging techniques, and especially multi-modality imaging, is preferred. Such choices, however, could be cost prohibitive and many insurance companies may not allow such utilization. Irrespective of imaging modality, CT has become the standard, as it is a low cost imaging modality that can be used for IMRT volume delineation.

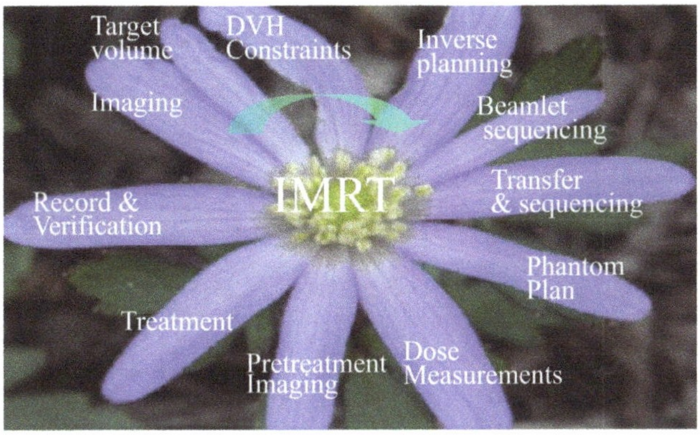

Figure 6.1. An illustration of the IMRT process where each petal of the flower represents a part of the IMRT process making a beautiful flower. In IMRT, a perfect treatment for a patient provides minimum dose to normal tissues. Animation available at https://iopscience.iop.org/book/978-0-7503-1335-3.

6.3 Target volume

As mentioned in the previous section, imaging is used to define the target volume and normal structures without which IMRT planning is not possible or is meaningless. Chapter 7 provides details of the contouring and segmentation process. The target volume is drawn by radiation oncologists with variable skills and training; hence, there is enormous volume variability, which has been discussed extensively in the literature for most disease sites [7, 8, 10, 11, 13, 17–32]. The target volume variability is the weakest link for outcomes of radiation treatment [33]. The variability in volume is so pronounced, as indicated above and in the various references [20, 34, 35], that most societies now offer contouring courses during their annual meetings or on selected occasions. The variability of the target volume can be reduced with multi-modality imaging, training, and the selection of the appropriate techniques. Apart from physician-drawn volumes, the variability in volumes is also associated with the treatment planning system and the selection of slice thickness [36, 37]. Figure 6.2 shows the variability of the target in various imaging techniques, where visualization is more pronounced to help in target volume delineation [38].

ICRU-83 recommended that every possible imaging modality should be used for IMRT [39]. It is granted that volumes are variable in different modalities [11, 14, 15, 29, 40]; hence, it is important to utilize every means to know the exact location of the tumor. This is especially important for soft tissues where CT does not provide adequate discrimination. MRI and PET imaging could be used in many situations. Image fusion provides suitable options in determining the target volumes based on the selectivity of the method as shown by many investigators [7, 38], where various modalities are used. MRI-based volumes have a greater variability and therefore multi-modality imaging is often the choice for delineating structures for radiation treatment [7].

Currently, there are many different types of contouring software for anatomy that can be used such as eContouring (http://www.imaios.com/en/e-Anatomy) and

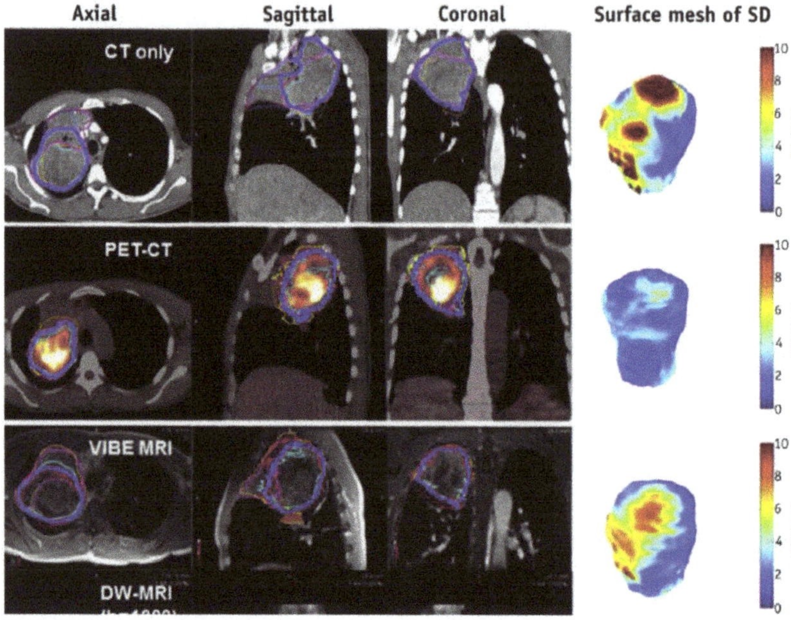

Figure 6.2. The variability of the target volume among seven physicians for a well visualized lung cancer. The standard deviation in the surface mass is also shown from CT, CT-PET, and MRI imaging. Adapted from Karki *et al* [7] with permission from Elsevier.

RTOG Contouring Atlases (http://www.rtog.org/CoreLab/ContouringAtlases.aspx); other vendors have also incorporated software that may yield support in delineation. Even now, most treatment planning systems have incorporated smart contouring packages that can help in drawing the volume.

6.4 DVH constraints

The DVH constraint is a wish list to a computer for executing an order in optimization; this will be discussed further in chapter 9. The constraints are derived from the clinical knowledge of the radiation tolerances in each type of tissue. In the old days (before the 1990s), this was compiled from a paper by Emami *et al* [41] that was collected in the 3DCRT era on the tolerances of tissues. Later, *Quantitative Analysis of Normal Tissue Effects in the Clinic* (QUATEC) published a special issue dealing with each disease site and its radiation effects [42]. The constraints provided by the user are entered into the system to create a cost function for minimization. Figure 6.3 provides an example of the constraints on a graphical interface or enter the dose-volume constraints numerically to achieve. These constraints are the boundary limit that the system may or may not fulfill depending upon the difficulty of the competing cost functions of other structures and the weight assigned to the constraints. These constraints can be entered numerically; that will translate into arrows in the system, as shown in figure 6.3. The user can enter as many data points with weight factors as desired. However, it is advisable that the user does not get

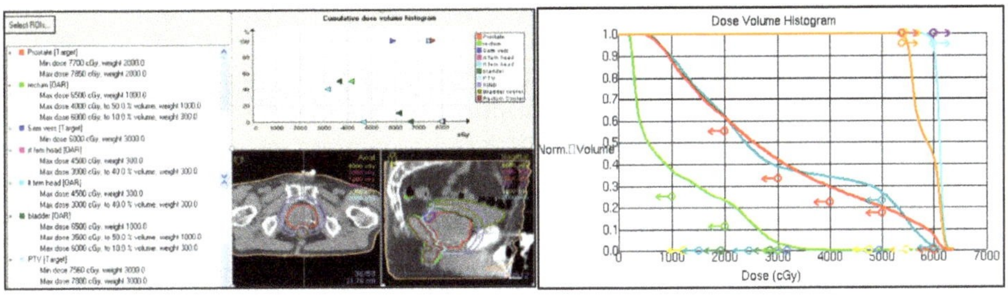

Figure 6.3. DVH constraints as entered in the planning system before the optimization. Arrows indicate where optimization-related dose distribution is desired. The left panel is from Oncentra treatment planning system (TPS) and the right is from Pinnacle TPS.

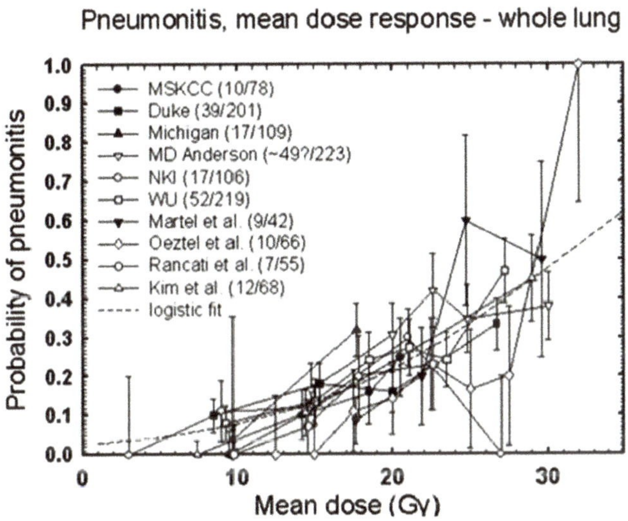

Figure 6.4. Lung toxicity (radiation pneumonitis) versus mean lung dose as reported by many group. Note the variation and spread of data points. Adapted from Marks *et al* [42] with permission from Elsevier.

confused with the DVH limits in the target and OAR, as they will never find an optimized plan due to possible contraindications.

Additionally, OAR constraints are relatively hard to agree upon among the radiation oncologists as there is no single value of dose that can be agreed upon for a given complication. For example data from Marks *et al* [42] on radiation pneumonitis compiled from multiple sources, as shown in figure 6.4, has a very large spread. This spread is due to many factors but mainly the dose computation. It is well-known that calculation algorithms have evolved that produce large differences in dose [43–53]. In such situations, personal knowledge and judgment is used to set clinical DVH constraints. These variations in each disease site are due to the origin of the data. For example, heart constraints are derived from multiple sources for the treatment of breast, Hodgkin, esophagus toxicity data and variation is large [54]. Similar variations are also noted in every site.

6.5 Inverse planning

Inverse planning is a long process including optimization based on DVH constraints as discussed in the previous section. Optimization is a set of minimization routines based on the cost function. Every TPS has its own set of robust programs for optimization that are user-friendly, efficient, and time-saving. Some systems even pick many of the cost functions and provide multiple options for dose distribution, which saves even more time.

This process includes optimization, as will be discussed in chapter 9, followed by dose calculation, as will be discussed in chapter 10. An example of the optimization is shown in figure 6.5. Please note: the computer creates a cost function based on the DVH constraints, and then global minimization takes place. In between iterations, it plots the arbitrary value of the cost function (see right upper panel). The value starts at a very large number and then begins falling rapidly. Later, it levels off and becomes a plateau (as shown in figure 6.5(b)), where one can stop optimization and move on to dose calculation.

After the optimization where the cost function reaches a plateau, as shown in figure 6.5(b), the user stops the module and moves to the dose calculation module. In dose calculations, there are many selectable options for algorithms such as pencil beam, collapsed cone, convolution superposition, Boltzman transport, and many others depending upon treatment planning system. The dose calculation aspect is dealt with in detail in chapter 10. It is advisable, however, that for inhomogeneity corrections in the IMRT calculations, a suitable dose calculation engine should be adopted. There are many publications that provide the merits of these algorithms, which can be evaluated to help choose a proper selection [45, 46, 52, 55–64]. However, it is now well-known that pencil beam algorithms are not suitable for a low-density medium like lung dose calculations and should be avoided [47, 49, 65], as they do not consider lateral electron transport, which is predominant in a low-density medium.

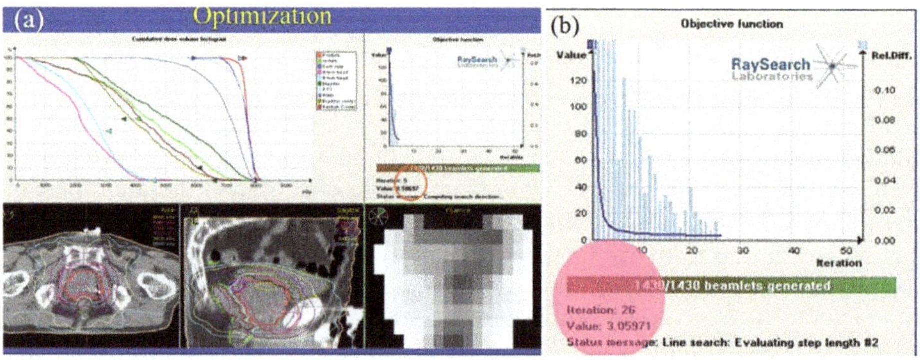

Figure 6.5. (a) Optimization panel is shown from Oncentra TPS. Similar views are also shown by most other TPS. Note the DVH constraints, cost function display, isodose, and fluence map. (b) Note the saturation of the cost function at 26 iterations. No improvement in dose distribution after this is achievable.

6.6 MLC sequencing

In MLC-based IMRT, the non-uniform field is initially converted into an intensity map that is represented as a matrix of beam intensities after the optimization and dose calculation. The intensity map is then decomposed into a series of beamlets or segments of uniform intensities for beam delivery. Even though the optimizer may have produced the ideal plan and dose distribution, it is not guaranteed that such a plan is deliverable due to constraints placed on the MLC. Hence, MLC sequencing plays an important role in the feasibility of the delivery of the plan. There are many ways of segmenting the beam intensity matrix, but a resulting subfield is only deliverable if it satisfies the constraints imposed by the individual MLC design and its constraints. Hence, a plan with optimum dose distribution can become distorted depending on the linear accelerator and its MLC design. The same plan on two different MLC designs will produce two entirely different final dose distributions [66–73]. Desai *et al* [74] provided a unique sequencing method for the tomotherapy unit that, in general, can be used in other machines. Another approach in leaf sequencing optimized algorithms was provided by Wistozky *et al* [73], who provided fast sequencing without providing under and over dose. This method has been proposed for tumor motion adaptability in fast MLC movements.

The initial dose distribution does not guarantee that the final MLC sequencing, due to its delivery constraints, will provide the same dose distribution. Therefore, in general, every plan is sent for sequencing and then a final dose calculation is performed. It is well-known that there is nearly 10% deterioration in the dose distribution in the final calculation. Some treatment planning or users are aware of such situations and they incorporate the effect of the MLC sequencing during the optimization process. To overcome this problem, direct aperture optimization (DAO) was introduced [75–82]. There had been significant improvement in the MLC sequencing algorithms to avoid wasting time in MLC movement, increase the quality in beam delivery, and reduce overall time of treatment. The MLC sequencing finally led to the VAMT, where some of the restrictive constraints in step-and-shoot IMRT can be eliminated.

A smart sequencer produces beamlets that are easily deliverable and combines them with iso-intensity maps that form the segment (figure 6.6). Remember, a segment is a collection of beamlets that have the same intensity or monitor unit. Additional constraints are imposed by users for a minimum size of beamlets, on average 2×2 cm^2, and a minimum fluence, generally >2 MU, since the beam quality at low MU is usually unstable [83–87]. However, with modern machines, beam delivery can be performed within ±2% accuracy even down to 1 MU, since MU is no longer an integer number.

The sequencing process is proprietary to the TPS. A study conducted shows the variation of the final results for a prostate cancer case. Figure 6.7 shows a multi-center study where the same CT data and DVH constraints were sent to various institutions to perform IMRT with a 6 MV beam with minimum (<1%) variation in beam quality. The final plan is summarized here for the prostate PTV. The variability gets magnified in complex treatments with multiple OAR, as in the

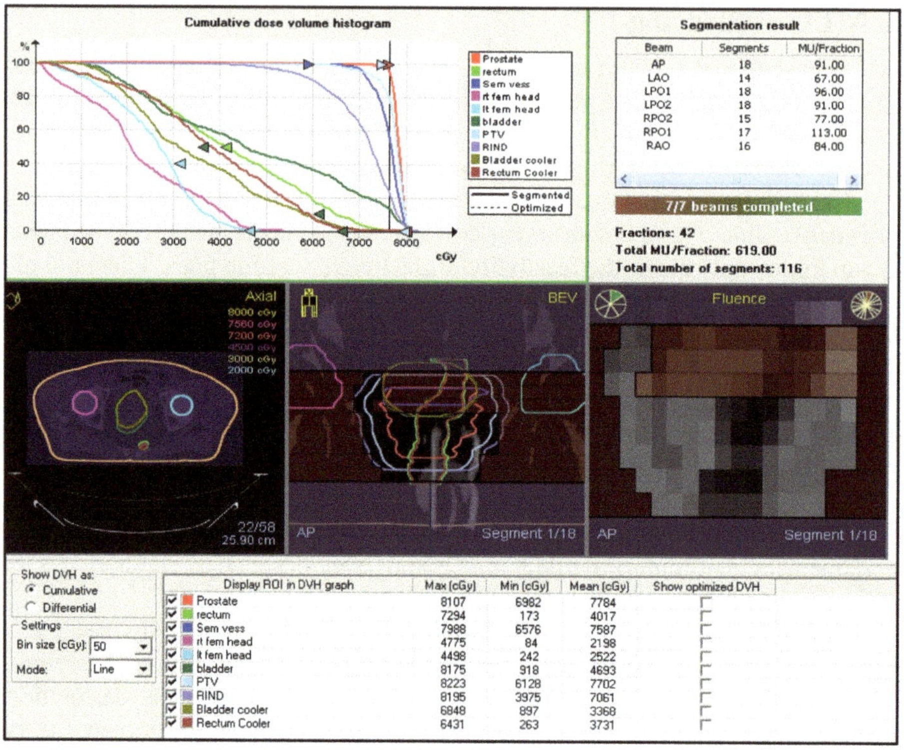

Figure 6.6. The outcome of MLC sequencing. Optimized and segmented dose distributions along with the segments in each beam.

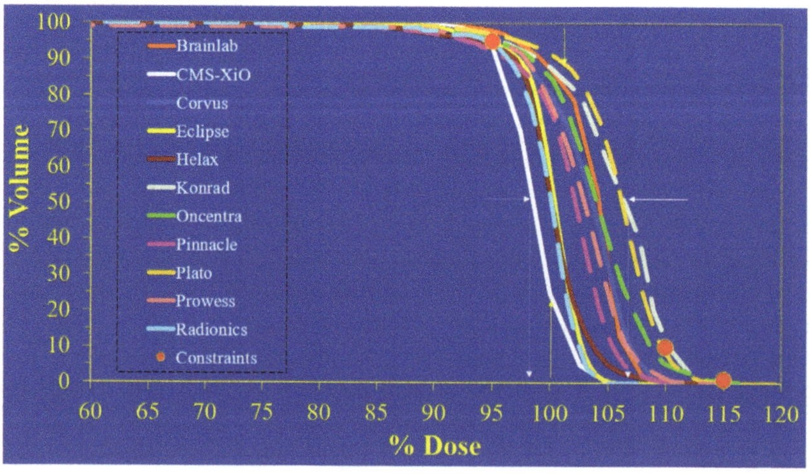

Figure 6.7. A multi-center planning exercise with 11 TPS for a prostate cancer. For the same constraints, the results are very different >10% at 50% which is due to the algorithms, MLC design, and optimization routine [88].

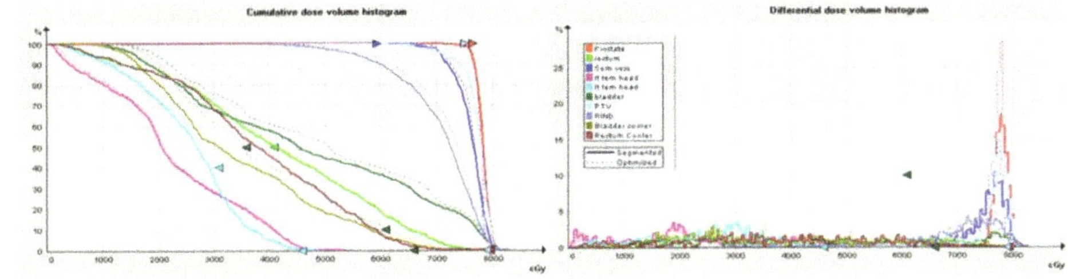

Figure 6.8. Calculated final DVH along with DVH constraints point. Right panel shows dDVH of the same prostate plan.

case of head and neck cancer. The treatment plan variability is further elaborated in chapter 11. With the same TPS, the same plan on two different MLCs will also produce two different results due to the MLC sequencing. Hence, the sequencer plays an important role in the IMRT planning.

The dose calculation after MLC sequence should be evaluated with its congruence with DVH constraints. When there are a large number of structures, the DVH evaluation visually gets very difficult and time consuming. In such a situation differential DVH (dDVH) should be evaluated as shown in figure 6.8. The advantage of dDVH is that for a perfect DVH, it produces a delta function. The spread in delta function shows the degree of disagreement between expected and planned DVH. At the present time, there are several software approaches that can compare user DVH constraints with final calculated DVH and flag with color code each structure green, yellow and red, indicating agreement, intermediate and failing. Such a display provides quick visulization of the IMRT/VMAT plan.

6.7 Transfer and treatment sequencing

After an IMRT plan has been evaluated for its quality and content and signed off by a physician, the plan is then transferred to the treatment machine for patient treatment. Due to the variation in machines, a plan is unique to a specific machine and cannot be interchanged unless the machines are identical in beam characteristics and the MLC characteristics are also the same. During the planning phase, no consideration is given to the beam angle and the sequence phase. In planning, plan quality and agreement with DVH constraints are the only considerations. These fields, in general, may not be suitable for delivery, as most machines can only travel 180° for their beam angle. Some beams cannot cross the limit, which adds a significant amount of time for gantry rotation.

Thus, the IMRT beam needs sequencing to reduce treatment time, which is a critical factor in throughput and patient comfort. Additionally, for non-coplanar treatment, the table and gantry movements need to be evaluated for correct sequencing, which is performed by the therapist before treatment. Based on the ease of delivery, at the time of treatment the therapist must manually sequence the beam so that there is a reduced time for the gantry and table rotation between each field. Such decisions are important because it saves time to move the gantry in a sequence rather than randomly moving the gantry back and forth, which would take more time. In modern machines, this sequencing can be performed *a priori* by the machine itself; however, in general, this process is still performed by a therapist before the treatment.

6.8 Phantom plan

It is essential to have the dose verification of the TPS generated plan. Since dosimetry in the patient is not possible, phantom measurements are required, which will be discussed in chapter 12. The planned IMRT segments may have some difficulties in the delivery of the beam due to MLC sequencing and gantry rotation. This needs to be checked before the patient is treated. The verification is performed for the quality of beam delivery and dosimetric accuracy (as will be discussed in the next section). In such situations, a phantom plan is required. In general, the phantom can be made of solid water or can be a commercially available phantom for QA, as will be discussed in section 6.9.

The Dicom file of the approved plan is sent to the machine for treatment, as described in section 6.7, and to the phantom. Depending on the institutional criterion, the dose calculation is performed on the phantom with same grid size as the case for patient treatment. It is, however, recommended that a smaller calculation grid size be used for better accuracy [89]. In this process, optimization is not required; rather, dose calculation is performed based on the plan segments, MU, gantry angle, and calculation algorithm. Here, the MLC motion is checked for a deliverable condition. The phantom calculation is then used for IMRT QA.

6.9 IMRT PSQA

In-vivo dose verification is not possible for most patients. Hence, the phantom plan as described in section 6.8 is performed. Chapter 12 will describe the details of PSQA, the methodology, the approaches, and the techniques that can be tailored to individual needs. The phantom plan includes 3D dose calculation. For IMRT verification, only a limited number of slices or planes are used. So a 2D plan is sent to the IMRT QA software for comparison with the measured plan. These two sets of data (calculated and measured) are then compared for the gamma index and DTA before the patient treatment. Variability in IMRT QA has been discussed by Pulliam *et al* [90], and if the criterion set does not meet the required goal, a new plan should be generated or QA should be repeated. Kry *et al* [91] have shown that even meeting the requirement does not provide an optimal plan. This has been echoed by Nelm *et al* [92, 93] that QA does not assure the quality of an acceptable plan. In general, AAPM TG-218 [94] should be followed for the methodology and acceptance criterion. At the present time, it is universally accepted that 90% of the points should meet the 3% gamma index and a 3 mm DTA for a 10% threshold.

6.10 Treatment verification

The IMRT process as described above has to be implemented for patient treatment. Therefore, for treatment accuracy, the isocenter or reference point needs to verified

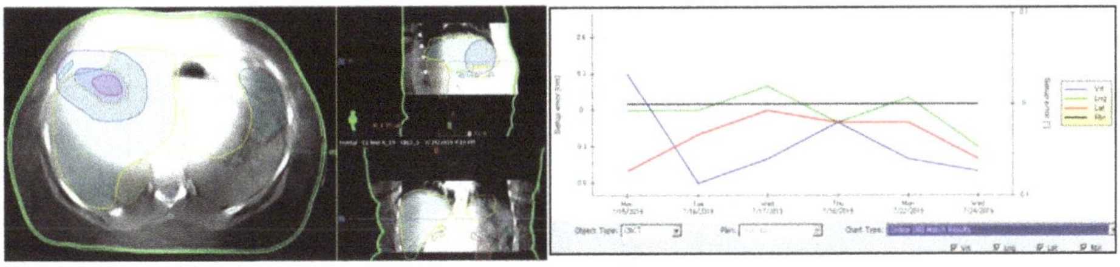

Figure 6.9. Pre-treatment imaging using CBCT of a liver lesion. The daily treatment shift is plotted in the right panel indicating the magnitude of error if the position is not corrected.

as having been transferred from the TPS. There are a multitude of devices for pre-treatment verifications, such as KV imaging [95], MV imaging [96, 97], cone beam CT (CBCT) [97–103], in room imaging [104], and CT on-rail [105, 106] for the isocenter and target volume verification. The evolution of image guided radiotherapy [97, 107–112] has provided a hallmark for accurate localization of the isocenter and tumor volume.

Accuracy in treatment is an important aspect of IMRT, since the dose gradient is usually very steep and any deviation in the isocenter location may have serious consequences. Before the patient is treated, imaging is essential. Excluding motion, the initial setup is performed though kV imaging or CBCT that provides an essential six degrees of freedom shift in patient coordinates. Figure 6.9 shows such an effort in a liver SBRT. For soft tissues, it is very difficult to visualize the location of the tumor and thus the isocenter. In this situation, small radio-opaque fiducial markers are implanted in the patient before planning. These markers are then used to align the isocenter, improving the accuracy in beam delivery [113–115].

6.11 Record and verification

IMRT is a complex process where MLC leaves, the gantry, the collimator, and the treatment table are all variables along with the dose rate and MU in each segment. These treatment parameters are dynamic and need to be recorded in real time. The genesis of the record and verify (RV) system is from Memorial Sloan Kettering Cancer Center [116]. The RV system is responsible for the reduction in radiation treatment error and has become an integral part of treatment delivery software. Every step of the beam delivery is recorded based on an RV system such as ARIA (Varian Medical System, Palo Alto) and Mosiaq (Elekta medical system, Sweden). The treatment parameters can be evaluated after the treatment through the RV or stored in a log file but this is more intrusive. As will be discussed in chapter 12, log files are used for PSQA. The treatment records provide an important safety measure for any litigation related to wrong treatment. Thus, the stored data in RV can be accessed and evaluated in future for its accuracy in treatment delivery.

References

[1] Smith A R and Purdy J A 1991 Three-dimensional photon treatment planning: report of the collaborative working group on the evaluation of treatment planning for external photon beam radiotherapy *Int. J. Radiat. Oncol. Biol. Phys.* **21** 1–265

[2] ICRU Report 62 1999 *Prescribing, Recording, and Reporting Photon Beam Therapy (Supplement to ICRU Report 50)* (Bethesda, MD: International Commission on Radiation Units and Measurements)

[3] ICRU Report 50 1993 *Prescribing, Recording, and reporting Photon Beam Therapy* (Bethesda, MD: International Commission on Radiation Units and Measurements)

[4] Drzymala R E, Holman M D and Yan D *et al* 1994 Integrated software tools for the evaluation of radiotherapy treatment plans *Int. J. Radiat. Oncol. Biol. Phys.* **30** 909–19

[5] Galvin J M 1994 The CT-simulator and simulator-CT: advantages, disadvantages, and future development *Radiation Therapy Physics.* ed A R Smith (New York: Springer) pp 19–32

[6] Coia L R, Schultheiss T E and Hanks G E 1995 *A Practical Guide to CT Simulation.* (Madison, WI: Advanced Medical Publishing)

[7] Karki K, Saraiya S and Hugo G D *et al* 2017 Variabilities of magnetic resonance imaging-, computed tomography-, and positron emission tomography-computed tomography-based tumor and lymph node delineations for lung cancer radiation therapy planning *Int. J. Radiat. Oncol. Biol. Phys.* **99** 80–9

[8] Wee C W, Sung W and Kang H C *et al* 2015 Evaluation of variability in target volume delineation for newly diagnosed glioblastoma: a multi-institutional study from the Korean Radiation Oncology Group *Radiat. Oncol.* **10** 137

[9] Steenbergen P, Haustermans K and Lerut E *et al* 2015 Prostate tumor delineation using multiparametric magnetic resonance imaging: inter-observer variability and pathology validation *Radiother. Oncol.* **115** 186–90

[10] Lim K, Erickson B and Jurgenliemk-Schulz I M *et al* 2015 Variability in clinical target volume delineation for intensity modulated radiation therapy in 3 challenging cervix cancer scenarios *Pract. Radiat. Oncol.* **5** e557–65

[11] Dalah E, Moraru I and Paulson E *et al* 2014 Variability of target and normal structure delineation using multimodality imaging for radiation therapy of pancreatic cancer *Int. J. Radiat. Oncol. Biol. Phys.* **89** 633–40

[12] Ulin K, Urie M M and Cherlow J M 2010 Results of a multi-institutional benchmark test for cranial CT/MR image registration *Int. J. Radiat. Oncol. Biol. Phys.* **77** 1584–9

[13] Hurkmans C W, Borger J H and Pieters B R *et al* 2001 Variability in target volume delineation on CT scans of the breast *Int. J. Radiat. Oncol. Biol. Phys.* **50** 1366–72

[14] Dubois D F, Prestidge B R and Hotchkiss L A *et al* 1998 Intraobserver and interobserver variability of MR imaging-and CT-derived prostate volumes after transperineal interstitial permanent prostate brachytherapy *Radiology* **207** 785–9

[15] Kagawa K, Lee W R and Schultheiss T E *et al* 1997 Initial clinical assessment of CT-MRI image fusion software in localization of the prostate for 3D conformal radiation therapy *Int. J. Radiat. Oncol. Biol. Phys.* **38** 319–25

[16] Khoo V, Adams E and Saran F *et al* 2000 A comparison of clinical volumes determined by CT and MRI for the radiotherapy planning of base of skull meningiomas *Int. J. Radiat. Oncol. Biol. Phys.* **46** 1309–17

[17] Furuya T, Phua J H and Ruschin M *et al* 2019 Assessing functionality and benefits of comprehensive dose volume prescriptions: an international, multi-institutional, treatment planning study in spine stereotactic body radiation therapy *Pract. Radiat. Oncol.* **9** 9–15

[18] Mercieca S, Belderbos J S A and De Jaeger K *et al* 2018 Interobserver variability in the delineation of the primary lung cancer and lymph nodes on different four-dimensional computed tomography reconstructions *Radiother. Oncol.* **126** 325–32

[19] Lee E, Park W and Ahn S H *et al* 2018 Interobserver variation in target volume for salvage radiotherapy in recurrent prostate cancer patients after radical prostatectomy using CT versus combined CT and MRI: a multicenter study (KROG 13-11) *Radiat. Oncol. J.* **36** 11–6

[20] Vinod S K, Min M and Jameson M G *et al* 2016 A review of interventions to reduce inter-observer variability in volume delineation in radiation oncology *J. Med. Imag. Radiat. Oncol.* **60** 393–406

[21] Hong T S, Bosch W R and Krishnan S *et al* 2014 Interobserver variability in target definition for hepatocellular carcinoma with and without portal vein thrombus: radiation therapy oncology group consensus guidelines *Int. J. Radiat. Oncol. Biol. Phys.* **89** 804–13

[22] Nijkamp J, de Haas-Kock D F and Beukema J C *et al* 2012 Target volume delineation variation in radiotherapy for early stage rectal cancer in the Netherlands *Radiother. Oncol.* **102** 14–21

[23] Louie A V, Rodrigues G and Olsthoorn J *et al* 2010 Inter-observer and intra-observer reliability for lung cancer target volume delineation in the 4D-CT era *Radiother. Oncol.* **95** 166–71

[24] Li X A, Tai A and Arthur D W *et al* 2009 Variability of target and normal structure delineation for breast cancer radiotherapy: an RTOG Multi-Institutional and Multiobserver Study *Int. J. Radiat. Oncol. Biol. Phys.* **73** 944–51

[25] Geets X, Daisne J F and Arcangeli S *et al* 2005 Inter-observer variability in the delineation of pharyngo-laryngeal tumor, parotid glands and cervical spinal cord: comparison between CT-scan and MRI *Radiother. Oncol.* **77** 25–31

[26] van de Steene J, Linthout N and Mey J *et al* 2002 Definition of gross tumor volume in lung cancer: inter-observer variability *Radiother. Oncol.* **62** 37–49

[27] Weltens C, Menten J and Feron M *et al* 2001 Interobserver variations in gross tumor volume delineation of brain tumors on computed tomography and impact of magnetic resonance imaging *Radiother. Oncol.* **60** 49–9

[28] Caldwell C B, Mah K and Ung Y C *et al* 2001 Observer variation in contouring gross tumor volume in patients with poorly defined non-small-cell lung tumors on CT: the impact of 18FDG-hybrid PET fusion *Int. J. Radiat. Oncol. Biol. Phys.* **51** 923–31

[29] Rasch C, Barillot I and Remeijer P *et al* 1999 Definition of the prostate in CT and MRI: a multi-observer study *Int. J. Radiat. Oncol. Biol. Phys.* **43** 57–66

[30] Dawson L, Mah K and Fransen E *et al* 1998 Target position variability throughout prostate radiotherapy *Int. J. Radiat. Oncol. Biol. Phys.* **42** 1155–61

[31] Cazzaniga L, Marinoni M and Bossi A *et al* 1998 Interphysician variability in defining the planning target volume in the irradiation of prostate and seminal vesicles *Radiother. Oncol.* **28** 293–6

[32] Leunens G, Menten J and Weltens C *et al* 1993 Quality assessment of medical decision making in radiation oncology: variability in target volume delineation for brain tumors *Radiother. Oncol.* **28** 169–75

[33] Njeh C F 2008 Tumor delineation: the weakest link in the search for accuracy in radiotherapy *J. Med. Phys.* **33** 136–40

[34] Esposito M, Maggi G and Marino C *et al* 2016 Multicentre treatment planning inter-comparison in a national context: the liver stereotactic ablative radiotherapy case *Phys. Med.* **32** 277–83

[35] Moustakis C, Blanck O and Ebrahimi Tazehmahalleh F *et al* 2017 Planning benchmark study for SBRT of early stage NSCLC: results of the DEGRO Working Group Stereotactic Radiotherapy *Strahlenther. Onkol.* (Accepted)

[36] Fogliata A, Nicolini G and Alber M *et al* 2007 On the performances of different IMRT treatment planning systems for selected paediatric cases *Radiat. Oncol.* **2** 7

[37] Srivastava S P, Cheng C W and Das I J 2016 The effect of slice thickness on target and organs at risk volumes, dosimetric coverage and radiobiological impact in IMRT planning *Clin. Transl. Oncol.* **18** 469–79

[38] Erdi Y E, Rosenzweig K and Erdi A K *et al* 2002 Radiotherapy treatment planning for patients with non-small cell lung cancer using positron emission tomography (PET) *Radiother. Oncol.* **62** 51–60

[39] ICRU Report 83 2010 *Prescribing, Recording, and Reporting Intensity-Modulated Photon-Beam Therapy (IMRT)(ICRU Report 83)* (Bethesda, MD: International Commission on Radiation Units and Measurements)

[40] Rasch C, Keus R and Pameijer F A *et al* 1997 The potential impact of CT-MRI matching on tumor volume delineation in advanced head and neck cancer *Int. J. Radiat. Oncol. Biol. Phys.* **39** 841–48

[41] Emami B, Lyman J and Brown A *et al* 1991 Tolerance of normal tissue to therapeutic irradiation *Int. J. Radiat. Oncol. Biol. Phys.* **21** 109–22

[42] Marks L B and Ten Haken R K 2010 K. MM Quantitative analyses of normal tissue effects in the clinic (QUANTEC) *Int. J. Radiat. Oncol. Biol. Phys.* **76** S1–160.

[43] Fogliata A, Nicolini G and Vanetti E *et al* 2006 Dosimetric validation of the anisotropic analytical algorithm for photon dose calculation: fundamental characterization in water *Phys. Med. Biol.* **51** 1421–38

[44] Fogliata A, Nicolini G and Clivio A *et al* 2011 Accuracy of acuros XB and AAA dose calculation for small fields with reference to RapidArc((R)) stereotactic treatments *Med. Phys.* **38** 6228–37

[45] Fogliata A, Nicolini G and Clivio A *et al* 2011 Dosimetric evaluation of Acuros XB advanced dose calculation algorithm in heterogeneous media *Radiat. Oncol.* **6** 82

[46] Fogliata A, Nicolini G and Clivio A *et al* 2011 On the dosimetric impact of inhomogeneity management in the Acuros XB algorithm for breast treatment *Radiat. Oncol.* **6** 103

[47] Akino Y, Das I J and Cardenes H R *et al* 2014 Correlation between target volume and electron transport effects affecting heterogeneity corrections in stereotactic body radiotherapy for lung cancer *J. Radiat. Res.* **55** 754–60

[48] Jones A O and Das I J 2005 Comparison of inhomogeneity correction algorithms in small photon fields *Med. Phys.* **32** 766–76

[49] Xiao Y, Papiez L and Paulus R *et al* 2009 Dosimetric evaluation of heterogeneity corrections for RTOG 0236: stereotactic body tadiotherapy of inoperable stage I-II non–small-cell lung cancer *Int. J. Radiation. Oncol. Biol. Phys.* **73** 1235–42

[50] Ojala J J, Kapanen M K and Hyodynmaa S J *et al* 2014 Performance of dose calculation algorithms from three generations in lung SBRT: comparison with full Monte Carlo-based dose distributions *J. Appl. Clin. Med. Phys.* **15** 4662

[51] Nielsen T B, Wieslander E and Fogliata A *et al* 2011 Influence of dose calculation algorithms on the predicted dose distribution and NTCP values for NSCLC patients *Med. Phys.* **38** 2412–8
[52] Ali I and Ahmad S 2013 Quantitative assessment of the accuracy of dose calculation using pencil beam and Monte Carlo algorithms and requirements for clinical quality assurance *Med. Dosim.* **38** 255–61
[53] Yamashita T, Akagi T and Aso T *et al* 2012 Effect of inhomogeneity in a patient's body on the accuracy of the pencil beam algorithm in comparison to Monte Carlo *Phys. Med. Biol.* **57** 7673–88
[54] Gagliardi G, Constine L S and Moiseenko V *et al* 2010 Radiation dose-volume effects in the heart *Int. J. Radiat. Oncol. Biol. Phys.* **76** S77–85
[55] Ahnesjö A, Andreo P and Brahme A 1987 Calculation and application of point spread functions for treatment planning with high energy photon beams *Acta Oncol.* **26** 49–56
[56] Bragg C M and Conway J 2006 Dosimetric verification of the anisotropic analytical algorithm for radiotherapy treatment planning *Radiother. Oncol.* **81** 315–23
[57] Panettieri V, Barsoum P and Westermark M *et al* 2009 AAA and PBC calculation accuracy in the surface build-up region in tangential beam treatments. Phantom and breast case study with the Monte Carlo code PENELOPE *Radiother. Oncol.* **93** 94–101
[58] Han T, Mourtada F and Kisling K *et al* 2012 Experimental validation of deterministic Acuros XB algorithm for IMRT and VMAT dose calculations with the Radiological Physics Center's head and neck phantom *Med. Phys.* **39** 2193–202
[59] Hoffmann L, Jorgensen M B and Muren L P *et al* 2012 Clinical validation of the Acuros XB photon dose calculation algorithm, a grid-based Boltzmann equation solver *Acta Oncol.* **51** 376–85
[60] Ojala J, Kapanen M and Sipila P *et al* 2014 The accuracy of Acuros XB algorithm for radiation beams traversing a metallic hip implant – comparison with measurements and Monte Carlo calculations *J. Appl. Clin. Med. Phys.* **15** 162–76
[61] Tsuruta Y, Nakata M and Nakamura M *et al* 2014 Dosimetric comparison of Acuros XB, AAA, and XVMC in stereotactic body radiotherapy for lung cancer *Med. Phys.* **41** 081715
[62] Aspradakis M M, Morrison R H and Richmond N D *et al* 2003 Experimental verification of convolution/superposition photon dose calculations for radiotherapy treatment planning *Phys. Med. Biol.* **48** 2873–93
[63] Al-Hallaq H A, Reft C S and Roeske J C 2006 The dosimetric effects of tissue heterogeneities in intensity-modulated radiation therapy (IMRT) of the head and neck *Phys. Med. Biol.* **51** 1145–56
[64] Vanderstraeten B, Reynaert N and Paelinck L *et al* 2006 Accuracy of patient dose calculation for lung IMRT: a comparison of Monte Carlo, convolution/superposition, and pencil beam computations *Med. Phys.* **33** 3149–58
[65] Kry S F, Feygelman V and Balter P *et al* 2020 AAPM Task Group 329: reference dose specification for dose calculations: dose-to-water or dose-to-muscle? *Med. Phys.* **47** e52–64
[66] Saw C B, Siochi R C and Ayyangar K M *et al* 2001 Leaf sequencing techniques for MLC-based IMRT *Med. Dosim.* **26** 199–204
[67] Seco J, Evans P M and Webb S 2001 Analysis of the effects of the delivery technique on an IMRT plan: comparison for multiple static field, dynamic and NOMOS MIMiC collimation *Phys. Med. Biol.* **46** 3073–87

[68] Crooks S M, McAven L F and Robinson D F *et al* 2002 Minimizing delivery time and monitor units in static IMRT by leaf-sequencing *Phys. Med. Biol.* **47** 3105–16

[69] Seco J, Evans P M and Webb S 2002 An optimization algorithm that incorporates IMRT delivery constraints *Phys. Med. Biol.* **47** 899–915

[70] Xia P, Hwang A B and Verhey L J 2002 A leaf sequencing algorithm to enlarge treatment field length in IMRT *Med. Phys.* **29** 991–8

[71] Kamath S, Sahni S and Li J *et al* 2003 Leaf sequencing algorithms for segmented multileaf collimation *Phys. Med. Biol.* **48** 307–24

[72] Suss P, Kufer K H and Thieke C 2007 Improved stratification algorithms for step-and-shoot MLC delivery in intensity-modulated radiation therapy *Phys. Med. Biol.* **52** 6039–51

[73] Wisotzky E, O'Brien R and Keall P J 2016 Technical note: a novel leaf sequencing optimization algorithm which considers previous underdose and overdose events for MLC tracking radiotherapy *Med. Phys.* **43** 132–6

[74] Desai D, Ramsey C R and Breinig M *et al* 2006 A topographic leaf-sequencing algorithm for delivering intensity modulated radiation therapy *Med. Phys.* **33** 2751–6

[75] Ahunbay E E, Chen G P and Thatcher S *et al* 2007 Direct aperture optimization-based intensity-modulated radiotherapy for whole breast irradiation *Int. J. Radiat. Oncol. Biol. Phys.* **67** 1248–58

[76] Bergman A M, Bush K and Milette M P *et al* 2006 Direct aperture optimization for IMRT using Monte Carlo generated beamlets *Med. Phys.* **33** 3666–79

[77] Bedford J L and Webb S 2007 Direct-aperture optimization applied to selection of beam orientations in intensity-modulated radiation therapy *Phys. Med. Biol.* **52** 479–98

[78] Milette M P and Otto K 2007 Maximizing the potential of direct aperture optimization through collimator rotation *Med. Phys.* **34** 1431–8

[79] Zhang G, Jiang Z and Shepard D *et al* 2006 Direct aperture optimization of breast IMRT and the dosimetric impact of respiration motion *Phys. Med. Biol.* **51** N357–69

[80] Niu Y, Zhang G and Berman B L *et al* 2012 Improving IMRT-plan quality with MLC leaf position refinement post plan optimization *Med. Phys.* **39** 5118–26

[81] Shepard D M, Earl M A and Li X A *et al* 2002 Direct aperture optimization: a turnkey solution for step-and-shoot IMRT *Med. Phys.* **29** 1007–18

[82] Earl M A, Afghan M K and Yu C X *et al* 2007 Jaws-only IMRT using direct aperture optimization *Med. Phys.* **34** 307–14

[83] Malet C, Ginestet C and Hall K *et al* 2000 A study of dose delivery in small segments *Int. J. Radiat. Oncol. Biol. Phys.* **48** 535–9

[84] Rajapakshe R and Shalev S 1996 Output stability of a linear accelerator during the first three seconds *Med. Phys.* **23** 517–9

[85] Buchgeister M and Nüsslin F 1998 Startup performance of the traveling wave guide versus standing wave linear accelerator *Med. Phys.* **25** 493–5

[86] Sharpe M B, Miller B M and Yan D *et al* 2000 Monitor unit settings for intensity modulated beams delivered using step-and -shoot approach *Med. Phys.* **27** 2719–25

[87] Das I J, Kase K R and Tello V M 1991 Dosimetric accuracy at low monitor unit settings *Br. J. Radiol.* **64** 808–11

[88] Das I J, Bieda M and Cheng C *et al* 2004 Dosimetric comparison of inverse treatment planning system for IMRT: a collaborative study *Med. Phys.* **31** 1750

[89] Srivastava S P, Cheng C W and Das I J 2017 The dosimetric and radiobiological impact of calculation grid size on head and neck IMRT *Pr. Radiat. Oncol.* **7** 209–17

[90] Pulliam K B, Followill D and Court L *et al* 2014 A six-year review of more than 13,000 patient-specific IMRT QA results from 13 different treatment sites *J. Appl. Clin. Med. Phys.* **15** 196–206

[91] Kry S F, Molineu A and Kerns J R *et al* 2014 Institutional patient-specific IMRT QA does not predict unacceptable plan delivery *Int. J. Radiat. Oncol. Biol. Phys.* **90** 1195–201

[92] Nelms B E, Zhen H and Tomé W A 2011 Per-beam, planar IMRT QA passing rates do not predict clinically relevant patient dose errors *Med. Phys.* **38** 1037–44

[93] Nelms B E, Chan M F and Jarry G *et al* 2013 Evaluating IMRT and VMAT dose accuracy: practical examples of failure to detect systematic errors when applying a commonly used metric and action levels *Med. Phys.* **40** 111722

[94] Miften M, Olch A and Mihailidis D *et al* 2018 Tolerance limits and methodologies for IMRT measurement-based verification QA: recommendations of AAPM Task Group No. 218 *Med. Phys.* **45** e53–83

[95] Lee Y H, Kim Y S and Lee H C *et al* 2015 Tumour volume changes assessed with high-quality KVCT in lung cancer patients undergoing concurrent chemoradiotherapy *Br. J. Radiol.* **88** 20150156

[96] Chen J, Morin O and Aubin M *et al* 2006 Dose-guided radiation therapy with megavoltage cone-beam CT *Br. J. Radiol.* **79** S87–98

[97] Ding G X, Alaei P and Curran B *et al* 2018 Image guidance doses delivered during radiotherapy: quantification, management, and reduction: report of the AAPM Therapy Physics Committee Task Group 180 *Med. Phys.*

[98] Jaffray D A, Siewerdsen J H and Wong J W *et al* 2002 Flat-panel cone-beam computed tomography for image-guided radiation therapy *Int. J. Radiat. Oncol. Biol. Phys.* **53** 1337–49

[99] Makimoto Y, Matsuzaki K and Yoshida S *et al* 1998 Early clinical experience on cone-beam CT *J. Digital Imag.* **11** 211–3

[100] Cho P S, Johnson R H and Griffin T W 1995 Cone-beam CT for radiotherapy applications *Phys. Med. Biol.* **40** 1863–83

[101] Ding G X, Duggan D M and Coffey C W *et al* 2007 A study on adaptive IMRT treatment planning using kV cone-beam CT *Radiother. Oncol.* **85** 116–25

[102] van Kranen S, van Beek S and Rasch C *et al* 2009 Setup uncertainties of anatomical sub-regions in head-and-neck cancer patients after offline CBCT guidance *Int. J. Radiat. Oncol. Biol. Phys.* **73** 1566–73

[103] Nielsen M, Bertelsen A and Westberg J *et al* 2009 Cone beam CT evaluation of patient set-up accuracy as a QA tool *Acta Oncol.* **48** 271–6

[104] Nagata Y, Negoro Y and Aoki T *et al* 2002 Clinical outcomes of 3D conformal hypofractionated single high-dose radiotherapy for one or two lung tumors using a stereotactic body frame *Int. J. Radiat. Oncol. Biol. Phys.* **52** 1041–6

[105] Wong J R, Gao Z and Uematsu M *et al* 2008 Interfractional prostate shifts: review of 1870 computed tomography (CT) scans obtained during image-guided radiotherapy using CT-on-rails for the treatment of prostate cancer *Int. J. Radiat. Oncol. Biol. Phys.* **72** 1396–401

[106] Wong J R, Grimm L and Uematsu M *et al* 2005 Image-guided radiotherapy for prostate cancer by CT-linear accelerator combination: prostate movements and dosimetric considerations *Int. J. Radiat. Oncol. Biol. Phys.* **61** 561–9

[107] Song W Y, Schaly B and Bauman G *et al* 2006 Evaluation of image-guided radiation therapy (IGRT) technologies and their impact on the outcomes of hypofractionated

prostate cancer treatments: a radiobiologic analysis *Int. J. Radiat. Oncol. Biol. Phys.* **64** 289–300
[108] Verellen D, De Ridder M and Linthout N *et al* 2007 Innovations in image-guided radiotherapy *Nat. Rev. Cancer* **7** 949–60
[109] Ling C C, Yorke E and Fuks Z 2006 From IMRT to IGRT: frontierland or neverland? *Radiother. Oncol.* **78** 119–22
[110] Dawson L A and Sharpe M B 2006 Image-guided radiotherapy: rationale, benefits, and limitations *Lancet Oncol.* **7** 848–58
[111] Dawson L A and Jaffray D A 2007 Advances in image-guided radiation therapy *J. Clin. Oncol.* **25** 938–46
[112] Caillet V, Booth J T and Keall P 2017 IGRT and motion management during lung SBRT delivery *Phys. Med.* **44** 113–22
[113] Jayachandran P, Minn A Y and Van Dam J *et al* 2010 Interfractional uncertainty in the treatment of pancreatic cancer with radiation *Int. J. Radiat. Oncol. Biol. Phys.* **76** 603–7
[114] Tanyi J A, He T and Summers P A *et al* 2010 Assessment of planning target volume margins for intensity-modulated radiotherapy of the prostate gland: role of daily inter- and intrafraction motion *Int. J. Radiat. Oncol. Biol. Phys.* **78** 1579–85
[115] Jonsson J H, Garpebring A and Karlsson M G *et al* 2012 Internal fiducial markers and susceptibility effects in MRI-simulation and measurement of spatial accuracy *Int. J. Radiat. Oncol. Biol. Phys.* **82** 1612–8
[116] Mohan R, Podmaniczky K C and Caley R *et al* 1984 A computerized record and verify system for radiation treatments *Int. J. Radiat. Oncol. Biol. Phys.* **10** 1975–85

IOP Publishing

Intensity Modulated Radiation Therapy
A clinical overview
Indra J Das, Nicholas J Sanfilippo, Antonella Fogliata and Luca Cozzi

Chapter 7

Contouring

To exploit the improved conformity achievable through intensity modulation techniques, the definition and subsequent delineation of both targets and OAR are essential in ensuring accurate reproducibility of the treatment as planned and to avoid any geographical misses.

This chapter summarizes the need for proper contouring for IMRT or VMAT planning.

7.1 Contouring for intensity modulation inverse planning

Inverse planning is a mathematical concept generating the optimal plan as described in previous chapters, using input information as dose–volume constraints, CT dataset, and delineated structures; this last information assumes a knowledgeable definition of OAR and targets. The optimal dose distribution obtained by this process for the intensity modulated plans is very conformal around the target, with abrupt dose gradients from the target to the healthy tissue and OARs. The clinical results of the optimization process depend crucially on the accuracy of input information, hence the accuracy of the definition and delineation of the structures is fundamental, and the inverse planning more sensitive to contouring than 3DCRT.

There are two types of structure to outline: the target(s) and the OAR, which are different in terms of strategy and dose to deliver. The target, in particular the clinical target volume (CTV), depends on the disease, the stage, patient status, is mostly determined according to specific guidelines, and should receive high dose levels with a good coverage; the OARs are anatomical structures, close if not adjacent to the target, where the delivered dose is a consequence of the tumor cure attempt and should be kept at the lowest possible level. For IMRT optimization, the close vicinity of these two types of outlines that receive very different dose levels, much stress is placed on dose gradients. However, as clearly described in the ICRU Report 83 [1], targets and OAR are purely oncological or anatomical concepts, and the volumes used in the planning process are *outlines* on a CT scan representing those

doi:10.1088/978-0-7503-1335-3ch7

concepts. Moreover, these representations should be considered as a snapshot of the anatomy at a given time. Motion or anatomical changes will be discussed in more detail in section 7.3.

Contouring plays an important role in both the 3DCRT or IMRT planning process. The variability of contouring is so rampant that most organizations such as ESTRO and ASTRO took the responsibility of training the radiation oncologists for accurate contouring. In every annual meeting there are contouring sessions where the experts give live demonstrations on each type of contouring. Of course, there is no gold standard but using multi-modality imaging enhances skills and knowledge can be propagated through training. A few examples of such problems in the head and neck area are discussed in the following section.

A very practical issue that should not be overlooked in the delineation of tiny structures is the CT dataset slice thickness and the reconstruction algorithm. This applies to both targets for particularly small lesions and OARs. The cochlea contouring, for example, would require scanning in a maximum of 1 mm slices; however, general CT scans for radiotherapy planning have larger slice spacing, e.g., 2.5 mm, hosting the cochlea outline in maybe only a couple of slices, making its volume highly inaccurate. Srivastava *et al* [2] evaluated the slice thickness effect on contoured volumes. For example, in the Varian Eclipse TPS, the value of the structure volume is based on rounding off the structure at the upper- and lower-most slices to half of the slice thickness, which is a pre-defined and not modifiable approximation of the craniocaudal structure edges. The percentage error in the volume estimation increases with slice thickness, and it is of great importance for small structures; for volumes of 1–3 cm^3 it was shown to be of ~20%, ~30%, ~40% for slice thicknesses of 1, 2, 3 mm, with the Eclipse TPS (the volume estimation is TPS dependent, although the trend remains the same for most planning systems [3]). The inaccuracy in the volume estimation could lead to significant clinical implications in order to reach protocol-specific dose–volume criteria, especially if these are to reflect the actual clinical meaning of the dose statistics from the dose–volume histograms, and ultimately estimate tumor control and normal tissue complication probabilities (TCP, NTCP). This special dose calculation related point is discussed in the dose calculation chapter of this book.

For the different anatomical structures, guidelines to delineate targets and OAR have been introduced over the years, especially since the advent of IMRT technology in clinical practice, but it is not within the scope of this book to go through them. Let us simply take the example of the head and neck tumors as a paradigmatic site to analyze the contouring problem and complexity in IMRT planning and treatments.

The non-homogeneous target volume selection and delineation has been the most important source of variations that threatens to downplay the advantages of IMRT planning, by increasing the risk either of geographical misleading to recurrence, or of normal tissue complication due to high doses delivered to non-target volumes. This point was also outlined by many clinical trials reporting the impact on the outcome of treatment delivery ([4–6]). To homogenize the treatments in the world radiotherapy community, international consensus guidelines have been proposed and updated, firstly for the delineation of the nodal regions to include in the CTV (starting in 2000 [7], followed by a consensus guideline in 2003 [8] for the delineation of the node-negative neck lymph node levels, enriched by the proposal for the nodal regions in the node-positive and post-operative neck [9] and ending with an updated consensus guideline in 2014 [10]). It is however only recently, in 2018, that international consensus guidelines were published for the delineation of the primary CTV in laryngeal, hypopharyngeal, oropharyngeal and oral cavity squamous cell carcinoma [11]. The nasopharyngeal carcinoma was in any case covered by another document, from Lee *et al* [12]. Although the guidelines help in reducing differences, the target delineation remains subject to interobserver variations.

A recent example can be found in van der Veen's published work [13] where results were reported from a survey conducted in Belgium in 2017, where centers were asked to delineate CTV for the primary and elective nodal neck. Despite all the centers referring to the published guidelines for nodal volumes, the median dice similarity coefficient ranged between 0.67 and 0.82. The authors thus suggest that the availability and implementation of guidelines alone are not sufficient in guaranteeing uniform delineation, and additional teaching or training is needed on this subject.

Of course, not only the head and neck region has been studied for the interobserver variability in structure delineation. The brain was explored by Weltens *et al* [14] using MR images as well, and by Wee *et al* [15] in a multi-institutional setting for glioblastoma patients. Target delineation in lung cancer was studied by Caldwell *et al* [16] also associated with PET imaging, van de Steene *et al* [17], Louie *et al* [18] and Mercieca *et al* [19] on 4DCT images. Again in the thorax region, breast contouring variations were analyzed by Hurkmans *et al* [20], and by Li *et al* [21] on a multi-institutional base. In the abdominopelvic region, interobserver variation to delineate targets and OARs were studied by Dalah *et al* for pancreatic tumors [22], Hong *et al* for hepatocellular carcinoma [23], Lim *et al* for cervix cancer [24], Nijkamp *et al* for early-stage rectal cancer [25], to cite just some of the published works. Moreover, the imaging modality also plays a fundamental role in delineation, as pointed out for example by Yeung *et al* [26], where the authors reported on prostate volumes outlined on CT imaging that appeared larger than the corresponding volumes on MRI.

However, interobserver variation is of concern in the IMRT process not only regarding target delineation, but also for OAR outlines. Although human anatomy is quite well understood, the dosimetric effects on the tissues are still evolving at the research level. A lot of work has been done, and many summaries based on meta-analysis have been published. The Emami data were the first published in 1991 [27], followed by the QUANTEC project in 2010, which concluded its work with a supplement issue published in the Red Journal [28]. These summarized, through in-depth review of the literature as well as meta-analysis, the possible correlations between toxicity and dosimetry for all the known OAR. This approach, that is commonly used in all radiotherapy centers, assumes and presumes a correct definition of the OAR that is not always obvious, often needing guidelines and recommendations on how to delineate critical structures.

Keeping to the head and neck OAR example, Brouwer *et al* [29] investigated the interobserver variability in their delineation, both in terms of magnitude and location by studying the contours of five experienced radiation oncologists on 12 patient CT scans, as shown in figure 7.1. They found the largest differences for the glottic larynx, with a mean concordance index (ratio of the intersection of the volumes and their union, where the unity indicates the perfect agreement) of 0.37 and range 0.11–0.81. This should not be surprising, due to the anatomical complexity of the laryngeal sub-structures together with a lack of clear definition of radiotherapy scope, but opens a more general question on all the dosimetric parameters in use in our clinical practices. The other organs analyzed in the Brouwer study were the parotid and submandibular glands, the spinal cord and the thyroid cartilage, ending with mean concordance indices in the range of 0.64–0.71. Their conclusion suggested the need to establish delineation guidelines in order to reduce the current interobserver variability in common practice and standardize patient treatments. Indeed, in 2015, a 'head and neck guidelines' document was published as a consensus guideline of many organizations (DAHANCA, EORTC, GORTEC, HKNPCSG, NCIC CTG, NCRI, NRG Oncology, and TROG) for a correct CT-based delineation of 25 OAR in the head and neck region [30]. In the document, a concise description of anatomical boundaries of each structure was given together with an atlas, as exemplified in figure 7.2.

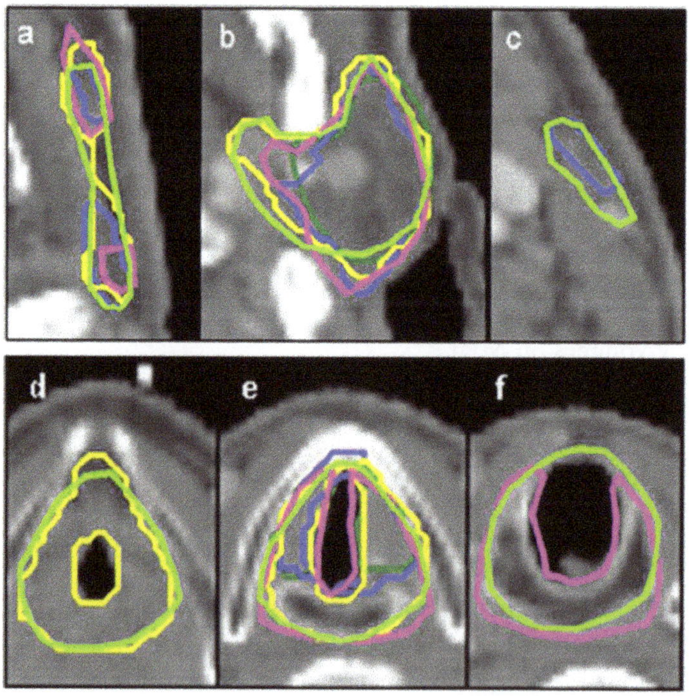

Figure 7.1. Variations in delineation of OARs: each color corresponds to one observer. Cranial, central, and caudal axial slices of a left parotid gland (a, b, c) and glottic larynx delineations (d, e, f). Reproduced from Brouwer *et al* [29]. Open access CC BY 2.0.

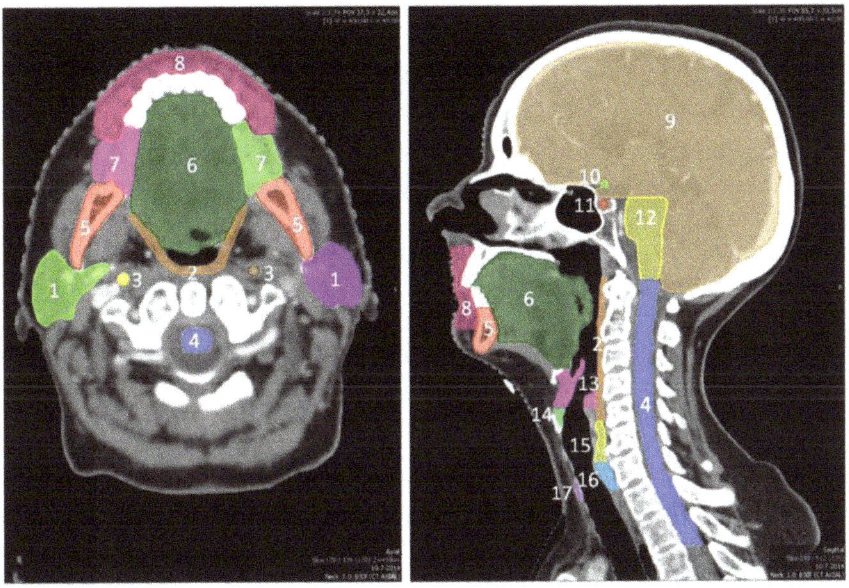

Figure 7.2. Axial (left) and sagittal (right) view of the consensus delineations of the parotid glands (1), pharyngeal constrictor muscles (2), carotid arteries (3), spinal cord (4), mandible (5), extended oral cavity (6), buccal mucosa (7), lips (8), brain (9), chiasm (10), pituitary gland (11), brainstem (12), supraglottic larynx (13), glottic area (14), cricopharyngeal inlet (15), cervical esophagus (16) and thyroid (17). From Brouwer *et al* [30], reproduced with permission from Elsevier.

The importance of improving and homogenizing the OAR delineation for planning is mostly linked to the possible dosimetric impact of the current interobserver variability. A systematic review of the studies related to the uncertainty of volume delineation was published in 2016 by Vinod *et al* [31], identifying 119 studies, of which only 25 reported the dosimetric consequences of interobserver variability. Two of them reported results in OAR for head and neck (oropharyngeal cancer) IMRT treatment for different contours, with different perspectives, as underlined here below.

Loo *et al* [32] evaluated the interobserver variation in the sole parotid gland delineation and its impact on IMRT plans, on 10 patients whose anatomy was compatible with parotid sparing of 24 Gy mean dose within 10%, delineated by four radiation oncologists and three radiologists who had also access to contrast-enhanced MRI as well as anatomical atlas. A conformity index was computed for each patient as the average of the possible Jaccard coefficients assessed for all the possible pairs of contours (the Jaccard coefficient is the ratio between the intersection and the union of two volumes). Interestingly, the mean conformity index was 0.66 (range 0.46–0.73) among radiologists, and 0.52 (range 0.26–0.61) among oncologists. Then a dosimetric assessment was based on the clinically delivered IMRT plan. Only half of all the parotid contours achieved the mean parotid dose within 10% of 24 Gy, and 20% had a mean dose exceeding 10% above 24 Gy. This translates to the fact that almost half of the contours were sufficiently different, and a different IMRT plan would have been produced in practice. Another interesting point was that the dosimetric variation of the mean parotid dose per patient was larger among the oncologist delineated contours than the radiologist delineated contours (that were more compatible). Also to be noted is that qualitative analysis showed the greatest degree of variations in the medial edge of the deep lobe, the anterior border of the superficial lobe, and the superior and inferior margins of the gland. In conclusion, the authors confirmed the importance of accurate delineation of the parotid gland, finding differences even between oncologists and radiologists and their impact on IMRT planning in many cases.

Nelms *et al* [33] reported the results of an international study on 32 datasets of the same test patient, received from different institutions, where the targets were pre-contoured, and the participants were asked to delineate OAR for IMRT planning. Variations were assessed against reference contours, and dosimetric differences according to the dose distributions planned by each participant on the reference structures. The Dice similarity coefficient ($2 \times [X \cup Y]/[|X| + |Y|]$) resulted in 0.76 ± 0.9 for the parotids, and 0.66 ± 0.2 for the brainstem, leading to a difference of the mean dose to the parotids between −18% to +56%, and the maximum dose to the brainstem between −2% and +23%. The authors concluded that there is significant variability in the contouring of the organs at risk, and its dosimetric impact in terms of differences in mean and maximum dose were large, depending on the degree of the contour differences and the dose gradients in the plan. These variances highlighted again the importance of the accuracy and consistency in OAR contouring (and not only target contouring) since the related contour-dependent dosimetric statistics are the key point in the plan evaluation phase.

An important related item considering the future perspectives of adaptive therapy is the effect of the variability of the OAR in terms of both interobserver and possible anatomical changes during treatment. From a pragmatic viewpoint, interobserver delineation variability and anatomical changes during treatment produce similar dosimetric consequences, except that in the first case the potential error systematically affects the whole treatment, while the second generates a continuous change in the dose actually delivered.

Feng *et al* [34] considered the effect of OAR variability on planning during head and neck treatments, exploring the dosimetric implications. They reported mean difference in OAR dose of 0.9 Gy (range 0.6–1.1 Gy) in three different sessions, averaged on 10 patients, evaluating the consequences of anatomical variations during the treatment, to correlate to a fractional overlap of 0.7 (range 0.4–0.9). They found that when contour differences fell within areas of homogeneous dose, the dosimetric differences were small. However, if these were within areas of rapid dose fall-off, dosimetric differences were larger.

Keeping to the head and neck anatomical treatment region, several studies have shown that the salivary glands undergo radiation-induced variations not only some time after ending radiotherapy [35] but also during the course of treatment. It has been proven that there is a treatment-induced reduction in the parotid, as well as changes in the HU pattern. The parotid volume change has been studied by many authors, showing a rather continuous reduction during the treatment, with an average rate of 1%–1.5% per day [36–39]. Over the whole head and neck IMRT treatment the parotid volume reduction was estimated in ~27% by Wang *et al* [40] and in a range of 25%–30% by Ren *et al* [38] on CT data, 31% by Marzi *et al* [41] on MRI, to 44% by Fiorentino *et al* [37] on CBCT data. The greatest change was shown to appear in the third treatment week [37, 38, 41]. The anatomical variations during treatment were described by Vasques Osorio and colleagues [42]: the lateral regions of the irradiated parotid glands moved inward in an average of 3 mm, and the medial regions tended to remain in the same position, as similarly reported by Barker *et al* [43]. Moreover, Xu *et al* [39] also reported a reduction in CT number of 17–18 HU during the whole therapy course, while Wang *et al* [40] reported a volume reduction significantly correlated with the mean parotid dose, having included in their 82-patient study about half of the cohort treated with IMRT and parotid sparing (average mean parotid dose 22.2 Gy), and the remaining with 3DCRT with no parotid sparing (average mean parotid dose 50.2 Gy). Conversely, no correlation between the mean parotid dose and its volume reduction was found by Marzi *et al* [41], on a cohort of 40 patients all treated with IMRT with an average mean parotid dose of 35.8 ± 8.9 Gy. The dosimetric impact of this anatomical variation was evaluated by several groups. Wu *et al* [44] reported that the anatomic and volumetric shrinkage in head and neck patients during radiotherapy did not result in a significant dosimetric difference in targets and critical structures, except for the parotid gland, for which the mean dose increases by ~10% on 35 patients treated with tomotherapy. Lee *et al* [45] reported an increased mean parotid dose in a range of 6 to 42% on 10 patients, and the dose difference was correlated with a migration of the parotids toward the high-dose region. Vasques Osorio *et al* [42], correlating the volume changes with the planned mean doses, found a highly significant relation for the parotid glands. Summarizing the proven parotid shrinkage and increase of mean dose, a re-planning [37, 44] on the third week of treatment is suggested; this can be considered an initial approach of adaptive IMRT.

To comment on this small discussion on the delivered dose variation due to anatomical changes and delineation uncertainties in the IMRT era, we could consider the clinical trial studies that determined the dose–volume relationships for the OAR. Keeping to the parotid case, the initial paper of Eisbruch *et al* [46] reported dose–volume correlations for the parotids of 88 patients, concluding that a parotid mean dose of ⩽26 Gy should be a planning goal for a substantial preservation of the salivary flow rate, and this value was similarly confirmed also later and summarized in the QUANTEC work [47]. However, clear indications or descriptions on how the glands were delineated were not provided in those works, leading to possible inaccurate dose–volume correlations simply derived by uncertainties in the gland contouring.

Accuracy of structure delineation could also depend on the imaging modality used to determine the contours. It is well known that multi-modality imaging can significantly improve structures definition: for example, MRIs better discriminate soft tissues, leading in most cases to enhanced target and OAR definitions as compared to CT images. Geets *et al* [48] evaluated the parotid delineations by different observers on both CT and MRI; in addition to the interobserver variation, they reported a systematic difference in the parotid volume, with MRI-based parotids showing smaller than CT-based ones, meaning that the imaging modality used for structure delineation could also induce variations, which, moreover, would have a dosimetric impact. Finally, the uncertainty of the image co-registration, as in the example CT/MR fusion, is also not to be forgotten.

An interesting aspect that may confound the dose–volume relationships, although not strictly correlated with the accurate contouring, is the physiological interaction between different organs. For example, the combined irradiation of lung and heart causes an intensification of cardiopulmonary toxicity, making the co-irradiation of heart and lung deleterious [49]. Multiorgan irradiation develops physiological mechanisms that could create confusion regarding the origins of radiation-induced damage to single organs and the dose–volume correlations of the single structures. Again referring to head and neck treatment, Orlandi *et al* [50] evaluated oral mucositis on a multifactorial base, considering the complex interplay factors related to the patient, the tumor, and the chemoradiation treatment, assessing possible clinical and dosimetric factors predictive for oral toxicity. They found, after a precise definition of the OAR delineation, that the oral cavity mean dose was found to impact the oral mucositis duration, while high toxicity grade was associated with a combined effect of the parotid gland mean dose and the hot spots received by the oral cavity.

This discussion shows that uncertainty still remains regarding which structures are best delineated in order to optimize IMRT so as to mitigate the severity of its toxicity as well as the impact on sequela and quality of life. The development and grade of mucositis are difficult to predict. Although with IMRT we tend to spare, whenever possible, the oral mucosa, there are at least two critical points: the delineation of the oral mucosa (or the extended oral mucosa according to the OAR delineation guidelines [30]) should be adapted to find better dose/anatomy relationships for toxicity prediction; and the physiological interactions of the multiorgan irradiation, at least oral cavity and parotid [50], would require further studies. For the first point, an attempt of a novel method for the oral mucosa delineation was proposed in 2015 by Dean *et al* [51], aiming to improve the toxicity modeling of oral mucositis. They proposed to contour the 3 mm thick surfaces of the oral mucosa in a realistic way. However, once defined this novel structure, named 'mucosal surface contour', they found that the simpler oral cavity (as described in the guidelines) should be preferred over the mucosal surface contour for NTCP modeling of severe mucositis [52], due to the complexity of the problem, and finally, they recommended that radiotherapy plans should prioritize the reduction of the volumes of oral mucosa receiving high and intermediate doses, rather than reducing the mean dose. In the QUANTEC work, however, there is no specific paper on the oral cavity which could serve the purpose of expanding knowledge regarding this particular structure; the only mention of it is in the parotid paper, due to possible correlation between xerostomia and oral cavity dose (that includes also submandibular and sublingual glands).

All these comments intend to underline how complex and critical conscious delineation and tolerance dose level definition with accurate toxicity predictive modeling still are today, particularly given the continuously increasing automation that is made available to the community in the intensity modulation frame, in terms of contouring, planning and adaptation. In the IMRT era, deeper knowledge of the interconnections between dosimetrics and toxicities, including the physiopathology of the various structures and sub-structures of complex organs and their interplay mechanisms are required, since we cannot simply rely on anatomical structure delineation in deciding upon treatment plan quality. However, we have to keep in mind that an inaccurate definition of the critical volumes, both OAR and targets, will affect all the downstream processes of the treatment: the optimization and planning, the dose–volume histogram analysis and plan evaluation.

7.2 Margins

The ICRU 83 Report [1] gave recommendations for the delineation of tumor and normal tissue structures, including the margins necessary to cover possible microscopic spread of the tumor, the organ motion, and the patient set-up uncertainties. Margins are required for both target (from CTV to PTV) and normal tissues (from OAR to PRV).

The previously described interobserver variation in outlining anatomical structures is a crucial source of uncertainty which must be considered a systematic error as it will influence all the sessions of treatment in the same way [53], and as such has to be included in the PTV margin. This makes the accuracy of the structure contouring of primary importance.

During the 2000s, van Herk and his group proposed recipes for dealing with the PTV margin taking into account different aspects [54–56]. There are many geometrical uncertainties in the radiotherapy process, as volume delineation, organ motion, and set-up accuracy; proper combination of all those uncertainties can describe the proper margin to apply to the structures. Geometric errors are separated into random errors, including patient set-up and organ motion, and systematic errors [57–59]. The former describes the day-by-day condition, with different errors for different fractions, and generally their assessment is managed by blurring the dose distribution; the latter is introduced during the treatment preparation (CT scan, delineation, planning) and influences the whole treatment in the same manner. This leads, in general, to a greater effect of systematic errors on dose than random errors.

The principal objective of the van Herk margin formula is to ensure, for 90% of patient population, a minimum CTV dose of 95% of the nominal prescribed dose. His recipe [54, 57] separated the systematic Σ and the random σ errors: Σ combines in quadrature the standard deviations of all the preparation errors—the position, set-up at the scanner, and delineation errors –, σ combines in quadrature the standard deviations of all the random errors—the organ motion and set-up errors, and the penumbra σ_P (dose fall-off) –; simplifying with the exclusion of the penumbra, valid for $\sigma_P = 3.2$ mm, the combined random error of only motion and set-up is σ' $\left(\sigma' = \sqrt{\sigma_{\text{motion}}^2 + \sigma_{\text{set-up}}^2}\right)$:

$$\text{margin} = 2.5\Sigma + 1.64(\sigma - \sigma_P) \approx 2.5\Sigma + 0.7\sigma' \tag{7.1}$$

The calculations did not account for rotation and shape variations, assumed ideal dose conformity and the treatment delivery in many fractions. In this formulation, the organ motion error is considered to have a Gaussian distribution, while it is not generally the case for periodic movements as the respiratory motion.

Monte Carlo based calculations evaluating the margin to be applied to CTV concerning tumor control, and refining the above formula to keep 90% of the population with a maximum of 1% of tumor control probability reduction due to both systemic and random uncertainties [55], which resulted in:

$$\text{margin} = \sqrt{2.7^2\Sigma^2 + 1.6^2\sigma^2} - 2.8\text{ mm} \approx 2.5\Sigma + 0.7\sigma' - 3\text{ mm} \qquad (7.2)$$

for, as in equation (7.1), $\sigma_P = 3.2$ mm. The 3 mm reduction of the margin resides in the equivalence between 1% TCP reduction and 84% minimum CTV dose, and 3 mm is the distance between 95% and 84% in the dose fall-off. This is also a confirmation that tumor control is not determined by the minimum dose to the target, rather by the mean dose [60], as reported from studies on biopsies by Levegrun *et al* [61], thus allowing a reduction of the PTV margin with an acceptable risk of TCP loss.

In a subsequent work [56] the fractionation effect was also evaluated, showing that the extra blurring in the dose distribution was rather small, being the random error divided by the square root of the number of fractions.

Having overviewed how to determine PTV margins, it has become clear that since systematic errors have a greater impact on final PTV volume, particular attention must be paid to contouring especially in the presence of very conformal dose distributions as is the case with intensity modulation technologies.

7.3 Motion and contouring

In this section we analyze how to consider organ motion in order to properly define margins. Already in the ICRU 62 Report [62], the CTV to PTV margin was considered to have two components: the internal and the set-up margin, the first being used to compensate for physiologic movements and variations in size, shape, and position, that could result from respiration, bladder, and rectum filling, swallowing, heartbeat, bowel movements. The CTV plus the internal margin is denoted as the internal target volume ITV. Similarly, uncertainties and variations in the OAR position during treatment are included in a margin that, added to the OAR, comprise the concept of *planning organ at risk volume* PRV. The margin approach, especially related to the target margin, would result in dose spills in healthy tissue located in the margin. In figure 7.3 the volumes and margins as defined in the ICRU 62 are reported.

A more realistic situation is shown in figure 7.4, also from ICRU Report 62, where different scenarios are presented in which a balance between CTV coverage and risk of complications due to an oversized PTV are sought.

In scenario A, a margin to GTV including subclinical invasion is added to determine the CTV. An internal margin (IM) is added for the variations in position and/or shape and size of the CTV to define the internal target volume (ITV).

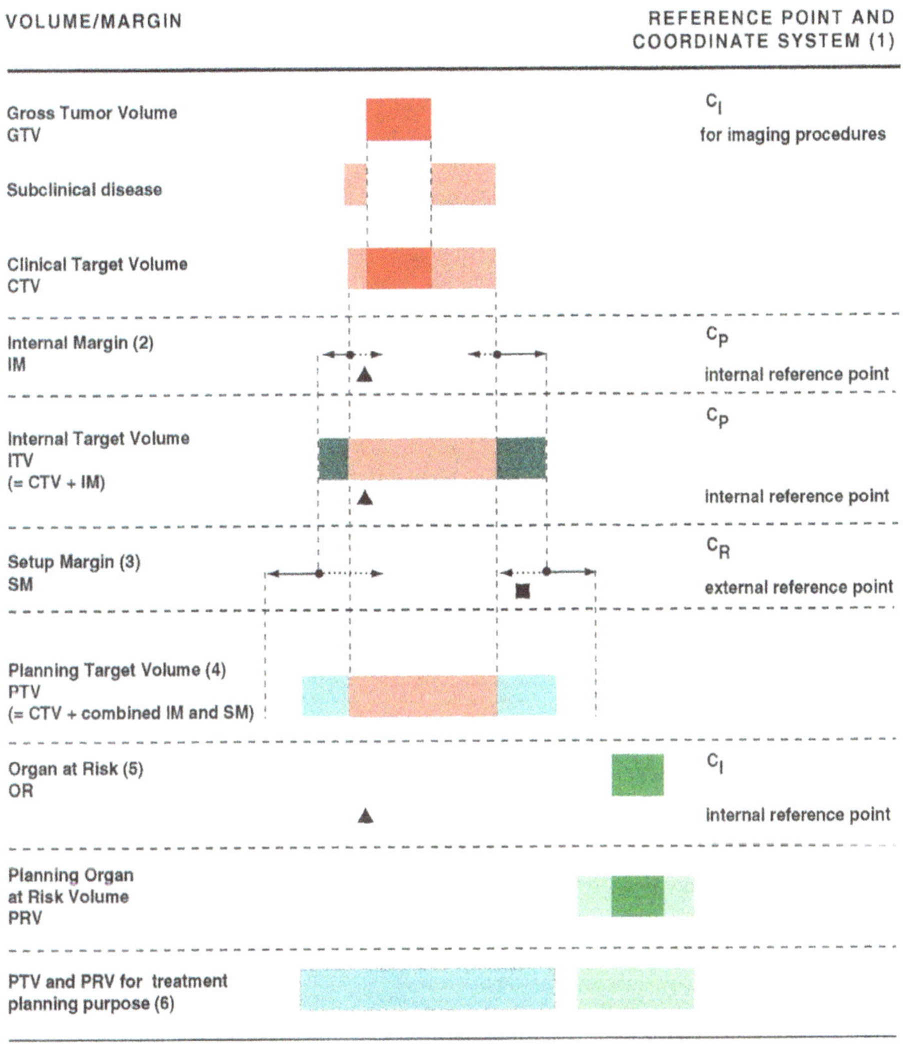

Figure 7.3. Schematic representation of the different volumes/margins. From ICRU Report 62 [62], reproduced with permission. Copyright 1999 Sage Publications.

A set-up margin (SM) is then added to take into account all the uncertainties in the patient positioning. The planning target volume (PTV) is the sum of CTV + IM + SM.

The simple linear summation of the above uncertainties often leads to excessively large PTV, incompatible with the tolerance dose levels of the surrounding normal tissues. In scenario B, instead of linearly adding IM and SM, a smaller PTV is accepted. However, a quantitative approach with a 'global' safety margin is only relevant if all uncertainties are known, that happens in few protocols.

In the majority of the clinical situations, a 'global' safety margin is adopted. This is scenario C in figure 7.4: in some cases, the presence of OAR reduces the width of the acceptable safety margin. However, since the incidence of subclinical invasion

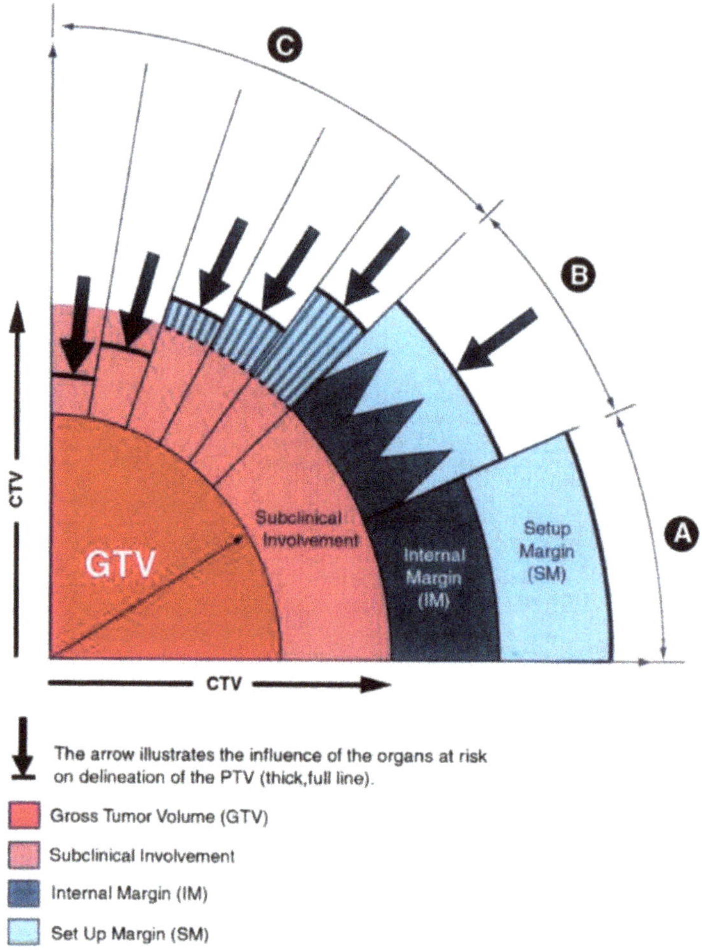

Figure 7.4. Schematic representation of the relations between the different volumes (GTV, CTV, PTV, and PRV) in different clinical scenarios. From ICRU Report 62 [62], reproduced with permission. Copyright 1999 Sage Publications.

may decrease with distance from the GTV, a reduction of the margin for subclinical invasion may hence be adopted.

Physiologic organ motion could refer to inter-fractional movement (as a consequence of possible weight loss, or radiation-induced organ changes), or intra-fractional motion as respiration, heartbeat or bladder filling. Since respiratory motion may have a predictable pattern, it can be managed so as to reduce the need for large margins in moving targets with regards to intra-fraction motion [63].

An important step in respiratory motion management was made in 2001, when the 4DCT image sorting concept was published in the seminal works of Li *et al* [64], Ford *et al* [65], Vedam *et al* [66], according to which it is possible to differentiate the respiratory cycle, generally monitored with an external surrogate, in different breathing phases.

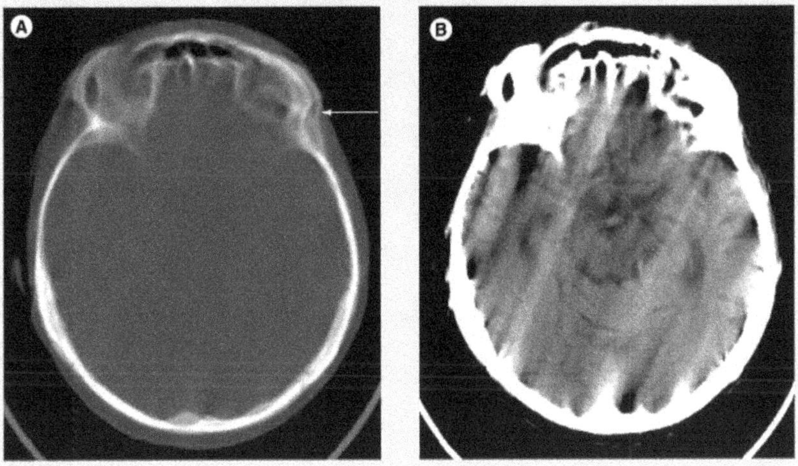

Figure 6. Motion artifact in a head CT. (A) Motion causes blurring and double images, **(B)** as well as long range streaks.

Figure 7.5. Motion-related artifacts. Reproduced from Boas *et al* [67]. Open access CC BY 4.0.

However, one of the major issues related to the acquisition of moving structures is the generation of artifacts, which depend on the scanner setting and timing, as well as on the characteristics of the specific respiration. The most common artifact is the blurring which occurs with rather slow CT scans relative to the breathing cycle. On one hand this effect could give a representation of an average position of the structure, but on the other hand, a blurred image makes the delineation of any structure more difficult. In figure 7.5 an example of motion-related artifacts is reported, showing blurring and image doubling, as well as streaks [67].

Another important artifact occurring in CT or even in 4DCT is partial projection [68–71], due to the residual motion of an object during a single scanner gantry rotation, that could distort the object reconstruction making it appear shortened, elongated, or even divided into different reconstructed volumes. It is a well known fact that when scanning regular objects in motion, their physical shape is not represented. For example, an apple in motion will appear pear-shaped when scanned. In figure 7.6 the surface renderings of a spherical object under regular motion are shown [71]: in the first row CT scans present the interplay between CT data acquisition and object motion, in the second row a 4DCT acquisition shows the residual motion artifacts.

In particular, there are large discrepancies in object reconstruction when large motion (>1.5 cm) occurs in combination with a short breathing period (<4 s). In cases of fast gantry rotations, long breathing periods or small breathing amplitude, the partial projection artifacts could be negligible [68]. Additional partial volume-type artifacts could be generated by irregular breathing over the time of the scan acquisition, where the reconstructed objects can easily present cuts and separate sub-volumes of the same unique object, as shown in figure 7.6. Some remaining artifacts

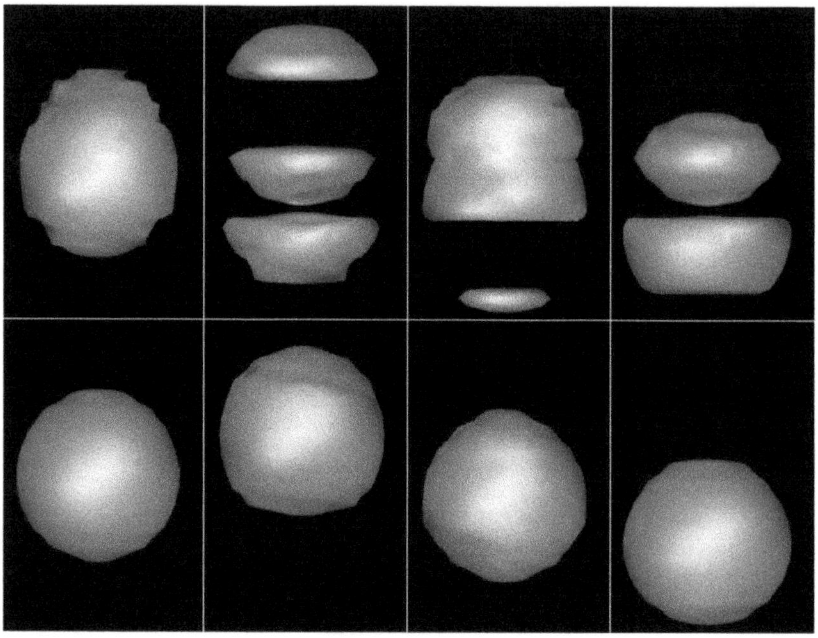

Figure 7.6. Surface rendering of a spherical object in periodic motion (amplitude 1 cm, period 4.4 s). On the top row: CT acquisition; on the bottom row: 4DCT acquisition. From Rietzel *et al* [71], reproduced with permission. John Wiley & Sons. Copyright 2005 American Association of Physicists in Medicine.

could also depend on cycle time, motion extent, scanner settings as the slice acquisition time or the pitch [71], beam collimation width, and also the choice of phases of the respiration cycle for reconstruction. However, a good understanding (and quantification) of the limitations in the 4DCT image reconstruction may permit the incorporating of appropriate margins to the target delineation on a patient-specific basis.

A single 3DCT reconstructed from the 4DCT acquisition can also be generated, as the average intensity projection AIP, or the maximum intensity projection MIP images. The AIP is an image where each voxel intensity is the average voxel intensity over all the respiratory phases [72] whereas, in the MIP image, each voxel intensity reports the highest value encountered over all the respiratory phases [73]. An example of AIP and MIP reconstructions is presented in figure 7.7.

Once the motion trajectory is determined with the time-resolved 4DCT scan, a delineation strategy is to be defined. Choices include delineation of the ITV as encompassing the tumor excursion during the breathing cycle; or the target volume restricted to a portion of the cycle then gated during the treatment; or again the mid-position approach where the time-weighted mean tumor position is defined, as described by Wolthaus *et al* [74].

The ITV approach. The ITV represents the volume encompassing the CTV and the internal margin [62]. It can be delineated in all the 4DCT reconstructed

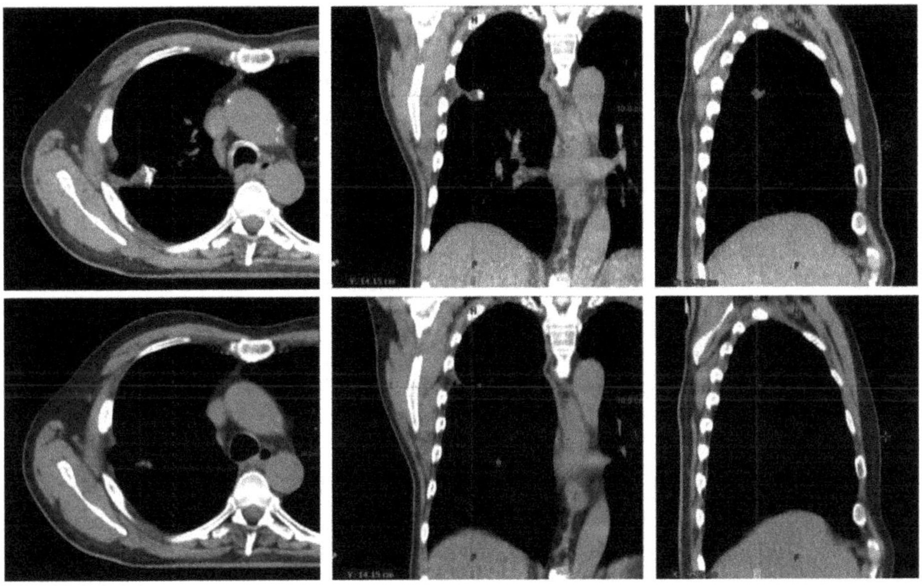

Figure 7.7. MIP (on the top) and AIP (on the bottom) reconstructions from the same 4DCT acquisition.

time-resolved phases, and subsequently enveloping them, or, alternatively, it can be delineated on the MIP image.

The gating approach. The target is irradiated only during part of the breathing cycle, and the corresponding reconstructed respiration phase is used to delineate the target. In general, apart from the case of deep inspiration breath-hold, the exhale phase (a passive phase) is used, being longer and more reproducible than the inhale phase. The time window width commonly used to gate the treatment is ~30% of the respiratory cycle, as a balance between motion and treatment time [75, 76].

The mid-ventilation and mid-position approaches. The mid-ventilation scan is the single 3DCT frame from a 4DCT representing the tumor closest to its mean position during the motion [77]. The time (%) in the breathing cycle representing the mean position of the tumor determines the mid-ventilation phase. However, the tumor moves asynchronously in more directions, drawing an elliptical trajectory (hysteresis of the tumor motion). This potential issue is accounted for in the mid-position approach [74].

The ITV concept translates the organ motion to the target delineation, covering the whole possible target position, and therefore considering it as a systematic error. In this way, the ITV approach could overestimate the dosimetric impact of the motion, with possibly a larger PTV that might prevent dose escalation and may increase toxicity due to a higher dose delivered to closely surrounding tissues [74]. In this respect, a mid-ventilation (or mid-position) approach could reduce the PTV volume size, including the organ motion in the van Herk formula, thus reducing the CTV to PTV margin, once the time-weighted average position is determined by the 4DCT scan acquisition. Although the ITV concept is most commonly used for target delineation, it has been proven that the mid-ventilation approach could have the advantage of a smaller PTV while keeping adequate target coverage.

The IMRT or VMAT delivered by gating the beam according to patient breathing during a selected respiratory phase within an associated threshold and based on an external surrogate has been proven to be technically feasible. Fixed beam IMRT with respiratory gating was studied by Duan *et al* [78], Keall *et al* [79] confirming the usability of such a technical solution while also pointing out the additional potential uncertainties that could arise, and suggesting particular attention on dose rate and leaf speed (the slower, the better) and the number of interruptions. The case of VMAT, where also the gantry has to stop its rotation and restart from the correct position together with the right MLC shape and dose rate, has been explored by Nicolini *et al* [80], finding, in a pre-clinical setting on a Varian Clinac, reliable and dosimetrically accurate deliveries even with a high number of interruptions. However, this could be considered an additional uncertainty, and gated intensity-modulators would require the application of adequate margins.

The organ motion was assessed and quantified by van Herk *et al* in their 2003 work [56] so as to be included in PTV margin formula. Since the internal and external sources of error are generally not correlated, it is not correct simply to linearly add the standard deviations coming from internal and external sources. The respiratory motion, with a regular pattern, caused an asymmetric deviation of the dose distribution, depending on the breathing amplitude A, showing a caudal and a cranial shift of $0.25A$ and $0.45A$, respectively, for amplitude larger than 1 cm; for narrower breathing there is no additional effect of the non-Gaussian blurring generated by the sinusoidal motion.

The anatomical site where the respiratory motion is evaluated is the lung, also with attention to the stereotactic lung treatment, due to the close vicinity of the critical structures to the moving target, thus increasing the risk of toxicity or treatment failure if the choice of the PTV margin is suboptimal.

Here the results of a few rather recent studies are reported. In 2014 Peulen *et al* [81], on 297 patients, applied on the mid-ventilation scans the patient-specific margins over the three main directions, evaluated from the 4DCT scan. They estimated that the PTV margin based on the ITV approach would have been larger in about half of the patients. With the ITV approach, the errors are summed up linearly, while they are summed up quadratically in the mid-ventilation approach. In 2017 Ehrbar *et al* [82] reported a reduction of the PTV volume for the mid-ventilation method relative to the ITV approach of 23%; the ITV method ensures the tumor coverage, together with exposing the lung tissue to higher doses, while the lung dose can be reduced with the mid-ventilation method, but at the price of a slightly reduced target coverage. In 2019 Thomas *et al* [83] found that for the mid-ventilation approach plus a margin evaluated according to the van Herk formula, the dose covering 95% of the CTV for 95% of the time was greater than using the ITV concept and 5 mm isotropic margin to PTV.

There are some possible reasons for the limited use of the mid-ventilation (or, even more, the mid-position) solution instead of the ITV outline. Firstly, there are currently no tools in the treatment planning systems to determine the reference mid-ventilation phase or to generate the mid-position image. Secondly, the non-Gaussian nature of the breathing motion would suggest that the respiration induced motion should be accounted for separately, by linearly adding a margin to the quadrature sum of the other contributing errors, and not included in the quadrature sum like that used in the actual concept [56, 84].

Additionally, the choice of image selection based on a motion approach for target delineation should also consider the possible issues related to artifact management. The mid-ventilation phase, once determined, is in a position of the breathing cycle where the tumor motion is fast and large, conditions presenting more partial projection artifacts. This effect is mitigated once the ITV concept is used.

The interplay effect between organ and MLC motions will be discussed more in detail in chapter 8 on treatment planning, while a section dedicated to the dosimetric consequences of organ motion is available in chapter 10 on dose calculation.

7.4 Auto-segmentation

The contouring phase has a fundamental role in the inverse planning process of IMRT, and an accurate outline of the targets and OAR is critical for maximizing tumor control and minimizing normal tissue complication probabilities. As outlined in the previous section, studies have shown high correlations between contouring variations (targets and organs at risk) and dosimetry, and between dosimetry and treatment outcome (tumor control and toxicity). However, the manual delineation of all the needed structures is time-consuming and labor-intensive, along with being prone to inter-(and intra-)observer variations.

Under these premises, great efforts have been made over the past two decades to develop solutions for automatic contouring (auto-segmentation, or auto-contouring), aimed specifically at reducing delineation time, increasing adherence to guidelines, and minimizing inter-observer variability.

Prior to any auto-contouring process, an ontology serving as a reference must be defined based on the previous knowledge of GTV, CTV, and organ at risk; these must pertain to specific image modalities that follow defined and precise guidelines which summarize imaging, anatomical, clinical and pathological information. Note that the actual references for contouring evaluation and comparison are the manual delineations by experts, presenting all the uncertainties of any observer-related criticalities.

Different auto-segmentation approaches were explored in the last two decades [85] and can be summarized in four generations, with increasing levels of algorithmic complexities. The first three are well summarized by Withey and Koles [86], giving a brief and schematic view of the medical image segmentation problems and methods. The main issues related to the images are *noise*, *intensity non-uniformity* and *partial volume averaging*. The first can modify the pixel intensity value making its classification uncertain. The second is the gradual variation of the intensity values of a single tissue class in the same image. The third regards the occurrence of the pixel volume containing a mixture of different tissue classes information, so that the resulting averaged intensity value is not consistent with any tissue class. To these technical problems must be added the possible segmentation uncertainties derived by tissue variability among individuals of the population. However, segmentation validity is still decided upon by the image interpretation of medical experts, with all the uncertainties linked to inter- and intra-observer variations.

7.4.1 First generation of auto-segmentation methods (model-based)

These are techniques where no or little prior knowledge is included, and are based on the analysis of the image content and properties, using voxel information such as intensity, directional change, and image gradient, and are thus subject to the three main segmentation problems summarized above. The main methods are *threshold*, *region growing*, and *edge tracking*. *Threshold* distinguishes objects according to similar intensity levels in the pixels. *Region growing* starts from a certain point of the segmented region and checks for pre-defined homogeneity criteria within adjacent pixels in a continuous manner, thus augmenting the region area with connected structures. For the *edge tracking* method, the edges of the object are detected by sequentially following the connectivity of adjacent neighbor pixels resulting in an object boundary. [87, 88]

7.4.2 Second generation of auto-segmentation methods

In this generation, uncertainty models and optimization methods were introduced, attempting to overcome the image segmentation problems. Among those, to cite just a few: the *deformable models*, the *graph search*, and the *neural networks*. The *deformable models* (as the *active contour* or the *active surface*) [89] are artificial, closed contours or surfaces that can contract or expand within an image to conform to specific image features. In the *graph search* methods (as the *graph cuts* [90]), nodes are defined and inter-connected to neighbors according to pixel associations in the image which use optimization algorithms in order to minimize the cost function. For example in *graph cut*, the removal of inter-connections between nodes generates a separation of the graph in two sets. With the *neural network* method, some neural networks have to be trained with suitable image data before being used to segment an image.

7.4.3 Third generation of auto-segmentation methods (atlas-based)

Only the introduction of high-level knowledge, as expert-defined rules and models (expert segmentation as ground truth), such as those included in these third generation models, can produce accurate auto-segmentation. The *shape* and *appearance models* and the *atlas-based segmentation* are the most popular methods, also applied to some auto-contouring software in the commercial planning systems. The *active shape model* follows the deformable models [91]. The object is represented statistically by identifying landmarks on the boundaries of an object and evaluating their variations according to selected training images; the method identifies objects of the same class within other images. The *active appearance model* is an extension of the shape model [92], where the intensity of the object rather than the shape, is included. The most applied method is the *atlas-based model*, which consists of pre-segmented objects in a pre-defined atlas. A mapping is then determined between the contoured atlas and the image to segment. *Single-atlas*-based techniques use a single dataset as prior knowledge, which is then propagated via a deformable registration [93–95]. However, since the patient population is hardly represented by a single-atlas case, *multi-atlas* methods combine datasets of multiple anatomies/atlases [96, 97]. In this case, multiple single-atlas segmentations are combined to generate average contouring, based on the multi-atlas population. Different techniques have been used to combine multiple atlases, mostly the simultaneous truth and performance level estimation (STAPLE) [98], where all the atlases have the same weight, or the similarity and truth estimation for propagated segmentations (STEPS) [99], where only the atlases with the highest anatomical similarity to the patient are used for the atlas-combination process.

Hybrid auto-segmentation methods, combining model-based and atlas-based approaches, ensured and enforced a robust adaptation to the structure boundaries. The shape or appearance models provide closed and anatomically correct surfaces represented by landmarks, surface meshes, vector fields, and voxel intensities, that are then combined with atlas-based segmentation to improve model initialization, possibly preventing trapping in local minima [100].

The atlas-based approach for auto-segmentation has some limitations [101]. Anatomical deformation could be estimated with insufficient accuracy by the image registration algorithm, and the boundaries of organs may not present sufficient contrast leading to deformation errors. The missing truth as reference could lead the algorithms to propagate random errors toward systematic errors. Finally, the image quality and the different protocols used for image acquisitions affect the segmentation that, again, may bring rise to inaccurate results.

7.4.4 Fourth generation of auto-segmentation methods (deep learning)

As suggested by Cardenas *et al* [102] in 2019 in their review on traditional auto-segmentation algorithms, the fourth generation of auto-segmentation methods probably arose with the application of deep learning algorithms, made available to medical imaging thanks to advances in GPU technology. Recent papers give an overview of the current status of deep learning techniques for medical image segmentation, covering different aspects: Litjens *et al* [103], Shen *et al* [104] and Hesamian *et al* [105]. Deep learning consists of machine learning algorithms, through application of artificial intelligence, by which systems are able to automatically learn and improve from their experience based on examples, instructions or human experience training, by looking for special patterns in the data. In particular, deep learning is based on a deep neural network DNN architecture, that is an improvement on artificial neural networks since it enables the constructions of networks with multiple (hidden) layers between input and output, which can discover hierarchical feature representations, learning only from data. However, the structural information among neighboring voxels is crucial for evaluating medical images. For example the convolution neural network CNN is designed to better utilize spatial and pattern information: the architectures are usually formed by stacking several types of layers (convolutional layers, pooling layers, fully-connected layers, etc) that transform the input (image) into the desired output providing local connectivity between neurons of adjacent layers exploiting spatially local correlations, allowing the network to learn the features both globally and locally. The fully-convolutional networks FCN, introduced by Long *et al* [106], have both an encoding (as the CNN) and a decoding path producing accurate segmentations.

Deep learning auto-segmentation does have some limitations, however [102]: it is a sort of black-box process, making interpretation of the features affecting the network training difficult. Secondly, it depends on the quality of the prior knowledge used to train the models, where 'garbage in, garbage out' holds true. Finally, similarly to the atlas-based methods, the image quality and the different protocols used for image acquisitions could affect the results of a deep learning approach.

The current status of auto-segmentation tools in most used treatment planning systems shows that algorithms are available in all major TPS, mostly atlas-based.

Varian provides the Smart Segmentation Knowledge-Based Contouring module in Eclipse, as well as the VelocityAI software, the first being a combined single-atlas and model-based approach for targets and organs at risk, the second an atlas-based model. In view of the adaptive radiotherapy with Ethos, Varian is including a deep learning approach based on the convolution neural network CNN method.

RaySearch, inside RayStation, implemented a multi-atlas-based segmentation module MABS.

Elekta adopted the single-atlas-based method with the ABAS software module, compatible with any treatment planning system.

Philips, in Pinnacle^3, has SPICE, a model-based module using probabilistic segmentations.

Brainlab included in their Elements a single-atlas knowledge-based anatomical segmentation.

Other atlas-based software for auto-contouring are available, not linked to any treatment planning system, as Mirada (Mirada Medical Ltd, UK) with its atlas-based ABAS WorkflowBox and deep learning DLCExpert approaches. Irrespective of computer-based contouring, it is important to caution that not every patient has standard anatomy and there are numerous variations such as the liver being on the left side or having only one of two organs.

Concerning the general behavior of different auto-contouring methods, many studies have been published, the vast majority of which pertain to the head and neck region, on both research and commercial solutions. Here is just a small report on some of those works. Voet *et al* [107] reported about the ABAS Elekta segmentation, using a dosimetric approach, which brought to light the need to edit the auto-contoured neck CTVs in order to avoid underdosing ($V_{95\%}$ reduced by up to ~7% and smaller CTVs by up to ~9% for average Dice similarity coefficients of 0.81), while editing of the parotids did not lead to significant dosimetric variations. The need to edit auto-contouring is suggested by almost all the studies based on the different segmentation methods, atlas-based or hybrid ([100, 108–114] on head and neck [115], on breast target) or deep learning approaches ([116–120] on head and neck [121], on lung). When the deep learning approach was compared to atlas-based solutions (e.g. [119–121]), the authors found the first outperformed the second.

A study was published on MRI for brain structures delineation—a quite complex anatomical site to contour—by Conson and colleagues [122], finding very valuable results with a STAPLE multi-atlas-based method. Another study, by Kieselmann *et al* [123], on MRI images on head and neck, using three different atlas-based methods, reported promising results, but a low correlation between geometric and dosimetric figures, suggesting that the geometric figures alone present on the segmentation results could be insufficient to predict the dosimetric impact of inaccuracies derived from auto-segmentation.

Let us now look into the clinical applications and related quality assurance regarding auto-segmentation methods, which are key points of the whole high precision treatment frame. Errors in structure delineation may have a serious impact on the dose and ultimately on patient treatment, as shown in the case of inter-observer variations. For that reason, all auto-segmentation systems should have an appropriate quality assurance program, from commissioning through to maintenance. Cardenas *et al* [102] suggested inclusion in the commissioning process of auto-segmentation, intensive testing with patient data from the local institution, to ensure that the software works as expected for their range of image types and patient anatomies. In addition, the information transfer, import/export process must also be checked for consistency.

Valentini *et al* [124] published recommendations for evaluating performances and benchmarks and described potentials and criticisms on the auto-segmentation software in radiotherapy. They discussed the indices used to evaluate auto-contouring performances (as the Dice similarity, area of intersection, conformation number, Hausdorff distance, Jaccard index) and to assess how an auto-segmentation software can adhere to the defined benchmark. It was shown that the indices hardly distinguish between random and systematic uncertainties, or between false positives and false negatives [125, 126], and for example, the reported Dice similarity coefficients are still well below unity in most of the anatomical regions, relative to manual contours delineated by experts. In view of evaluating and validating the auto-contouring software, there is a need for reliable sets of structures to use as a referral contour to benchmark. However, the impossibility of having a complete overlap between two manual outlines, even from physicians with a high degree of expertize, makes this task far from being solved.

Another interesting comment in Valentini *et al* [124] is the possible educational benefit offered by auto-contouring, which gives trainees the availability of expert outlined structures to consult, study and test on, without directly referring to experienced people. This is an interesting view, considering the increasing demands together with the shortage of adequately trained staff. Moreover, the example of the possibility of delineating very complex brain structures thanks to auto-segmentation on MRI, as shown by Conson *et al* [122], is not prosecutable with manual tools in radiotherapy clinical practice, while it could potentially provide new knowledge on dose-related features of those complex structures. On the other hand, there is the risk of a decrease in actual teaching efforts by assigning the task almost solely to artificial intelligence which could result in a reduction of deep (human) knowledge. It is left to future generations to find the most intelligent way of properly using and benefiting from automation without losing human knowledge.

Technological advances in the intensity modulation era indeed stem from the capabilities of the auto-segmentation technique in the field of adaptive therapy. The concept of adaptive radiotherapy was initially expressed by Makie *et al* [127], Mohan *et al* [128]; however, an adaptive radiotherapy concept can be applied on-line only if automatic segmentation is possible, thus acquiring all the beneficial evidence [129]. It is known that any adaptation of radiation treatment for biological or anatomical changes during therapy requires very rapid re-optimization and re-planning, based on the modified anatomy; clearly, the time needed for manual delineation of all the involved structures prevents on-line adaptive radiotherapy from being implemented. It is only thanks to the fast computer capabilities allowing quick and reliable auto-segmentation that we are today standing on the threshold of a transformation of routine radiotherapy planning via the use of artificial intelligence [101].

References

[1] ICRU Report 83 2010 *Prescribing, Recording, and Reporting Intensity-Modulated Photon-Beam Therapy (IMRT)* (Bethesda, MD: International Commission on Radiation Units and Measurements)

[2] Srivastava S P, Cheng C W and Das I J 2016 The effect of slice thickness on target and organs at risk volumes, dosimetric coverage and radiobiological impact in IMRT planning *Clin. Transl. Oncol.* **18** 469–79

[3] Das I, Bieda M and Cheng C *et al* 2004 Dosimetric comparison of inverse treatment planning systems for intensity modulated radiation therapy: a collaborative study *Med. Phys.* **31** 1750

[4] Eisbruch A, Harris J and Garden A S *et al* 2010 Multi institutional trial of accelerated hypofractionated intensity-modulated radiation therapy for early-stage oropharyngeal cancer (RTOG 00–22) *Int. J. Radiat. Oncol. Biol. Phys.* **76** 1333–8

[5] Peters L J, O'Sullivan B and Giralt J *et al* 2010 Critical impact of radiotherapy protocol compliance and quality in the treatment of advanced head and neck cancer: results from TROG 02.02 *J. Clin. Oncol.* **28** 2996–3001

[6] Wuthrick E J, Zhang Q and Machtay M *et al* 2015 Institutional clinical trial accrual volume and survival of patients with head and neck cancer *J. Clin. Oncol.* **33** 156–64

[7] Grégoire V, Coche E, Cosnard G, Hamoir M and Reychler H 2000 Selection and delineation of lymph node target volumes in head and neck conformal radiotherapy. Proposal for standardizing terminology and procedure based on the surgical experience *Radiother. Oncol.* **56** 135–50

[8] Grégoire V, Levendag P and Ang K K *et al* 2003 CT-based delineation of lymph node levels and related CTVs in the node-negative neck: DAHANCA, EORTC, GORTEC, NCIC, RTOG consensus guidelines *Radiother. Oncol.* **69** 227–36

[9] Grégoire V, Eisbruch A, Hamoir M and Levendag P 2006 Proposal for the delineation of the nodal CTV in node-positive and the post-operative neck *Radiother. Oncol.* **79** 15–20

[10] Grégoire V, Ang K and Budach W *et al* 2014 Delineation of the neck node levels for head and neck tumors: a 2013 update. DAHANCA, EORTC, HKNPCSG, NCIC CTG, NCRI, RTOG, TROG consensus guidelines *Radiother. Oncol.* **110** 172–81
[11] Grégoire V, Evans M and Le Q T *et al* 2018 Delineation of the primary tumour Clinical Target Volumes (CTV-P) in laryngeal, hypopharyngeal, oropharyngeal and oral cavity squamous cell carcinoma: AIRO, CACA, DAHANCA, EORTC, GEORCC, GORTEC, HKNPCSG, HNCIG, IAG-KHT, LPRHHT, NCIC CTG, NCRI, NRG Oncology, PHNS, SBRT, SOMERA, SRO, SSHNO, TROG consensus guidelines *Radiother. Oncol.* **126** 3–24
[12] Lee A W, Ng W T and Pan J J *et al* 2018 International guideline for the delineation of the clinical target volumes (CTV) for nasopharyngeal carcinoma *Radiother. Oncol.* **126** 25–36
[13] van der Veen J, Gulyban A and Nuyts S 2019 Interobserver variability in delineation of target volumes in head and neck cancer *Radiother. Oncol.* **137** 9–15
[14] Weltens C, Menten J and Feron M *et al* 2001 Interobserver variations in gross tumor volume delineation of brain tumors on computed tomography and impact of magnetic resonance imaging *Radiother. Oncol.* **60** 49–59
[15] Wee C W, Sung W and Kang H C *et al* 2015 Evaluation of variability in target volume delineation for newly diagnosed glioblastoma: a multi-institutional study from the Korean Radiation Oncology Group *Radiat. Oncol.* **10** 137
[16] Caldwell C B, Mah K and Ung Y C *et al* 2001 Observer variation in contouring gross tumor volume in patients with poorly defined non-small-cell lung tumors on CT: the impact of 18FDG-hybrid PET fusion *Int. J. Radiat. Oncol. Biol. Phys.* **51** 923–31
[17] Van de Steene J, Linthout N and Mey J *et al* 2002 Definition of gross tumor volume in lung cancer: inter-observer variability *Radiother. Oncol.* **62** 37–49
[18] Louie A V, Rodrigues G and Olsthoorn J *et al* 2010 Inter-observer and intra-observer reliability for lung cancer target volume delineation in the 4D-CT era *Radiother. Oncol.* **95** 166–71
[19] Mercieca S, Belderbos J S A and De Jaeger K *et al* 2018 Interobserver variability in the delineation of the primary lung cancer and lymph nodes on different four-dimensional computed tomography reconstructions *Radiother. Oncol.* **126** 325–32
[20] Hurkmans C W, Borger J H and Pieters B R *et al* 2001 Variability in target volume delineation on CT scans of the breast *Int. J. Radiat. Oncol. Biol. Phys.* **50** 1366–72
[21] Li X A, Tai A and Arthur D W *et al* 2009 Variability of target and normal structure delineation for breast cancer radiotherapy: an RTOG multi-institutional and multiobserver *Int. J. Radiat. Oncol. Biol. Phys.* **73** 944–51
[22] Dalah E, Moraru I, Paulson E, Erickson B and Li X A 2014 Variability of target and normal structure delineation using multimodality imaging for radiation therapy of pancreatic cancer *Int. J. Radiat. Oncol. Biol. Phys.* **89** 633–40
[23] Hong T S, Bosch W R and Krishnan S *et al* 2014 Interobserver variability in target definition for hepatocellular carcinoma with and without portal vein thrombus: radiation therapy oncology group consensus guidelines *Int. J. Radiat. Oncol. Biol. Phys.* **89** 804–13
[24] Lim K, Erickson B and Jurgenliemk-Schulz I M *et al* 2015 Variability in clinical target volume delineation for intensity modulated radiation therapy in 3 challenging cervix cancer scenarios *Pract. Radiat. Oncol.* **5** e557–65
[25] Nijkamp J, de Haas-Kock D F and Beukema J C *et al* 2012 Target volume delineation variation in radiotherapy for early stage rectal cancer in the Netherlands *Radiother. Oncol.* **102** 14–21

[26] Yeung A R, Vargas C E and Falchook A *et al* 2008 Dose-volume differences for computed tomography and magnetic resonance imaging segmentation and planning for proton prostate cancer therapy *Int. J. Radiat. Oncol. Biol. Phys.* **72** 1426–33

[27] Emami B, Lyman J and Brown A *et al* 1991 Tolerance of normal tissue to therapeutic irradiation *Int. J. Radiat. Oncol. Biol. Phys.* **21** 109–22

[28] 2010 Quantitative analyses of normal tissue effects in the clinic (QUANTEC) *Int. J. Radiat. Oncol. Biol. Phys.* **76** supplement

[29] Brouwer C L, Steenbakkers R J H M and van den Heuvel E *et al* 2012 3D variation in delineation of head and neck organs at risk *Radiat. Oncol.* **7** 32

[30] Brouwer C L, Steenbakkers R J H M and Bourhis J *et al* 2015 CT-based delineation of organs at risk in the head and neck region: DAHANCA, EORTC, GORTEC, HKNPCSG, NCIC CTG, NCRI, NRG Oncology and TROG consensus guidelines *Radiother. Oncol.* **117** 83–90

[31] Vinod S K, Jameson M G, Min M and Holloway L C 2016 Uncertainty in volume delineation in radiation oncology: a systematic review and recommendations for future studies *Radiother. Oncol.* **121** 169–79

[32] Loo S W, Martin W M C, Smith P, Cherian S and Roques T W 2012 Interobserver variation in parotid gland delineation: a study of its impact on intensity-modulated radiotherapy solutions with a systematic review of literature *Br. J. Radiol.* **85** 1070–7

[33] Nelms B E, Tomé W A, Robinson G and Wheeler J 2012 Variations in the contouring of organs at risk: test case from a patient with oropharyngeal cancer *Int. J. Radiat. Oncol. Biol. Phys.* **82** 368–78

[34] Feng M, Demiroz C, Vineberg K A, Eisbruch A and Balter J M 2012 Normal tissue anatomy for oropharyngeal cancer: contouring variability and its impact on optimization *Int. J. Radiat. Oncol. Biol. Phys.* **84** e245–9

[35] Nöymar A, Lell M, Sweeney R, Bautz W and Lukas P 2001 MRI appearance of radiation-induced changes of normal cervical tissues *Eud. Radiol.* **11** 1807–17

[36] Castadot P, Lee J A, Geets Z and Grégoire V 2010 Adaptive radiotherapy for head and neck cancer *Semin. Radiat. Oncol.* **20** 84–93

[37] Fiorentino A, Caivano R and Metallo V *et al* 2012 Parotid gland volumetric changes during intensity-modulated radiotherapy in head and neck cancer *Br. J. Radiol.* **85** 1415–9

[38] Ren G, Zu S P and Du L *et al* 2015 Actual anatomical and dosimetric changes of parotid glands in nasopharyngeal carcinoma patients during intensity modulated radiation therapy *BioMed Res. Int.* 670327

[39] Xu S, Wu Z and Yang C *et al* 2016 Radiation-inducted CT number changes in GTV and parotid glands during the course of radiation therapy for nasopharyngeal cancer *Br. J. Radiol.* **89** 20140819

[40] Wang Z H, Yan C and Chang Z Y *et al* 2009 Radiation-induced volume changes in parotid and submandibular glands in patients with head and neck cancer receiving postoperative radiotherapy: a longitudinal study *Laryngoscope* **119** 1966–74

[41] Marzi S, Farneti A and Vidiri A *et al* 2018 Radiation-induced parotid changes in oropharyngeal cancer patients: the role of early functional imaging and patient-/treatment-related factors *Radiat. Oncol.* **13** 189

[42] Vásquez Osorio E M, Hoogeman M S and Al-Mamgani A *et al* 2008 Local anatomic changes in parotid and submandibular glands during radiotherapy for oropharynx cancer and correlation with dose, studied in detail with nonrigid registration *Int. J. Radiat. Oncol. Biol. Phys.* **70** 875–82

[43] Barker J L, Garden A S and Ang K K *et al* 2004 Quantification of volumetric and geometric changes occurring during fractionated radiotherapy for head-and-neck cancer using an integrated CT/linear accelerator system *Int. J. Radiat. Oncol. Biol. Phys.* **59** 960–70
[44] Wu Q W, Chi Y and Chen P Y *et al* 2009 Adaptive replanning strategies accounting for shrinkage in head and neck IMRT *Int. J. Radiat. Oncol. Biol. Phys.* **75** 924–32
[45] Lee C, Langen K M and Lu W *et al* 2008 Assessment of parotid gland dose changes during head and neck cancer radiotherapy using daily megavoltage computed tomography and deformable image registration *Int. J. Radiat. Oncol. Biol. Phys.* **71** 1563–71
[46] Eisbruch A, Ten Haken R K, Kim H M, Marsh L H and Ship J A 1999 Dose, volume, and function relationships in parotid salivary glands following conformal and intensity-modulated irradiation of head and neck cancer *Int. J. Radiat. Oncol. Biol. Phys.* **45** 577–87
[47] Deasy J O, Moiseenko V and Marks L *et al* 2010 Radiotherapy dose-volume effects on salivary gland function *Int. J. Radiat. Oncol. Biol. Phys.* **76** Suppl. S58–63
[48] Geets X, Daisne J F and Arcangeli S *et al* 2005 Inter-observer variability in the delineation of pharyngo-laryngeal tumor, parotid glands and cervical spinal cord: comparison between CT-scan and MRI *Radiother. Oncol.* **77** 25–31
[49] Ghobadi G, van der Veen S and Bartelds B *et al* 2012 Physiological interaction of heart and lung in thoracic irradiation *Int. J. Radiat. Oncol. Biol. Phys.* **84** e639–46
[50] Orlandi E, Iacovelli N A and Rancati T *et al* 2018 Multivariable model for predicting acute oral mucositis during combined IMRT and chemotherapy for locally advanced nasopharyngeal cancer patients *Oral Oncol.* **86** 266–72
[51] Dean J A, Welsh L C, Gulliford S L, Harrington K L and Nutting C M 2015 A novel method for delineation of oral mucosa for radiotherapy dose-response studies *Radiother. Oncol.* **115** 63–6
[52] Dean J A, Welsh L C and Wong K H *et al* 2017 Normal tissue complication probability (NTCP) modelling of severe acute mucositis using a novel oral mucosal surface organ at risk *Clin. Oncol.* **29** 263–73
[53] van Herk M 2004 Errors and margins in radiotherapy *Semin. Radiat. Oncol.* **14** 52–64
[54] van Herk M, Remeijer P, Rasch C and Lebesque J V 2000 The probability of correct target dosage: dose-population histograms for deriving treatment margins in radiotherapy *Int. J. Radiat. Oncol. Biol. Phys.* **47** 1121–35
[55] van Herk M, Remeijer P and Lebesque J V 2002 Inclusion of geometric uncertainties in treatment plan evaluation *Int. J. Radiat. Oncol. Biol. Phys.* **52** 1407–22
[56] van Herk M, Witte M, van der Geer J, Schneider C and Lebesque J V 2003 Biologic and physical fractionation effects of random geometric errors *Int. J. Radiat. Oncol. Biol. Phys.* **57** 1460–71
[57] Hunt M A, Kutcher G J and Burman C *et al* 1993 The effect of set-up uncertainties on the treatment of nasopharynx cancer *Int. J. Radiat. Oncol. Biol. Phys.* **27** 437–47
[58] Hunt M A, Schultheiss T E, Desobry G E, Hakki M and Hanks G E 1995 An evaluation of setup uncertainties for patients treated to pelvic sites *Int. J. Radiat. Oncol. Biol. Phys.* **32** 227–33
[59] Stroom J P, de Boer H C J, Huizenga H and Visser A G 1999 Inclusion of geometrical uncertainties in radiotherapy treatment planning by means of coverage probability *Int. J. Radiat. Oncol. Biol. Phys.* **43** 905–19
[60] Goitein M and Niemierko A 1996 Intensity modulated therapy and inhomogeneous dose to the tumor: a note of caution *Int. J. Radiat. Oncol. Biol. Phys.* **36** 519–22

[61] Levegrün S, Jackson A and Zelefsky M J *et al* 2000 Analysis of biopsy outcome after three-dimensional conformal radiation therapy of prostate cancer using dose-distribution variables and tumor control probability models *Int. J. Radiat. Oncol. Biol. Phys.* **47** 1245–60

[62] ICRU Report 62 1999 *Prescribing, Recording, and Reporting Photon Beam Therapy (Supplement to ICRU Report 50)* (Bethesda, MD: International Commission on Radiation Units and Measurements)

[63] Korreman S S 2012 Motion in radiotherapy: photon therapy *Phys. Med. Biol.* **57** R161–91

[64] Li R, Lewis J H, Cerviño L I and Jiang S B 2009 4D CT sorting based on patient internal anatomy *Phys. Med. Biol.* **54** 4821–33

[65] Ford E C, Mageras G S, Yorke E and Ling C C 2003 Respiration-correlated spiral CT: a method of measuring respiratory-induced anatomic motion for radiation treatment planning *Med. Phys.* **30** 88–97

[66] Vedam S S, Keall P J and Kini V R *et al* 2003 Acquiring a four-dimensional computed tomography dataset using an external respiratory signal *Phys. Med. Biol.* **48** 45–62

[67] Boas F E and Fleischmann D 2012 CT artifacts: causes and reduction techniques *Imag. Med.* **4** 229–40

[68] Watkins W T, Li R and Lewis J *et al* 2010 Patient-specific motion artifacts in 4DCT *Med. Phys.* **37** 2855–61

[69] Chen G T Y, Hung J H and Beaudette K P 2004 Artifacts in computed tomography scanning of moving objects *Semin. Radiat. Oncol.* **14** 19–26

[70] Nakamura M, Narita Y and Sawada A *et al* 2009 Impact of motion velocity on four-dimensional target volumes: a phantom study *Med. Phys.* **36** 1610–7

[71] Rietzel E, Pan T and Chen G T 2005 Four-dimensional computed tomography: image formation and clinical protocol *Med. Phys.* **32** 874–89

[72] Glide-Hurst C K, Hugo G D, Liang J and Yan D 2008 A simplified method of four-dimensional dose accumulation using the mean patient density representation *Med. Phys.* **35** 5269–77

[73] Underberg R W M, Lagerwaard F J, Slotman B J, Cuijpers D P and Senan S 2005 Use of maximum intensity projections (MIP) for target volume generation in 4DCT scans for lung cancer *Int. J. Radiat. Oncol. Biol. Phys.* **63** 253–60

[74] Wolthaus J W, Sonke J J and van Herk M *et al* 2008 Comparison of different strategies to use four-dimensional computed tomography in treatment planning for lung cancer patients *Int. J. Radiat. Oncol. Biol. Phys.* **70** 1229–38

[75] Keall P J, Mageras G S and Balter J M *et al* 2006 The management of respiratory motion in radiation oncology report of AAPM Task Group 76 *Med. Phys.* **33** 3874–900

[76] Mageras G S and Yorke E 2004 Deep inspiration breath hold and respiratory gating strategies for reducing organ motion in radiation treatment *Semin. Radiat. Oncol.* **14** 65–75

[77] Wolthaus J W H, Schneider C and Sonke J J *et al* 2006 Mid-ventilation CT scan construction from four-dimensional respiration-correlated CT scans for radiotherapy planning of lung cancer patients *Int. J. Radiat. Oncol. Biol. Phys.* **65** 1560–71

[78] Duan J, Shen S and Fiveash J B *et al* 2003 Dosimetric effect of respiratory-gated beam on IMRT delivery *Med. Phys.* **30** 2241–52

[79] Keall P, Vedam S and George R *et al* 2006 The clinical implementation of respiratory-gated intensity-modulated radiotherapy *Med. Dos.* **31** 152–62

[80] Nicolini G, Vanetti E, Clivio A, Fogliata A and Cozzi L 2010 Pre-clinical evaluation of respiratory-gated devliery of volumetric modulated arc therapy with RapidArc *Phy. Med. Biol.* **55** N347–57
[81] Peulen H, Belderbos J, Rossi M and Sonke J J 2014 Mid-ventilation based PTV margins in stereotactic body radiotherapy (SBRT): a clinical evaluation *Radiother. Oncol.* **110** 511–6
[82] Ehrbar S, Jöhl A and Tartas A *et al* 2017 ITV, mid-ventilation, gating or couch tracking—a comparison of respiratory motion-management techniques based on 4D dose calculations *Radiother. Oncol.* **124** 80–8
[83] Thomas S J, Evans B J and Harihar L *et al* 2019 An evaluation of the mid-ventilation method for the planning of stereotactic lung plans *Radiother. Oncol.* **137** 110–6
[84] McKenzie A L 2000 How should breathing margin be combined with other errors when drawing margins around clinical target volumes? *Br. J. Radiol.* **73** 973–7
[85] Sharp G, Fritscher K D and Pekar V *et al* 2014 Vision 20/20: perspectives on automated image segmentation for radiotherapy *Med. Phys.* **41** 050902-1–13
[86] Withey D J and Koles X J 2007 Medical image segmentation: methods and software *Proc. NFSI ICFBI* 140–3
[87] Pitas I 1993 *Digital Image Processing Algorithms* (Englewood Cliffs, NJ: Prentice-Hall)
[88] Pratt W K 1991 *Digital Image Processing* (Hoboken, NJ: Wiley)
[89] McInerney T and Terzopoulos D 1996 Deformable models in medical image analysis: a survey *Med. Image Anal.* **1** 91–108
[90] Boykov Y and Funka-Lea G 2006 Graph cuts and efficient N-D image segmentation *Int. J. Comput. Vision* **70** 109–31
[91] Cootes T F, Cooper D, Taylor C J and Graham J 1995 Active shape models: their training and application *Comput. Vis. Image. Understand.* **61** 38–59
[92] Cootes T F, Edwards G J and Taylor C J 2001 Active appearance models *IEEE Trans. Pattern Anal. Mach. Intell.* **23** 681–5
[93] Wells I, William M and Viola P *et al* 1996 Multi-modal volume registration by maximization of mutual information *Med. Image Anal.* **1** 35–51
[94] Commowick O and Malandain G 2007 Efficient selection of the most similar image in a database for critical structures segmentation *Proc. of the Medical Image Computing and Computer-Assisted Intervention – MICCAI 2007* Pt. 2 *Brisbane, Australia* **4792** 203–10
[95] Klein S, van der Heide U A and Lips I M *et al* 2008 Automatic segmentation of the prostate in 3D MR images by atlas matching using localized mutual information *Med. Phys.* **35** 1407–17
[96] Hartmann S L, Parks M H, Martin P R and Dawant B M 1999 Automatic 3-D segmentation of internal structures of the head in MR images using a combination of similarity and free-form transformations: part II. Validation on severely atrophied brains *IEEE Trans. Med. Imaging* **18** 917–26
[97] Sabuncu M R, Yeo B T T, Van Leemput K, Fischl B and Golland P 2010 A generative model for image segmentation based on label fusion *IEEE Trans. Med. Imag.* **29** 1714–29
[98] Warfield S K, Zou K H and Wells W M 2004 Simultaneous truth and performance level estimation (STAPLE): an algorithm for the validation of image segmentation *IEEE Trans. Med. Imag.* **23** 903–21
[99] Cardoso M J, Leung K and Modat M *et al* 2013 STEPS: similarity and truth estimation for propagated segmentations and its application to hippocampal segmentation and brain parcelation *Med. Image. Anal.* **17** 671–84

[100] Qazi A A, Pekar V and Kim J *et al* 2011 Auto-segmentation of normal and target structures in head and neck CT images: a feature-driven model-based approach *Med. Phys.* **38** 6160–70
[101] Kosmin M, Ledsam J and Romera-Paredes B *et al* 2019 Rapid advances in auto-segmentation of organs at risk and target volumes in head and neck cancer *Radiother. Oncol.* **135** 130–40
[102] Cardenal C E, Yang J, Anderson B M, Court L E and Brock K B 2019 Advances in auto-segmentation *Semin. Radiat. Oncol.* **29** 185–97
[103] Litjens G, Kooi T and Bejnordi B E *et al* 2017 A survey on deep learning in medical image analysis *Med. Image. Anal.* **42** 60–88
[104] Shen D, Wu G and Suk H I 2017 Deep learning in medical image analysis *Annu. Rev. Biomed. Eng.* **19** 221–48
[105] Hesamian M H, Jia W, He X and Kennedy P 2019 Deep learning techniques for medical image segmentation: achievements and challenges *J. Dig. Imag.* **32** 582–96
[106] Long J, Shelhamer E and Darrell T 2015 Fully convolutional networks for semantic segmentation *Proc. IEEE Comput. Soc. Conf. Comput. Vis. Pattern Recognit.* pp 3431–40
[107] Voet P W, Dirkx M L and Teguh D N *et al* 2011 Does atlas-based autosegmentation of neck levels require subsequent manual contour editing to avoid risk of severe target underdosage? A dosimetric analysis *Radiother. Oncol.* **98** 373–7
[108] Sims R, Isambert A and Grégoire V *et al* 2009 A pre-clinical assessment of an atlas-based automatic segmentation tool for the head and neck *Radiother. Oncol.* **93** 474–8
[109] Awan M, Kalpathy-Cramer J and Gunn G B *et al* 2013 Prospective assessment of an atlas-based intervention combined with real-time software feedback in contouring lymph node levels and organs-at-risk in the head and neck: quantitative assessment of conformance to expert delineation *Pract. Radiat. Oncol.* **3** 186–93
[110] Daisne J F and Blumhofer A 2013 Atlas-based automatic segmentation of head and neck organs at risk and nodal target volumes: a clinical validation *Radiat. Oncol.* **8** 154
[111] Walker G V, Awan M and Tao R *et al* 2014 Prospective randomized double-blind study of atlas-based organ-at-risk autosegmentation-assisted radiation planning in head and neck cancer *Radiother. Oncol.* **112** 321–5
[112] Thomson D, Boylan C and Liptrot T *et al* 2014 Evaluation of an automatic segmentation algorithm for definition of head and neck organs at risk *Radiat. Oncol.* **9** 173
[113] Haq R, Berry S L, Deasy J O, Hunt M and Veeraraghavan H 2019 Dynamic multiatlas selection-based consensus segmentation of head and neck structures from CT images *Med. Phys.* **46** 5612–22
[114] Fung N T C, Hung W M, Sze C K, Lee M C H and Ng W T 2020 Automatic segmentation for adaptive planning in nasopharyngeal carcinoma IMRT: time, geometrical, and dosimetric analysis *Med. Dosim.* Accepted
[115] Simões R, Wortel G and Wiersma T G *et al* 2019 Geometrical and dosimetric evaluation of breast target volume auto-contouring *Phys. Imag. Radiat. Oncol.* **12** 38–43
[116] Tong N, Gou S, Yang S, Ruan D and Sheng K 2018 Fully automatic multi-organ segmentation for head and neck cancer radiotherapy using shape representation model constrained fully convolutional neural networks *Med. Phys.* **45** 4558–67
[117] van Rooij W, Dahele M and Brandao H R *et al* 2019 Deep learning-based delineation of head and neck organs at risk: geometric and dosimetric evaluation *Int. J. Radiat. Oncol. Biol. Phys.* **104** 677–84

[118] Men K, Geng H and Cheng C *et al* 2019 Technical note: more accurate and efficient segmentation of organs-at-risk in radiotherapy with convolutional neural networks cascades *Med. Phys.* **46** 286–92
[119] van der Veen J, Willems S and Deschuymer S *et al* 2019 Benefit of deep learning for delineation of organs at risk in head and neck cancer *Radiother. Oncol.* **138** 68–74
[120] van Dijk L V, Van den Bosch L, Aljabar P, Peressutti D, Both S and Steenbakkers R J H M *et al* 2020 Improving automatic delineation for head and neck organs at risk by deep learning contouring *Radiother. Oncol.* **142** 115–23
[121] Lustberg T, van Soest J and Goodling M *et al* 2018 Clinical evaluation of atlas and deep learning based automatic contouring for lung cancer *Radiother. Oncol.* **126** 312–7
[122] Conson M, Cella L and Pacelli R *et al* 2014 Automated delineation of brain structures in patients undergoing radiotherapy for primary brain tumors: from atlas to dose-volume histograms *Radiother. Oncol.* **112** 326–31
[123] Kieselmann J P, Kamerling C P and Burgos N *et al* 2018 Geometric and dosimetric evaluations of atlas-based segmentation methods of MR images in the head and neck region *Phys. Med. Biol.* **63** 145007
[124] Valentini V, Boldrini L, Damiani A and Muren L P 2014 Recommendations on how to establish evidence from auto-segmentation software in radiotherapy *Radiother. Oncol.* **112** 317–20
[125] Hanna G G, Hounsell A R and O'Sullivan J M 2010 Geometrical analysis of radiotherapy target volume delineation: a systematic review of reported comparison methods *Clin. Oncol. (R Coll. Radiol.)* **22** 515–25
[126] Fotina I, Lütgendorf-Caucig C, Stock M, Pötter R and Georg D 2012 Critical discussion of evaluation parameters for inter-observer variability in target definition for radiation therapy *Strahlenther. Onkol.* **188** 160–7
[127] Mackie T R, Kapatoes J and Ruchala K *et al* 2003 Image guidance for precise conformal radiotherapy *Int. J. Radiat. Oncol. Biol. Phys.* **56** 8–105
[128] Mohan R, Zhang X and Wang H *et al* 2005 Use of deformed intensity distributions for on-line modification of image-guided IMRT to account for interfractional anatomic changes *Int. J. Radiat. Oncol. Biol. Phys.* **61** 1258–66
[129] Zhang T, Chi Y, Meldolesi E and Yan D 2007 Automatic delineation of on-line head-and-neck computed tomography images: toward on-line adaptive radiotherapy *Int. J. Radiat. Oncol. Biol. Phys.* **68** 522–30

IOP Publishing

Intensity Modulated Radiation Therapy

A clinical overview

Indra J Das, Nicholas J Sanfilippo, Antonella Fogliata and Luca Cozzi

Chapter 8

Treatment planning

The treatment planning process involves different steps:

- Suitable immobilization
- CT/MRI imaging
- Target and OAR delineation
- Dose volume constraints
- Optimizations
- Leaf sequencing
- Dose calculations
- Evaluation

This chapter summarizes the main key points of treatment planning with IMRT or VMAT in terms of beams delivery, field geometries, and dosimetric consequences.

8.1 Beam (and arc) geometry

Treatment planning starts with a beam arrangement, which is a fundamental part of the planning process. The choice of the number of fields and their entrance has been an area of research since clinical implementation of IMRT began. Bortfeld and Schlegel [1] in 1993 investigated the problem of optimizing beam orientations for multiple fixed beams. It is a complex, non-convex optimization problem, and a fast gradient descent method could be trapped in a local minimum. For this reason, the authors used the simulated annealing optimization method, and they found that apart from inconvenient entrances due to critical structures, evenly distributed beams can be considered good geometry. Except in cases of only two or three fields, where beam orientation must be well determined with a sufficiently large number of fields, the choice of beam direction is less significant, showing similar dose distributions for optimized or not optimized beam orientations. With a number of seven to nine beams, an even distribution of beam orientations seemed adequate for

doi:10.1088/978-0-7503-1335-3ch8

irradiation with IMRT even in the presence of an organ at risk (OAR), that can, however, be shielded through the fluence modulated intensity [2].

There are some golden rules to follow when placing fixed beam directions for an IMRT plan, similar to those used for 3DCRT.

- First of all, opposing fields should be avoided, by setting at least a 5 degree difference in directly opposing beams. During optimization, opposing beamlets would compete, whereas all points would contribute to optimization without competing with one another with non-opposing beams.
- Secondly, beam entrance, together with proper jaws and collimator rotation settings, should avoid critical structures, particularly in the case where they are located before the target in the beam path.
- The third point to consider is the target volume location, central or lateral. For central targets the solution of evenly distributed beams could be preferable, while for non-central targets, the beams should be located so as to avoid entrance through any contralateral structure: short beam paths are to be preferred. This could be the case of breast, lung, and any peripheral lesion.
- Finally, beam entrance from any movable part within the body contouring should be avoided.

This could be the case of a non-fixed bite in the mouth of the patient (for example to lower the tongue during the treatment), which cannot be in the same identical position during CT scan acquisition and each treatment session, or the arms along the body with no immobilization masks, or again the movable non-indexed rails of the treatment couch (figure 8.1). The fluence will be optimized considering the position of the movable piece, according to the CT images, resulting in an incorrectly optimized fluence for the piece positions during the treatment, and consequently unacceptable delivery error. In general, beam entrance through any anatomy subject to unexpected or uncontrollable motion during treatment should be avoided.

For treatment with a very high dose per fraction (stereotactic radiotherapy treatment, or hypofractionation) the entrance dose of individual beams should be restricted to prevent acute skin reaction. In the report of AAPM Task Group 101 on stereotactic body radiotherapy [3], the dose is suggested to restrict each single beam

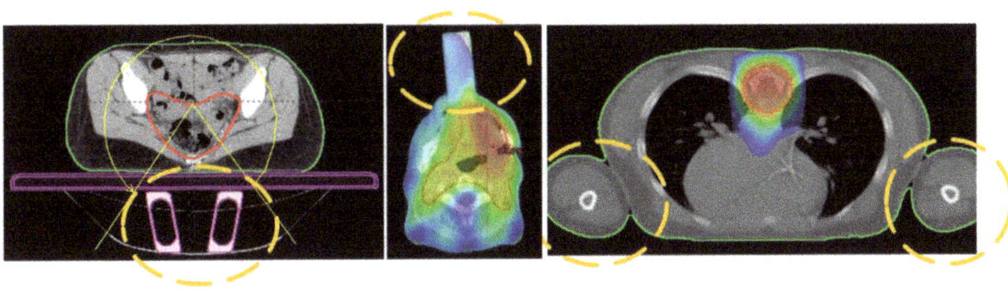

Figure 8.1. Examples of possibly movable regions where the beam entrance should be avoided: (a) non-indexed couch bars; (b) bite to lower the tongue; (c) non-immobilized arms along the body.

dose to less than 30% of the cumulative avoiding beam overlaps. Although there is no absolute dose value indication, spreading the entrance dose over a large surface is desirable. An example of high-grade acute skin toxicity (necrosis) was reported in 2008 by Hoppe *et al* [4], following stereotactic lung treatment with three IMRT fields within a narrow angular range. In particular, the authors found that distance from the tumor to the skin on the patient's back <5 cm, treatment with only three beams, and a maximum back skin dose >50% of the prescribed dose were significantly associated with the development of grade 2 or higher skin reactions. Additional bolus and chemotherapy treatments also contributed significantly to skin complications in IMRT.

In general, more complex cases may benefit from an increased number of fields. A greater number of fields could yield better target dose conformity and better OAR sparing. Moreover, when the number of beams is sufficiently high, the choice of beam direction is less significant. Note that though it may be preferable to limit the number of beams for practical reasons (shortening treatment time), a greater number of beams provides improved delivery accuracy and potential radiobiological benefit. The most appropriate number of fields has to be adapted accordingly [2].

Over the years, beam angle optimization has been subject to a number of studies [5–9] aiming at applying optimization algorithms through implementations in treatment planning systems for clinical use. They reported promising results for IMRT applications. As an example, Gaede *et al* [7] concluded that with optimized beam directions, it was possible to achieve better target dose uniformity and critical organ sparing with fewer numbers of beams than standard equally spaced beam plans. However, those algorithms, whenever used, have been mostly devoted to finding class solutions for specific anatomical sites, more than on a single patient basis.

Similar considerations to those made for fixed beams IMRT can be applied to VMAT in order to avoid entrance through OARs or movable objects.

Descriptions of clinical beam arrangements that determine the importance of the choice of beam entrances have been the subject of many publications. Grosshans *et al*'s [10] 2012 publication analyzed four different beam arrangements for IMRT planning, seeking to lower the heart dose in patients presenting distal esophageal carcinoma. They found that *a posterior*-lateral beam arrangement can significantly reduce the cardiac dose (of about 9–10 Gy as mean heart dose) with a minimal increase of the lung dose as compared to arrangements including anterior beams.

Yirmibersoglu *et al* [11] studied the beam geometry for patients affected by a parotid gland tumor, with a lateral target location, by comparing seven equally spaced beams with four coplanar ipsilateral fields or four non-coplanar, ipsilateral entrances. The main result of this study proved that ipsilateral field entrances should be preferred for lateral targets to avoid unnecessary dose to contralateral or more central critical structures, as were the contralateral parotid and oral cavity in their work.

A study comparing 7–9 equally spaced beams against optimized beam geometry using the optimizer implemented in the treatment planning system (Beam Angle Optimizer in the Eclipse system, Varian) was published by Shukla *et al* [12].

Analyzing head and neck, prostate and esophageal cancer patients, they found an improved OAR sparing and reduced MU when the automatic beam optimization was used, keeping similar target coverage and homogeneity to equispaced beams.

A work aiming to determine the appropriate arc arrangement for VMAT treatment was conducted by Ishii *et al* [13] for centrally located lung tumors. Three different arc approaches were explored, one full coplanar, two partial coplanar, and two partial non-coplanar arcs. It was found that the contralateral mean lung dose increased with the full arc by more than 10%, while its beneficial results were similar to those of the two partial arc cases, confirming the benefits gained by avoiding beam entrance through the critical and contralateral structures.

In 2017, Fu and coauthors [14] studied IMRT settings in the planning of upper esophageal carcinoma in simultaneous integrated boost, evaluating plans with four, five, and seven IMRT fields (the five and seven beams were equispaced, while the four beams had two opposed anteroposterior fields). The increased number of fields improved the target dose (conformity and homogeneity), and reduced the volume of lung receiving at least 30 Gy (for a 63.8 Gy prescription); however, the lung volume receiving at least dose levels equal or lower than 20 Gy was higher in the five and seven fields setting, as well as the mean lung dose. With this study, it was shown that a larger number of fields could increase the low dose bath relative to plans with fewer beam entrances.

Similarly, Tian and colleagues [15] evaluated the functional volume receiving at least a certain dose level, in different IMRT field settings (four, five, and seven beams, rather ipsilateral entries) for lung cancer patient planning. The study, prescribing 60 Gy, showed a reduction of the functional lung volume receiving 20 or 30 Gy when increasing the number of fields from four to seven, while an increase of the volume was assessed for 5 and 13 Gy dose level.

8.2 The collimator rotation

The collimator rotation in fixed beam IMRT planning should be selected to avoid critical structures, as should the gantry position choice. However, it is different in the case of rotational IMRT, as VMAT. For these treatments, the collimator angle should prevent the interleaf planes (MLC leaf motion) from being parallel to the gantry rotation plane. In this way any interleaf tongue and groove effect, physically unavoidable, is smeared out inside the patient volume, becoming negligible. Practically, the collimator rotation should be set different from zero for the standard linacs and MLCs. For example, dual-layer MLC, like on Halcyon treatment units, does not show this potential problem since the interleaf radiation from one layer is shielded by the leaves of the other layer. Also, tomotherapy units do not have classical collimators and rotation is not allowed. However, this is not the only reason for rotating the collimator. The leaf motion in a direction not parallel to the gantry rotation plane allows an increased modulation, with possible 'multiple apertures' as shown in figure 8.2, where the entrance dose beam on an axial section of a patient (on the right of the picture), parallel to the gantry rotation plane, is 'split' into five pseudo-subfields by the MLC shape (as depicted in the left side of the picture),

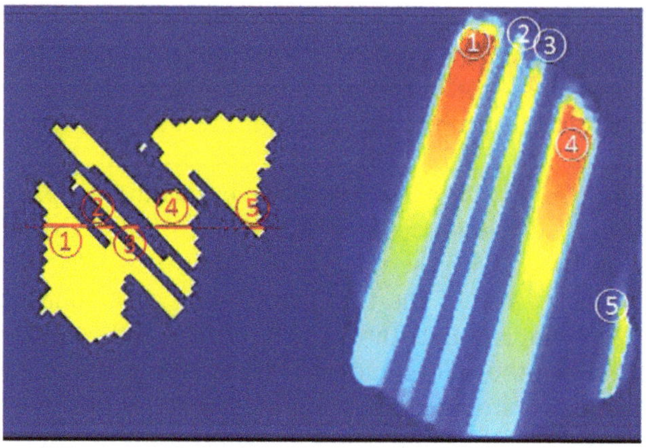

Figure 8.2. Instantaneous gantry position during a VMAT plan delivery. On the left: beam's-eye-view; on the right: axial instantaneous dose image relative to the red line position shown on the left. The circled numbers refer to the apertures generated by the MLC position on that slice.

generating modulation. The pseudo-subfield generation is maximized for increasing collimator angles, up to the limit of 90 degrees, where the pseudo-subfields can be as small as the leaf width.

The collimator angle setting in VMAT planning has been widely studied, as exemplified in the numerous publications summarized below.

An interesting example was published in 2010, where Mancosu and colleagues [16] analyzed spinal cord sparing for vertebral metastases treatment and proved that the collimator set with the leaf motion parallel to the cord presented the best cord sparing, with $D_{1\mathrm{ccm}}$ of 8.4 Gy for a 5 × 4 Gy prescription, while this parameter increased up to 10.8 Gy for other collimator settings.

Another planning challenge for VMAT treatment is the collimator angle for multiple brain targets. In this case, the best collimator angle is the one that allows closing the leaves in the intra-targets space, reducing the bridging dose between two lesions. However, also visible in the beam's-eye-view, the best collimator angle changes for different gantry positions during the arc, since the mutual position of the lesion changes, as shown in figure 8.3.

The difficulty arises from the inability to simultaneously rotate gantry and collimator (as is the case in the commercial TPS). Automatic collimator angle optimization exists, or a manual split of the arc into subarcs with different collimator angles could be easily pursued, at the cost of increasing the treatment time. Kim *et al* [17] explored the dosimetric influence of the collimator angle on the dose distribution for multiple brain lesions. They selected as optimal collimator angles those which minimized the area size difference between the integrated MLC aperture and the collimator settings, finding differences on MUs and most of the OARs doses, in favor of the optimized collimator angle.

An automatic tool is implemented in the Varian Eclipse TPS for the HyperArc technique, which is a fixed set of five non-coplanar half arcs for multiple brain metastases treatments. The 'Collimator Angle Optimizer' tool allows an improved

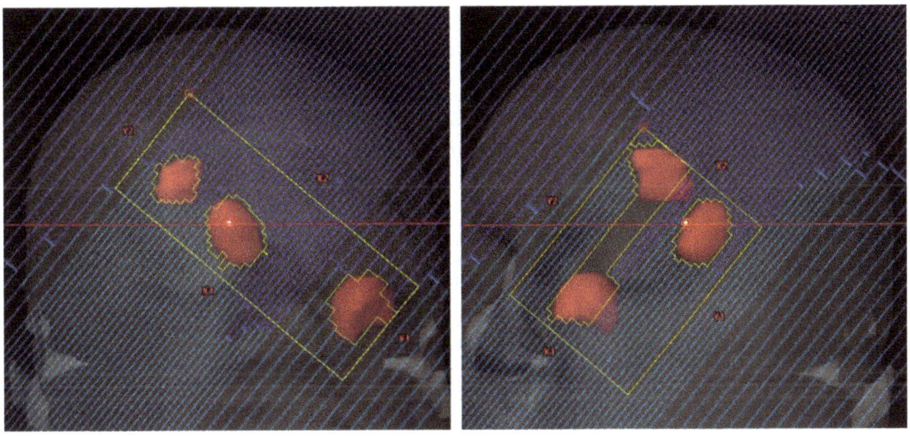

Figure 8.3. Collimator angle fixed during the gantry rotation of a single arc for a VMAT plan to treat multiple brain metastasis. On the left (gantry at 195 degrees), the collimator angle and the leaf motion fit well with the lesion positions; on the right (gantry at 35 degrees), the collimator angle is not optimal for the leaf motion, and a leaf opening is shown between two lesions, generating undesired bridging dose.

dose fall-off and significantly lowers the bridging dose. Ohira *et al* [18] reported significantly improved in V_{4Gy}, V_{12Gy}, V_{14Gy}, V_{16Gy}, with MLC complexity pattern, MU compared to the plans optimized without the Collimator Angle Optimizer tool.

The study published by Li *et al* [19] on an algorithm, based on simulated annealing, which simultaneously optimized the collimator angles and jaw positions for pancreatic tumor to be treated with VMAT stereotactic therapy is interesting. The OARs were significantly better spared with optimized plans (relative to standard template planning) for example the mean dose to the stomach was reduced by 6%, the near to max dose to the duodenum by 2% and the mean dose to the liver by 5%; optimized collimator angle plans also showed lower modulation complexity, suggesting a better capability of handling complex shapes and sparing critical structures.

Prostate treatment, although anatomically not complex, has also been explored for collimator angle adjustment. The simple geometry of this anatomical site is less prone to large dosimetric variations, as pointed out by Isa *et al* [20], Tas *et al* [21], Li *et al* [22], where, although in some cases statistically significant, only small improvements were found with different collimator angles, for single or double arc VMAT. Similarly, other anatomical sites have been studied, with the same conclusions: for example Sharma *et al* [23] with IMRT for parotid cancer, Ahn *et al* [24] with VMAT for irregularly shaped targets in the abdomen, head and neck and chest, Kim *et al* [25] with VMAT for head and neck treatments evaluating the delivery accuracy.

VMAT plans do not currently include dynamic collimator nor couch rotation, although it is clear that the optimal collimator angle often changes according to the gantry position. Some groups, however, investigated the possibility of dynamically rotating the collimator during the arc by optimizing the collimator-gantry trajectory to improve dose conformity. Zhang *et al* [26] explored it for paraspinal SBRT, confirming improvements in target coverage and spinal cord sparing. Other studies include a 2016 publication by the University of Bern [27], which used research scripting implemented in the planning system, and a 2018 publication of the University of California Los Angeles, which proposed optimization with dynamic collimator rotation [28], both of which proved the dosimetric benefit in collimator trajectory optimized plans.

8.3 Non-coplanarity

With the common C-arm linacs, the patient couch rotation allows the beams or arcs to enter the patient from directions different from the axial plane. This 'non-coplanar' technique has been widely used for decades in stereotactic radiotherapy, especially in the brain. Many non-coplanar entrances could deliver sharper dose gradients outside the target volume, and minimize the surrounding dose. An example is shown in figure 8.4, where the color wash for a coplanar arc, a coplanar arc plus half arc with 90 degree couch kick, and nine non-coplanar half arcs are depicted, with color wash from 10% dose level, showing a drastic reduction of the volume receiving low dose; on the right-hand side of figure 8.4, the profiles in the

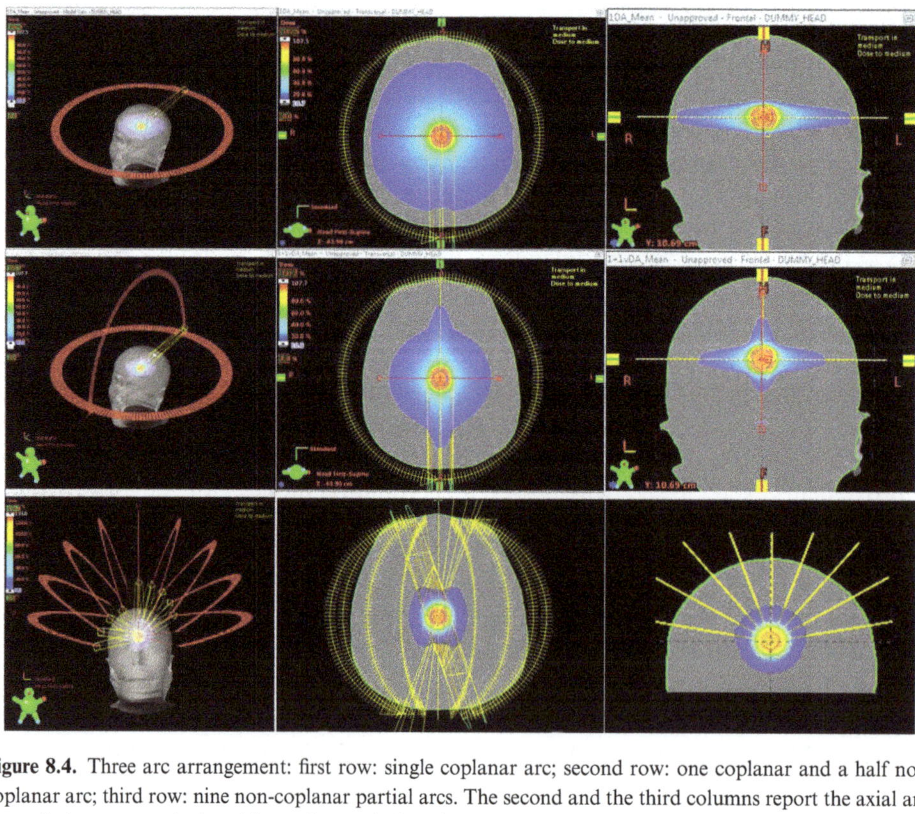

Figure 8.4. Three arc arrangement: first row: single coplanar arc; second row: one coplanar and a half non-coplanar arc; third row: nine non-coplanar partial arcs. The second and the third columns report the axial and coronal views, respectively, with a color wash dose from 10% of the isocenter dose.

main directions are shown for the three arc configuration, presenting the variations in the dose gradient.

A review of clinical applications of this concept has been reported by Smyth *et al* [29]. They reported the non-coplanarity applied to static IMRT beams as well as to rotational VMAT, and showed how different groups proposed to translate the advantages of additional degrees of freedom obtainable with couch rotation into clinical practice, so as to reduce the dose to OARs and healthy tissues, and potentially allowing a target dose escalation to improve TCP.

IMRT beam orientation optimization methods have been studied mainly by two groups: the University of California, Los Angeles (UCLA), and the Erasmus, Rotterdam. The maximal extension for the non-coplanar setting with fixed IMRT beams is achieved with the so-called 4π radiation therapy, a technique that simultaneously optimizes the static IMRT beam orientations and the fluences map attaining the optimal non-coplanar plan. The starting conditions include more than a thousand non-coplanar entries distributed throughout the entire 4π solid angle space (Dong *et al* [30, 31] started with 1162 beams with 6° separation between two adjacent beams), and eliminating those that would lead the gantry to collide with the couch or the patient. This 4π concept maximizes the possible degree of freedom and improves the dose distribution, especially by decreasing the 50% isodose and increasing the dose gradient. The initial works studying the clinical applicability of non-coplanar IMRT and 4π technique concerned the liver [30] and lung [31] SBRT planning, where 14 to 22 non-coplanar beams were explored, allowing higher target dose while reducing the OARs doses. Then the concepts extended to glioblastoma [32] aiming to escalate the target dose, head and neck [33], prostate [34, 35], liver [36], and brain [37, 38].

However, in organs different from the brain, when the number of IMRT fields is not as high as in the 4π method, non-coplanarity is not always advantageous, as reported by Chang *et al* [39] regarding pancreatic cancer: here the authors found an improvement in the kidney doses with the non-coplanar setting, but at the cost of higher doses in other organs, such as liver or stomach, and the surrounding healthy tissue, which suggests the use of this technique only in patients with risk factors for treatment-related kidney dysfunction.

Also, VMAT has been the subject of studies for non-coplanar arc settings, thus mimicking the 4π concept. The actual clinical implementation regards different static couch orientations. Sites explored in the literature are, among others, sinus cancer [40], liver [41], and head and neck [42, 43]. However, the most common non-coplanar VMAT clinical use is in brain tumors, especially intracranial stereotactic radiotherapy [44, 45]. A setting of mono-isocentric five half arcs (two coplanar, and three non-coplanar, with couch at 90, 45 and 315 degrees) was proposed by Thomas *et al* [46] for multiple brain metastases, similar to the arc setting for cone- and frame-based brain radiosurgery [47]. They found that such a non-coplanar VMAT setting gave similar dose distributions, especially in terms of dose fall-off and $V_{12\mathrm{Gy}}$ as opposed to Gamma Knife treatments. This same arc setting has been implemented on the Eclipse TPS and TrueBeam-platform linacs by Varian, as the HyperArc technique.

Improved dosimetric results were also published by Panet-Raymond *et al* [48] in high-grade glioma, for both IMRT and VMAT in a non-coplanar setting. In 2017, Uto *et al* [49] presented a planning study for craniopharyngiomas with non-coplanar VMAT to reduce hippocampal doses, resulting in a reduction of 40% of their doses, relative to coplanar VMAT setting.

Similarly to the dynamic collimator trajectory plans, a dynamically rotating couch has also been explored by researchers, especially from The Royal Marsden NHS in the UK. Smyth *et al* [50–52] proposed a trajectory optimization method for non-coplanar VMAT with dynamic couch rotation by combining ray tracing with a graph search algorithm: and a cost map reflecting the number of OAR voxels intersected for each potential source position was generated. The dose to specified OARs was reduced in plans otherwise comparable to coplanar VMAT strategy. Different anatomical cases were studied: partial breast, where the mean heart dose was reduced by 53%; brain, with maximum lens doses reduced by 61%–77% and globes by 37%–40%; and prostate treatment where a 15% reduction in mean bowel dose was registered. The group from Bern in Switzerland [53], using the Eclipse scripting in the Varian TPS developed a dedicated optimization framework for simultaneous collimator and couch dynamic rotation in VMAT deliveries. They demonstrated that mean and maximum OAR doses were lowered up to 16% and 38% compared to the VMAT plans for similar target coverage and dose homogeneity and presented accurate dose delivery.

However, dynamic couch and collimator rotations are not yet clinically implemented due to collision issues and are the subject of future research.

8.4 Flattened and unflattened beams

In the last decades, flattening filter free (FFF) beams have been made available on C-arm linacs (before they were applied to CyberKnife and tomotherapy units only), aiming to increase the dose rate allowing faster high dose per fraction treatments. The FFF beam profiles present a shape peaked on the central axis, especially visible in large fields, hence yielding useless beams for conformal deliveries. When combined with intensity-modulated techniques, the particular FFF beam shape can be ‘corrected’ by the modulation of the intensity, with IMRT (or VMAT).

The FFF beams started to be clinically used on C-arm linacs for stereotactic treatments only, taking benefit from the fast delivery. However, FFF beams present characteristics that are interesting also for standard fractionated treatments, as the reduced scattering (the flattening filter is the largest source of head scattering), leading to lower out-of-field dose and sharper gradients. Those points could make the FFF beams, associated with IMRT, interesting for many locations.

FFF-VMAT, in comparison with standard flattened beams, was analyzed for stereotactic treatments in liver by Reggiori *et al* [54], in prostate by Chung *et al* [55], in lung by Ong *et al* [56] and Liu *et al* [57], single brain metastasis by Lai [58], in breast by Spruijt *et al* [59] and Koivumäki [60], in advanced nasopharyngeal carcinoma by Jia [61], in prostate cancer [62, 63], in advanced esophageal cancer

[64], in chest wall [65], head and neck and prostate IMRT [66], prostate, brain, head and neck, and lung IMRT [67].

The potentiality of the FFF beams in intensity modulation for pediatric treatments is also interesting. An example was published by Cashmore *et al* [68]. In their study, the authors reported results supported by measurements on an anthropomorphic pediatric phantom, showing a peripheral dose reduction of 20%–30% in the thoracic region, and 62%–70% in the pelvic/abdominal region when FFF IMRT was used in place of standard flattened beams for five intracranial pediatric patient treatments. Additionally, the integral dose of FFF beams is lowered thanks also to a reduced neutron production from the missing flattening filter which is discussed in the following section of this chapter.

8.5 Modulation degrees and delivery accuracy

The plan complexity and modulation, following the initial suggestions of avoiding excessive fluence modulations to achieve accurate deliveries, has been the subject of renewed interest in recent years for both IMRT and VMAT. Importance has hence also been given to assessing possible identifiers for plan delivery accuracy at the planning level, as a tentative alternative solution to the actual measurement-based approach, which is quite time-consuming and requires dedicated linac occupancy.

IMRT fields can be highly modulated due to a large number of degrees of freedom of the optimization process, and MLC can efficiently deliver such highly modulated fields, i.e., the fluence of which can change abruptly within a small space, producing sharp fluence peaks and valleys in millimetric spatial scale. This concept of modulation was pointed out by Mohan *et al* in 2000 [69], by terming the fluence 'complexity' to subjectively describe the frequency and amplitude of fluctuation in the modulation intensity. They demonstrated in a head and neck case that complex anatomy and strong optimization constraints produce complex intensity patterns. In those cases, the average MLC apertures tend to be smaller and the number of MU consequently larger. Moreover, the accuracy of the estimated dose relative to the delivered dose is affected by the increased complexity. Over the years, different authors recommended solutions to reduce the fluence complexity including smoothing procedures as part of the optimization process. A measure of the smoothness in the beam fluence was defined by Llacer *et al* [70] and called fluence map complexity, FMC:

$$\mathrm{FMC} = \frac{1}{\sum_j a_j}\sqrt{\sum_j\left(a_j - \lambda_k \sum_{k\in N_j} a_k\right)^2} \tag{8.1}$$

where a_j is the fluence of the beamlets j, $k \in N_j$ is the neighborhood of pencil beam j, λ_k are the weight parameters for the neighboring beam fluences (equal to 1 in the periphery, 0.5 elsewhere). This metric is included in the Dynamically Penalized Likelihood algorithm for inverse planning.

In 2001, Webb [71] also suggested including two terms in the cost function, the first of which should incorporate fluence changes in adjacent pixels, and the second related to a minimum number of allowed field sizes in order to minimize the consequences of a high modulation degree. In 2003, the same Webb [72] proposed, as a general rule for good IMRT practice, that excessive complexity should be avoided and thus introduced the concept of Modulation Index (MI), a parameter that evaluates deviations between adjacent bixels relative to the standard deviation of the intensity fluence map, to assess it. The MI concept was based on a frequency spectrum (Z) analysis, in a single direction (the MLC motion direction):

$$\mathrm{MI} = \int_0^F Z(f)df = \int_0^F \frac{1}{n-1} N_{I_x}(f;\, \Delta I_x > f\sigma_I) \tag{8.2}$$

Possible correlation between the MI, adapting the original MI proposed by Webb by including two directions (parallel, x, and perpendicular, y, to the leaf motion) and their diagonal, xy, were investigated by Nicolini *et al* [73], with integration limits from 0.1 to 1.0, in head and neck and chest wall cases

$$\mathrm{MI} = \int_0^F Z(f)df = \int_0^F \frac{\left[Z_{I_x}(f) + Z_{I_y}(f) + Z_{I_{xy}}(f)\right]}{3} \tag{8.3}$$

They suggested that an MI threshold <19 (using an integration limit $F = 1.0$) could ensure that the planned fluences are safely and accurately delivered within stringent quality criteria (95% gamma evaluation agreement with 3 mm and 3% distance-to-agreement and dose-difference criteria).

Park *et al* in 2014 elaborated further the concept of MI, named MI_t, adapted from the previous for VMAT, including the speed and acceleration analysis of MLC, gantry rotation and speed dose rate comprehensively [74].

$$\begin{aligned} \mathrm{MI}_t = \sum_{l=1}^{N_{\mathrm{leaf}}} \int_0^F \left(\frac{1}{N_{\mathrm{CP}} - 2}\right) \sum_{i=1}^{N_{\mathrm{CP}}} \\ \times \left\{ N_i\left(f;\, \mathrm{MLC}_{\mathrm{speed}_i} > f\sigma_{\mathrm{MLC}_{\mathrm{speed}}} \text{ or } \mathrm{MLC}_{\mathrm{accel}_i} > \alpha f\sigma_{\mathrm{MLC}_{\mathrm{accel}}}\right) \cdot \right. \\ \left. W_{\mathrm{GA},i+1} \cdot W_{\mathrm{MU},i+1} \right\} df \end{aligned} \tag{8.4}$$

where N_{leaf} and N_{CP} are the numbers of leaves and control points, respectively. MI_t showed good performance for the evaluation of the modulation degree of VMAT plans using integration limits F similar to those used by Nicolini *et al* [73]. The AUC (area under the curve) from the ROC (relative operating characteristics) analysis performed with passing rates of local gamma at 90% from measurements (2 mm and 2% distance-to-agreement and dose-difference criteria) for MI_t was of 0.824 with $F = 1.0$ (1.0 specificity and 0.50 sensitivity). This indicated that MI_t could be considered as a good indicator to evaluate VMAT modulation degree. Also, they demonstrated that the most dominant modulating parameter influencing the deliverability of a VMAT plan is the MLC motion. However, the MI_t parameter considered only the mechanical uncertainty of VMAT. In 2015, the same group [75] proposed an extension of this parameter, a comprehensive modulation index MI_c, considering both mechanical uncertainty and dose calculation uncertainty generated by possible excessive modulation, by combining the MI_t with a weighting factor analyzing the size and irregularity of field aperture at each CP

$$\mathrm{MI}_c = \sum_{n=1}^{N_{\mathrm{leaf}}} \int_0^F \left(\frac{1}{N_{\mathrm{CP}} - 2}\right) \sum_{i=1}^{N_{\mathrm{CP}}} \times \left\{ N_i\left(f;\ \mathrm{MLC}_{\mathrm{speed}_i} > f\sigma_{\mathrm{MLC}_{\mathrm{speed}}} \text{ or } \mathrm{MLC}_{\mathrm{accel}_i} > \alpha f \sigma_{\mathrm{MLC}_{\mathrm{accel}}}\right) \cdot W_{\mathrm{GA},i+1} \cdot W_{\mathrm{MU},i+1} \cdot W_{\mathrm{AI},i} \right\} df \tag{8.5}$$

where the new weighting factor W_{AI} which is based on the thinning algorithm applied to the field shape of each CP to consider dose calculation uncertainty due to irregular or small field apertures. The MI_c ($F = 0.5$) higher than 60 (in their study on prostate and head and neck plans) indicated clinically unacceptable VMAT plans, suggesting the MI_c as a reliable modulation index to predict plan delivery accuracy.

In 2010 McNiven and colleagues [76] developed a new metric, the modulation complexity score, MCS, which incorporated plan information in terms of leaf position p, field shape irregularity, segment weight, and area. It combined two parameters, the leaf sequence variability LSV, and the aperture area variability AAV, and finally weighted each segment contribution with its relative monitor units MU; the modulation complexity is equal to the unity for non-modulated fields. The ability of MCS to provide information about the accuracy of dose delivery was assessed, considering pre-treatment quality assurance with a 90% gamma pass rate for 1 mm and 2% criteria. MCS and MU threshold criteria were determined to achieve specificity of 1.0. An MCS threshold of >0.8 was found with a sensitivity of 0.36. MU had a sensitivity of 0.23 for the threshold <50 MU.

$$\mathrm{MCS} = \sum_{k=1}^{N_{\mathrm{segment}}} \mathrm{AAV}_k \cdot \mathrm{LSV}_k \cdot \frac{\mathrm{MU}_k}{\mathrm{MU}}, \tag{8.6}$$

$$\mathrm{AAV}_k = \left(\frac{\sum_{l=1}^{N_{\mathrm{leaf}}} \left(p_{l,\text{left bank}} - p_{l,\text{right bank}}\right)}{\sum_{l=1}^{N_{\mathrm{leaf}}} \left(\max\left(p_{l,\text{left bank}}\right) - \max\left(p_{l,\text{right bank}}\right)\right)}\right)_k \tag{8.7}$$

$$\mathrm{LSV}_k = \left(\frac{\sum_{l=1}^{N_{\mathrm{leaf}}} \left[p_{\max} - \left(p_l - p_{l+1}\right)\right]}{N_{\mathrm{leaf}} \times p_{\max}}\right)_{\text{left bank},k} \left(\frac{\sum_{l=1}^{N_{\mathrm{leaf}}} \left[p_{\max} - \left(p_l - p_{l+1}\right)\right]}{N_{\mathrm{leaf}} \times p_{\max}}\right)_{\text{right bank},k} \tag{8.8}$$

where N_{segment} is the number of segments in the field.

An adaptation of the MCS for VMAT plans was proposed by Masi *et al*, considering the control points CP instead of the segments [77]:

$$\mathrm{MCS}_V = \sum_{i=1}^{N_{\mathrm{CP}}-1}\left(\frac{\mathrm{AAV}_i + \mathrm{AAV}_{i+1}}{2} \cdot \frac{\mathrm{LSV}_i + \mathrm{LSV}_{i+1}}{2}\right) \cdot \frac{\mathrm{MU}_{i,i+1}}{\mathrm{MU}_{\mathrm{arc}}} \tag{8.9}$$

$$\mathrm{AAV}_{\mathrm{CP}} = \left(\frac{\sum_{n=1}^{N_{\mathrm{leaf}}}\left(\langle p_n\rangle_{\text{lef tbank}} - \langle p_n\rangle_{\text{right bank}}\right)}{\sum_{n=1}^{N_{\mathrm{leaf}}}\left(\langle \max(p_n)\rangle_{\text{left bank}\in\text{arc}} - \langle \max(p_n)\rangle_{\text{right bank}\in\text{arc}}\right)}\right)_{\mathrm{CP}} \tag{8.10}$$

$$\mathrm{LSV}_{\mathrm{CP}} = \left(\frac{\sum_{n=1}^{N_{\mathrm{leaf}}-1}\left[p_{\max} - |(p_n - p_{n+1})|\right]}{(N_{\mathrm{leaf}} - 1) \times p_{\max}}\right)_{\text{left bank,CP}} \times \left(\frac{\sum_{n=1}^{N_{\mathrm{leaf}}-1}\left[p_{\max} - |(p_n - p_{n+1})|\right]}{(N_{\mathrm{leaf}} - 1) \times p_{\max}}\right)_{\text{right bank,CP}} \tag{8.11}$$

An interesting practical application of the MCS on a multi-institutional basis was conducted by McGarry *et al* [78] to evaluate the plan modulation in different conditions. In their study, the authors stratified the results in two groups: the first included centers where the TPS and linac manufacturer was the same, whereas they differed in the second. The results showed poorer quality, higher MU and MCS (indicating less efficiency) for this second group.

In 2014, a set of IMRT plan accuracy metrics, geometry-based, was proposed by Kairn *et al* [79], aiming to find predictors of QA failure. The study was based on BrainLab iPlan TPS plans computed with pencil beam algorithm and delivered with a Varian Clinac iX equipped with a Brainlab m3 microMLC, and the parameters included:

- mean field area (MFA), the average open area of each segment;
- mean aperture displacement (MAD), the average distance between the midway point between each pair of leaves and the central axis;
- cross axis score (CAS), the proportion of open leaf pairs when one leaf crossed the central axis;
- closed leaf score (CLS), the proportion of closed leaf pairs;
- small aperture score (SAS), the proportion of open leaf pairs that are separated by less than a given threshold distance.

Predictors of QA failure (defined as gamma pass rate of 90% for 2 mm, 2% criteria, or 95% for 3 mm, 3% criteria) in the study were: the MFA provided a threshold for an equivalent field size smaller than 2.2×2.2 cm^2; the SAS threshold of 10 mm when averaged over all beams, despite its weak correlation.

Similarly, Du *et al* [80], based on the beam aperture and MU weights for all segments or CP of IMRT or VMAT plans, investigated the beam area BA (weighted on the MU per segment), the beam irregularity BI, the beam modulation BM, and the corresponding plan related indices, PA, PI, PM, to finally identify correlations between metrics and QA results on several different anatomical sites (prostate, head, and neck, spine SBRT)

$$\mathrm{BA} = \frac{\sum_j (\mathrm{MU}_j \cdot \mathrm{AA}_j)}{\mathrm{MU}} \tag{8.12}$$

where AA_j is the aperture area,

$$\mathrm{BI} = \frac{\sum_j (\mathrm{MU}_j \cdot \mathrm{AI}_j)}{\mathrm{MU}} \tag{8.13}$$

where $\mathrm{AI_j}$ is the aperture irregularity $\mathrm{AI}_j = \left(\mathrm{AP}_j^2/4\pi \mathrm{AA}_j\right)_j$, AP is the aperture perimeter,

$$\mathrm{BM} = 1 - \frac{\sum_j (\mathrm{MU}_j \cdot \mathrm{AA}_j)}{\mathrm{MU} \cdot \bigcup_j (\mathrm{AA}_j)} \tag{8.14}$$

and

$$\mathrm{PA} = \frac{\sum_i (\mathrm{BA}_i \cdot \mathrm{MU}_i)}{\mathrm{MU_{plan}}},\ \mathrm{PI} = \frac{\sum_i (\mathrm{BI}_i \cdot \mathrm{MU}_i)}{\mathrm{MU_{plan}}},\ \mathrm{PM} = \frac{\sum_i (\mathrm{BM}_i \cdot \mathrm{MU}_i)}{\mathrm{MU_{plan}}} \tag{8.15}$$

are the corresponding plan indices, where the sums are on all the fields *i*. However, different results were found for different sites and specific techniques.

Crowe *et al* [81] analyzed all the above-described parameters, the complexity metrics from Llacer (FMC) and Webb (MI), the deliverability metrics from McNiven (MCS), and the accuracy metrics from Kairn, looking for possible thresholds able to determine undeliverable plans (failing quality assurance QA). They evaluated IMRT and VMAT plans on different anatomical sites, planned with a Varian Eclipse TPS, calculated with the AAA dose calculation algorithm, delivered with a Varian Clinac iX linear accelerator, and QA was performed with Epiqa software based on EPID images and GLAaS image to dose conversion algorithm. They concluded that deliverable IMRT plans can be obtained with MI < 0.02, MCS > 0.4 and CAS < 0.7. Moreover, SAS < 0.2 (with MLC aperture <10 mm) identified passing beams with 1.0 specificity. Regarding VMAT, no definitive significant relationships between QA and modulation metrics were identified, possibly indicating that VMAT arcs were less modulated and used fewer small and asymmetric apertures than IMRT plans.

In 2018, Park *et al* [82] also aimed to find a correlation between gamma passing rates and modulation indices for IMRT plans, analyzing MI_c [74], MCS [76], and PA, PI and PM [80]. They found that the plan averaged beam irregularity PI [80] showed moderately strong correlations with every plan delivery accuracy measure and can be considered as a predictor of IMRT delivery accuracy. The subsequent logical step has been published by the same Park and colleagues [83], evaluating six textural features calculated from fluence maps of IMRT beams, in a sort of radiomics analysis, finding the correlation and the variance as potential predictors for IMRT delivery accuracy.

A systematic historical review was published in 2019 by Antoine *et al* [84] to gather different plan complexity metrics published over the years, and discuss their ability in identifying possible patient-specific pre-treatment quality assurance. In their review, they identified a total of 163 publications on the subject of plan complexity, an indicator of its importance, and they evaluated 19 of those studies, for a total of 30 different plan complexity metrics. For now, plan complexity metrics should be seen as a planning procedure quality indicator although pre-treatment QA failure identifier results are mitigated. Yet, addressing the general pre-treatment QA failure prediction case could be possible with big data or machine learning help.

All the above summarized proposals for calculating specific modulation parameters and their associated results show how complex the modulation issue is and how difficult it is to determine the best way to understand the merit of the plans with the proposed parameters. We can conclude that there is a definite need to avoid over-modulation, by, e.g., lowering the MUs or avoiding small peaks of high fluence, to ensure better accuracy between the plan as presented by the TPS and its delivery, since the plan quality is not limited to the computed dose distribution, and the most important step in the whole chain is the treatment delivery together with its consistency with all the previous steps.

8.6 The feathering: large field splitting and multi-isocentric setup

IMRT is used for small and large targets. It is usually easy to plan small targets but often challenging for large targets. Whenever the beam needed to entirely cover the target is not sufficiently extended, solutions to safely deliver homogeneous doses are necessary. This could be the case in the longitudinal direction due to beam length limitation (maximum field size), but also in the lateral direction since the maximum field width is forced to be small by inherent design limitations of the multileaf collimator. In the first case, a multi-isocentre is the technical solution, while in the second case the IMRT field split and multiple carriage position delivery is best indicated.

In the conformal treatment, the solution for planning target volumes bigger than the largest field size came with the beam junction: two adjacent fields placed side by side on a geometrically well-defined plane. This technique presents the risk of dose gap or overlap during treatment delivery, due either to leaf positional errors, or, more frequently, to the patient and/or organ motion between the two fields' deliveries: this is especially true for medulloblastoma where beams are feathered with compromise dose uniformity as shown by Cheng *et al* [85].

With intensity modulation, field matching has been superseded by the concept of field overlapping. Two adjacent fields overlap (do not match on a plane), and each field fluence is optimized in the overlapping region to deliver the desired amount. A gradual decrease from one field to the other would minimize the field junction problems as shown in figure 8.5. This concept is named the feathering approach,

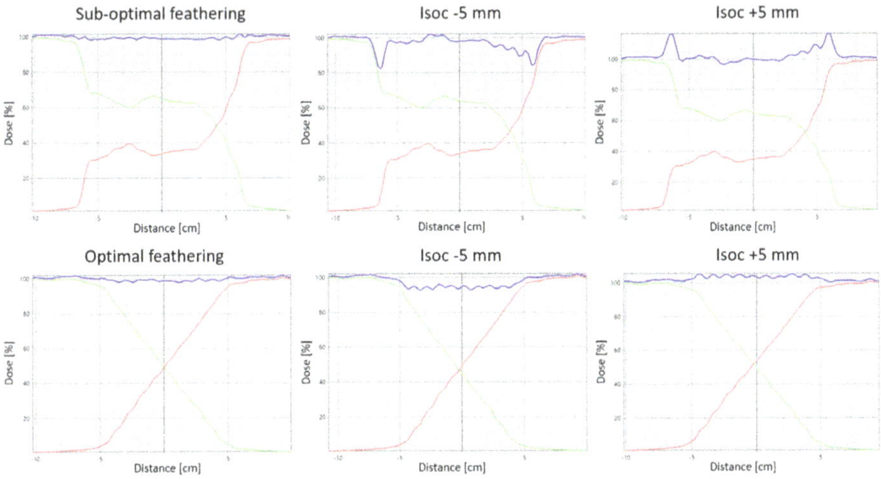

Figure 8.5. Feathering: the first row shows sub-optimal feathering, the second row good feathering. The three columns present, in order, the dose profiles (green and red the upper and lower field dose, blue the summation) with the correct distance between the upper and lower isocenters, 5 mm closer, and 5 mm more distant than planned. In the first row, with the sub-optimal feathering, peaks of ~15% of the desired dose are shown.

taking the name from the technique used in computer graphics to smooth or blur the edges of a feature.

8.6.1 Overlap in the lateral direction (large volumes)

In 2000, Wu *et al* [86] proposed a dynamic feathering method of splitting large intensity-modulated fields. With this technique, the component beams overlap each other by a defined amount, and the intensity in the overlap region gradually decreases/increases for one/the other field component. The sum of the intensities remains equal to the original beam intensity. They found that one split is adequate for fields as large as 25 cm, with a 4 cm overlap.

Malhotra *et al* [87] evaluated, on a phantom, large target volumes planning with IMRT using either multiple carriage delivery or multiple isocenters. With the dual carriage plan, the blending of the dose distribution did not present hot or cold spots. The dual isocenter plans were found to be clinically acceptable if they have at least a 3 cm overlap.

The large IMRT field splitting is a procedure generally accomplished by the treatment planning system, which automatically generates the two (or more) fields with reasonable overlap. Sometimes computer-based beam splitting may not always be suitable as shown by Srivastava *et al* [88].

8.6.2 Overlap in the longitudinal direction (long volumes)

Long volumes can be treated with multiple isocenters, with IMRT or VMAT. In both cases an overlap region to host the upper and lower field/arc is advisable. Most planning systems use a base plan and then optimize the dose in the gap region with

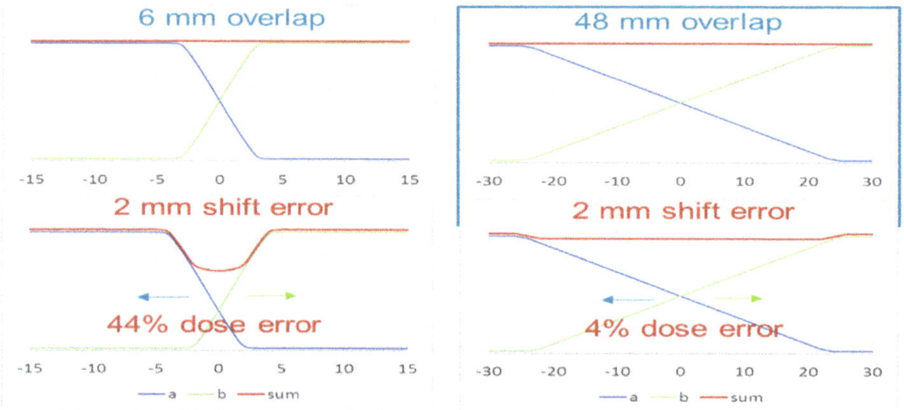

Figure 8.6. Overlap area with ideal feathering: first column: 6 mm overlap; second column: 48 mm overlap. In the second row, the dose summation (red profile) a 2 mm error in the two isocenters is shown, with the associated dose error in the overlapping region, of 44% in the 6 mm, and 4% in the 48 mm overlap area cases, respectively.

the other plans. In general, the smoothing effect of feathering increases as the size of the overlap region increases, because the slope of the dose gradient becomes less sharp. It is therefore recommended to use as large an overlap area as possible, as shown in figure 8.6.

The cranio-spinal axis irradiation can be considered as a paradigmatic case of the multiple isocentric technique and the feathering problem. Many papers have been published over the years specifically for this treatment site, some of which are summarized below. A few papers referred to IMRT with fixed beams, while the majority focused on the VMAT technique, focusing attention on the overlapping fields/arcs. However, all the technical and dosimetric considerations arising from this site planning and treatment can be translated to any other anatomical site when multiple isocenter settings for large target volumes is applied.

Initially, the field-in-field technique with forward planning was introduced and had been proposed for example by Yom *et al* [89], South *et al* [90], and Wilkinson *et al* [91] to overcome the cranial-spinal field junction. Feathering IMRT has been used, but with the cranial and spinal fields matched geometrically as shown by several investigators [92–94]. A mix between geometric field matching and inverse planning was proposed by Zeng *et al* [95]. They exploited an extended dose gradient throughout an overlap region of 4 to 6 cm to minimize the impact of field match errors on a junction dose. The gradient was controlled by dividing the overlap region into subregions 1–1.5 cm long and assigning decreasing dose objectives from 80 to 20% of the prescribed dose. The technique was shown on lower extremity treatments, proving that a ±3 mm shift between the two isocentres generated, in the overlapping region, inhomogeneities in an average of ±5%, with localized differences of about 10%. Cao *et al* [96] proposed a jagged-junction IMRT field for a three-isocenter field setting which overcomes the problems associated with field junction and beam edge matching. To avoid an undesirably sharp dose gradient, field edges belonging to the same isocenter were staggered in 1.1 cm steps. With seven fields in the cranial isocenter and three fields for each spine isocenter, the net result was a 9.9 cm long overlap between the cranial and spinal field sets, and a 5.5 cm overlap between the two spinal field sets. The optimization process hence smoothly integrated the dose inside the overlapped junction.

Similarly, Hadley *et al* [97] described a technique to generate a single gradient junction (on an minimum 4 cm long overlapping region) to replace multiple junction shifts as usually applied with conformal treatments between cranial and spinal volumes. With a mixed manual and automatic optimization, they adjusted the fluences of the classical fields to generate an intensity-modulated stepped gradient dose in the overlapping region.

However, a full inverse IMRT planning procedure was proposed by Seppälä *et al* in 2010 [98] to handle the gap issues. They investigated dynamic split field IMRT (sfIMRT) without interfraction feathering or field edge matching at any junction area. For the IMRT treatment plans the same classical conformal field setup was used, except that the fields were set to overlap each other at least by 4 cm. One single plan was required since the intra-fraction feathering was performed with the dynamic MLC, obtained by the inverse planning with a fluence optimization process. The accuracy of the dose distributions of sfIMRT was investigated by an intentional longitudinal error of ±3 mm of the treatment couch, resulting in a dose inhomogeneity in the cranial-spinal junction of ±11% with their sfIMRT, to compare with ±37% in the 3D conformal case.

The use of VMAT for the cranio-spinal axis has been widely explored. In 2011 a report on the first patients treated in five different European institutions was published [99]; the cranial and axial arcs were overlapped on a region 2 to 12 cm long (mean 7.5 cm, median 7.7 cm), avoiding field matching and leaving the dose transition distribution to the optimizer. In 2012, Chen *et al* [100] reported treatment planning results of two cranio-spinal axis irradiation patients, a 9-year-old child, and a 24-year-old adult, planned with VMAT, where the authors reported an overlapping region of 8 to 10 cm planned with the Varian Eclipse treatment planning system from Varian. Similarly, Lee *et al* [101] reported VMAT planning of five patients, applying 10 cm long overlapped volumes, planned with Philips Pinnacle system with the SmartArc module.

The above-mentioned VMAT studies reported on the overlapped region for the upper and lower arc, while having the optimizer produce the feathering solution. In 2013, Myers *et al* [102] dosimetrically evaluated the effect of inaccurate patient positioning in the junction area, by proposing a 'gradient-optimization technique' in Pinnacle. With this method, the target volume in the junction area was contoured as four equally long sections, the optimization being then run in two steps: firstly, the superior arc was optimized to deliver decreasing doses (80%, 60%, 40%, and 20%) to the four junction areas moving inferiorly down the target; the second step started after the superior arc optimization, by optimizing the inferior arc. At the end, in the overlapped area, the dose was optimized to gradual decreases in one arc, and complemented by a gradual increase from the other arc. This procedure guaranteed the smooth (or small stepwise) dose variation in the 'junction area'.

Similarly, Strojnik *et al* [103] used the Eclipse planning system: to assure a ramp-like dose in the overlap region, the upper spinal part was optimized first, with the dose enforcing a ramp-like dose profile in a transitional region of 10.8 cm subdivided into nine subregions, each 1.2 cm long, requiring the dose to gradually decrease to the periphery. The cranial part was then optimized taking into account the upper spinal arc dose.

The techniques described by Myers and Strojnik were made necessary due to a possible imperfect optimization implementation in the overlapping region, where the final dose sum corresponded to the requested amount, but the gradual dose decrease/increase was not ideal. Efforts are needed to ensure automatic feathering in the optimization procedures. As an example, in the Eclipse planning system, a recent feature called 'auto-feathering', that creates smooth dose gradients in plans with multiple isocenters with overlapping fields or arcs (IMRT or VMAT), has been implemented for some treatment units by specifically adding a set of spatial optimization objectives in the preprocessing step of the optimization algorithm. Those objectives are included in the total cost function to generate the dose gradient. The larger the size of the overlap region, the lesser the slope of the dose gradient, making a safer and more robust dose delivery. In figure 8.4 an example of the dose gradients in cases without and with the use of the auto-feathering option is shown: in the first row the auto-feathering was not adopted leading to a sub-optimal dose gradient, while in the second row auto-feathering was adopted and the dose gradient is smoothly decreasing in the overlap region.

8.7 Artifact handling

CT images of patients with metal implants such as hip prostheses or dental fillings suffer from artifacts generally in the form of bright streaks (high electron density), dark voids (low electron density), cupping and capping. Even the small marker bearing ball or wires used during the CT scan for planning produces artifacts. These artifacts are mostly due to quantum noise, scattered radiation, and beam hardening [104]. Both the metal artifacts and the beam attenuation from the metallic materials could lead to an inaccurate patient dose calculation, as shown in the cases of hip replacements on prostate treatment [105–107]. In the case of planning CT affected by artifacts, this might influence the fluence optimization and the dose calculation, inducing cold or hot spots.

To exemplify and demonstrate the impact of artifacts CT, let us consider a homogeneous dose requested on a volume affected by streaking artifacts, generated by metal inserts, of very high and very low densities. The effect of the incorrect high densities region on the dose estimation is quite clear, while the effect of incorrect low densities in the inverse planning process could be more subtle. To deliver enough dose in the low-density streaks (at the limit of air), the optimizer will plan a very high fluence in that region, a homogeneous dose distribution will be computed, while a very high fluence will be delivered to the patient. This will translate as a delivered dose level which is much higher than expected and planned, possibly leading to unexpected toxicity for the patient. The artifact problem has to be handled in any inverse planning process as IMRT or VMAT dose optimization. The anatomical sites where the artifact problem is mostly present are the head and neck treatment due to dental metal artifacts, and the pelvic treatment due to hip replacements. Several publications reported below refer to the dosimetric errors that could occur in the IMRT or VMAT planning processes, and CT correction solution.

The guidance document on planning IMRT [108], suggested planning how to handle contrast agents or streaking artifacts that may assign undesired CT numbers to voxels and inappropriately influence the dose calculations. For example, specific more appropriate densities can be assigned to regions with artifacts, and plans could be run with and without the corrections to determine the dosimetric magnitude of any effects.

In 2006, Kim *et al* [109] quantified the cold or hot spots induced in IMRT head and neck plans on 5 patients due to the presence of metal dental artifacts in CT images. They evaluated the dose distribution by using uncorrected images, homogeneous uncorrected (assigning homogeneous water), sinogram completion correction, minimum value correction, and minimum value correction and subsequent application of a streak artifact reduction algorithm, considering the last corrected image dataset as the most similar to the actual patient. The plans were optimized for IMRT in the different sets and recalculated on the most similar 'actual patient' to estimate hot and cold spots in targets and OARs. For example, the target dose was estimated to receive in general cold spots of a few percent, but in non-negligible volumes (~20%), while the parotids had hot spots in around 30% of the structure volume. The possible clinical effect was assessed with the TCP and NTCP evaluation [110], resulting in a parotid NTCP increase of 3.2% and TCP reduction of 1.9% when the original uncorrected CT dataset was used. Those results showed the importance of using artifact correction methods for planning purposes.

In the head and neck region using IMRT technique, Webster *et al* [111] found that an extended CT density table (including high densities of ~3 g cm^{-3}) and an additional simple manual bulk density correction of the artifacts areas (density 1.0 g cm^{-3} for tissue, and 1.8 g cm^{-3} for teeth) reduced the dosimetric impact of dental artifacts to acceptable levels. The dosimetric impact of dental implants in head and neck planning with the VMAT technique was explored by Lin *et al* [112] evaluating different implant materials with Monte Carlo dose calculations. The main effect of the dental implant was the severe attenuation in the downstream. The 1 cm^3 dental implant can lower the downstream dose by 10% (Ti) to 51% (Au) for a 3×3 cm^2 field. For the VMAT patient dose calculation, the target coverage was significantly degraded. However, with the use of the material's electron density ratio (AAA dose calculation algorithm, in this case) the dose calculation accuracy was within a clinically acceptable level.

To improve the CT image quality, some metal artifact correction algorithms have been studied, as reviewed in [113]. Within this framework, the dose calculation algorithm (and consequently the optimization processes) also benefited. An example of the benefit of a metal artifact reduction algorithm (MAR) on the dose calculation accuracy was published by Maerz *et al* [114], reporting data on a scanned phantom with a metallic implant, and virtually reconstructed according to the known densities.

IMRT and VMAT plans were computed and measured. The dose calculation accuracy relative to measurements was significantly better for the corrected rather than artifacts CT data ($p = 0.015$), with better agreement for VMAT ($p = 0.011$) than IMRT ($p = 0.029$) plans, proving on one hand the advantage of using the metal artifact reduction, and on the other hand that VMAT is preferable when CT planning is affected by artifacts.

Spadea *et al* [115] evaluated the dosimetric impact of uncorrected or MAR-corrected CT images against ground truth images of a phantom with low-Z (Ti, 4.54 g cm^{-3}) and high-Z (Cerrobend, 9.76 g cm^{-3}) inserts, with plans of 5-field IMRT (entrances avoided the metal along their path). Monte Carlo calculations showed errors in dose calculation up to ~25% inside the target in the high-Z material case for uncorrected images; the error was reduced to <0.4% for MAR-corrected data. No dosimetric impact was conversely found for low-Z inserts (<0.3% for uncorrected images). The same group, in a subsequent study, [116] assessed the impact for higher-Z materials (Au, 19.28 g cm^{-3}), finding a maximal difference between uncorrected and MAR-corrected patient images of 51% inside the metal, 13% adjacent to the insert, and 12% propagated downstream.

The impact of artifacts, and the possible benefit from MAR correction algorithms, depends on the material, but also on the position, being more relevant in regions close to the metal insert, or downstream. Lin *et al* [117], using CT images of six head and neck patients with dental implants, delineated target volumes with sizes and locations arbitrarily determined; the artifact regions were corrected by CT number assignment close to water. Different VMAT arc arrangements were explored (half, one and two arcs). The same plans were compared with the gamma index (2 mm, 2%) between corrected and uncorrected CT datasets. The target size was not correlating with artifact dosimetric impact when the target location was far from the implant; for targets close to the metal, higher dose discrepancy was found in larger targets. Also, a larger implant size presented larger dose differences. Finally, they found that the greatest impact was found for the half arc setting. In summary, small targets, large high-Z metallic implant and a short distance in between can cause severe dosimetric impact.

The iMAR (iterative MAR) algorithm was tested by Bär *et al* [118], reporting dose differences of up to ±5% for an IMRT plan on a head and neck patient with dental fillings, for uncorrected and iMAR-corrected images. Ziemann [119] evaluated, for VMAT plans, different MAR correction algorithms on a pelvic phantom with steel rods to mimic hip replacement and air cavity in the rectal position: the Linear Interpolation (LI) approach, and the Augmented Likelihood Image Reconstruction (ALIR). Dose accuracy was also estimated for manually corrected images. Uncorrected images lead to a dose error up to 8.4%; manual, LI and ALIR reduced the error to 4.1%, 3.2%, and 2.7%, respectively.

Additionally, the artifacts make the volume delineation difficult and it is often useful to manually mask the artifact with soft tissue if artifact reduction software is not available. The visible line artifact (for example in the breast) generated by the bearing balls or wires positioned during the CT scan acquisition can easily be overridden with soft tissue CT number assignments. It is thus recommended that preprocessing of the image either manually or with software is needed before proceeding with volume delineation and planning.

In conclusion, an overview of the artifact related dose calculation issue is provided but it is important to keep in mind that in the dose calculation, uncertainties have the greatest impact on the optimization process when dealing with inverse planning for IMRT or VMAT. The dose estimation in this phase of planning (earlier than the final dose computation) generates fluences according to the desired dose distribution based on the CT images: uncorrected images will produce incorrect fluences. This point makes the artifact correction procedures a fundamental step in all the intensity-modulated planning. Not to forget, the fluence generated on a CT dataset with bright and dark streaks could present over-modulation, with abrupt changes in a short space, to compensate for the abrupt changes in densities. Such unnecessarily increased complexity would also lower the delivery accuracy, as described in section 8.5, enforcing the importance of artifact correction.

8.8 The interplay effect

Intensity-modulated fields are composed of many segments or control points defined by the leaf positions as a function of time. During the treatment delivery (intra-fraction), the organs inside the patient move due to respiration, and the volume supposedly inside an open segment may move outside. This interplay between the organ and the leaf motions makes the delivered dose distribution different from the planned one and may generate undesired hot and cold spots. The organ motion affected the static 3DCRT fields only at the field boundaries generating a dose blurring that can be described as a convolution of the dose distribution with the motion pattern and can be managed by the CTV to PTV margin concept. However, margins are not sufficient to account for the interplay effects.

The interplay effect is a known problem, and it has been studied since the beginning of the IMRT era. In 1998, Yu *et al* [120] showed that, for clinically realistic parameters, the magnitude of intensity variations in the target can be greater than 100% of the desired intensity, and depends on the leaf speed relative to the target/organ motion speed, and on the segment size relative to the target/organ motion amplitude. However, with fractionated treatment, most of the intensity variations will smooth out, reducing the interplay effect. Tomotherapy deliveries are also affected by the interplay effect: Yang *et al* [121] reported that the patient breathing frequency, gantry rotational speed, field size and degree of modulation are all factors affecting the interplay effect.

Bortfeld and colleagues [122] theoretically and statistically evaluated the interplay problem and then reported on simulation for a clinical case. They found that the biggest deviations are at dose gradients that are oriented in the direction of the organ motion, and the main effect of organ motion in IMRT is an averaging of the dose distribution without motion over the path of the motion. Moreover, again, the effect of fractionation will be an averaging over the session by session treatment, and the cumulative error after several fractions will be smaller than the single day error. The fine assessment of the interplay effects dependencies was a subject of many studies over many years, both theoretically, through motion simulations to properly estimate the dose distribution including the motion, and through measurements.

Court *et al* [123, 124] investigated IMRT fields with the intent of evaluating the possibility to provide planning guidelines by predicting whether a given MLC sequence could give large (>10%) daily dose variations related to the motion. They found that a maximum leaf speed of 0.1 cm s^{-1} and a maximum dose rate of 300 MU/min keep a maximum dose discrepancy below 10%; however, these parameters also depend on the motion period (for regular, e.g., breathing motion), the MLC separation and the parallel or perpendicular organ motion relative to the MLC motion. Furthermore, they reported an increased interplay effect with increased plan complexity, breathing amplitude and regular target shape.

The interplay effect has seen a renewed interest in the last decade due to the rapid growth of the stereotactical treatments using IMRT and especially VMAT since in those cases the treatment is delivered in few, if not a single fraction, thus prejudicing the dose variation reduction due to fractionation. The site mostly studied is the lung SBRT [125–131], but also liver SBRT [132, 133] and pancreas [134] were analyzed.

Various factors were found to be responsible for the interplay effect, aiming to find the best patient, planning and machine characteristics to reduce the motion-induced dose variation. The breathing pattern showed reduced interplay for small amplitude and long period [125, 129, 133, 135]. For VMAT treatment, the single arc plan revealed more interplay effect than multiple arc setting [125, 127, 134, 135], as well as a high dose rate like FFF beams [127]. Concerning the plan, the high modulation (in terms of MU or complexity) was found to be significantly correlated with interplay effect [125, 132, 133, 135–137]. The discussion in Ecclestone *et al* [133] showed an increased interplay effect for lower modulation, in contrast with results from other studies; however, the high modulation generated a slower gantry speed, resulting in a longer delivery time, possibly responsible for the reduced interplay. This example provides the complexity of the interplay effect, where different characteristics combine, sometimes confounding the results of the single factors. Kubo *et al* [131] for example introduced parameters as a combination of different characteristics that were not found individually significant for interplay: the combination of tumor motion and MCSv (TMMCSv, ratio between MCSv and breathing amplitude), and the interplay effect variable score (ITV, product between the TMMCSv and the number of breaths). The increase of IVS and TMMCSv was associated with lower dose variation.

An interesting work has been published by Edvardsson *et al* [138], based on the thesis work of the same Edvardsson of Lund University [139], with a comprehensive evaluation of the dosimetric effects for VMAT on breathing motion by analyzing several patient- and machine-related parameters. In their work, the authors proposed a method to simulate the breathing motion from 4DCT images, to calculate the dose distribution with and without motion under different conditions. The method was validated against measurements. The interplay effect was evaluated as the relative dose differences in the two conditions with and without motion, to 98% and 2% of the CTV volume: $\Delta D_{98\%}$ and $\Delta D_{2\%}$. Considerable interplay effects were observed for individual fractions, with the minimum $\Delta D_{98\%}$ and maximum $\Delta D\%$ as −16.7% and 16.2%, respectively. The extent of interplay effects, for individual treatment fractions, was larger for: increasing breathing amplitudes up to approximately 20 mm, longer period times (slow breathing), FFF compared to flattened beams and lower dose levels (both parameters shorten the delivery time and possibly increase the MLC speed) and for more complex treatment plans (increased number of MU/Gy). Also, the interplay effects varied considerably with the initial breathing phase, and larger variations were observed for smaller CTV sizes. Only small differences were observed for varying collimator angles. However, these effects were substantially reduced for multiple fractions due to averaging effects.

In conclusion, to mitigate the interplay effects, we suggest reducing the plan complexity, lowering the dose rate and using targets based on MIP. However, lowering the dose rate prolongs the treatment time, increasing the patient's motion likelihood during the delivery. Moreover, care should be taken for patients experiencing breathing patterns with large amplitude and long period. The treatment machine characteristics also need to be evaluated, as presented in the study described by Netherton and colleagues [135] on the Varian Halcyon unit, a bore designed linac with high-speed MLC and gantry rotation performances (up to five times faster than the more classical c-arm linacs). They found dose deviations in case of motion are greater than those reported for conventional c-arm linear accelerators, due to the special speed characteristics, increasing the interplay effects due to the higher MLC and gantry speed, and the shorter delivery time. To compensate, additional efforts in terms of reduced plan complexity and tumor motion should be considered. Also, the dose deviation convergence with the number of fractions on the Halcyon unit is slower than that reported for conventional linear accelerators.

The last aspect underlined by many authors, as well as the IMRT pioneers, concerns the multi-fraction treatment, where the interplay effect is smoothed out, making the dose variation clinically acceptable in most cases [120, 122, 127, 128, 136]. This is an important aspect to take into consideration in the clinical practice of single-dose IMRT or VMAT SBRT where motion is of concern.

8.9 The neutron production and the whole body dose: beam quality

The medical linear accelerators deliver photon energy beams in a range of 4 to 25 MV. The choice of the best energy had been long discussed in detail by various investigators [140–142], however with IMRT techniques it depends on different factors: on one hand the dosimetric plan quality in terms of penumbra (lateral scattering) and healthy tissue and OARs doses, on the other hand the very low doses generated by leakage and neutron production that would increase the second cancer induction risk [143].

From the dosimetric viewpoint, higher energies could present some advantages for deep-sited tumors or large patients thanks to their greater penetration depth and increased skin-sparing effect. However, when a large number of beams is used the significance of beam energy is diminished as shown by Pirzkall *et al* [2]. Regarding the non-target dose, a higher entrance dose is expected for lower energies, and higher exit dose for higher energies [144], and this is valid for any technique. However, with IMRT, the dose conformality improves and the OARs doses are lower than non-IMRT plans, possibly decreasing the dose-related toxicities; the cost of the improved IMRT plan quality is an increase of the normal tissue exposed to low doses, and especially an increase of the delivered MU. The greater MU required with IMRT makes leakage through the collimator and scatter from the gantry an important component for the low dose bath. In addition, for photon beams generated by electrons of energies higher than ~7–8 MeV, (γ,n) reactions generate neutrons that concur to increase the patient integral dose. The biological effectiveness of neutrons (quality factor) is about 10 times that of photons. The neutron production depends mainly on the photon beam energy but it also depends on the high atomic number materials in the accelerator head.

The linac components within the gantry that may contribute to the neutron yield are mainly the collimators, the flattening filter and the accessories (mechanical wedge filters). Low energy photons, intended <8–10 MV, are below the threshold for neutron production, and this contamination component is not of concern. In high energy photon beams, the most important effect of the low doses from leakage coupled with the neutron production is the increased risk of second cancer induction. As early as 1997, Followill *et al* [145] estimated the likelihood of a fatal second cancer due to a 70 Gy treatment, for 3DCRT with wedges, IMRT (conventional linac) and tomotherapy IMRT of 0.6%, 1.0%, 2.8% for a 6 MV photon beam, respectively, and 2.5%, 4.5%, 13.1% for a 18 MV beam. Consistent with Followill's results, Chibani *et al* [146] found that for a 70 Gy treatment delivered with a 15 or 18 MV from Varian Clinac, the dose equivalent from neutron contamination at 50 cm off-axis distance translated into a 1.1 or 2.0% likelihood of a fatal second cancer. Based on A-bomb survivor data, Hall *et al* [147], in cases of the number of MU with IMRT increased by a factor of two to three relative to the 3DCRT, estimated that the risk of second malignancies is almost doubled for IMRT. Kry *et al* [148] reported the number of MU for IMRT plans 3.5–4.9 times the MU required for 3DCRT. This produced, for an 18 MV beam, a risk of secondary malignancy of 1.7% and 5.1%, respectively, for conformal and intensity-modulated beam. They also evaluated different beams from Siemens and Varian linear accelerators, where they found a slightly higher risk for the Siemens unit. Interesting are the IMRT cases of 6 and 10 MV (where the neutron production is not of concern), showing lower MU in the 10 MV case, yielding in a lower risk (2.1% to compare to 2.9% for the 6 MV), while higher energies showed an increased second cancer risk to 3.4% and 5.1% for 15 and 18 MV, respectively, due to neutron productions.

Another important point related to the photoactivation of elements in the linac hardware for high energy photon beams is the radiation exposure of the therapy staff, other than the patients. Rawlinson *et al* [149] estimated that, with an 18 MV beam with a workload of 60 000 MU/week, the therapy staff would receive about 60 μSv/week with 3DCRT treatment, compared with about 330 μSv/week for IMRT deliveries.

Over the years different groups have reported about photoneutrons for various treatment units from different vendors, pointing to the differences between conformal and IMRT techniques, as well as the effects on therapy staff (e.g., [146, 150–159]). Various studies also presented comparisons in dosimetric terms for different anatomical sites between low and high energy beams, showing very small or even not significant differences in using different qualities [144, 160–164].

It is commonly assumed that the neutron dose equivalent scales with the number of MUs. However, Hälg *et al* [165] reported, from measurements, that it does not scale with the ratio of IMRT applied MUs relative to those for open field irradiation. Outside the treatment volume, and at large depths, 35% less neutron dose equivalent is delivered than expected, leading the predicted increase of second cancer induction rates from IMRT to be overestimated when the neutron dose is simply scaled with MUs.

The FFF beams, removing one of the sources of neutron production (the flattening filter), reduces the integral dose. This was reported by Li *et al* [166] for 10 MV in standard (600 MU/min) and FFF mode (2400 MU/min) from a Varian TrueBeam accelerator where they found that the neutron cumulative dose in standard mode was almost threefold as large as that in FFF mode. Dawn *et al* [167] evaluated the in-field neutron production for standard and FFF 10 MV beams from a Varian TrueBeam, and for a 15 MV from NovalisTx and TrueBeam units, where they reported that the FFF beam drastically decreases the neutron production, and it is lower for TrueBeam than NovalisTx units.

All these aspects on the neutron production and the whole body dose on the beam energy choice for IMRT deliveries could be summarized in the suggestion of using low energy beams (e.g., 6 MV) for IMRT treatments to both lower second cancer risk for patients and improve radiation safety for therapy personnel. The FFF could also be a viable and interesting option for the future in this respect. Also consider that the ability of VMAT to deliver high-quality plans more efficiently than IMRT, with a significantly reduced number of MUs, could make the VMAT technique the treatment of choice given the lower neutrons and a lower integral dose.

8.10 Conclusions on treatment planning

In this chapter, some of the points related to the intensity-modulated treatment planning process are analyzed.

Beam geometry is the comprehensive choice of all the beam geometrical parameters: the gantry entrances (fixed for IMRT, arc span for VMAT), the collimator and the couch rotation and the beam quality. Their choice is mostly in the planners' hands (apart from some optimization tools not yet much used in today's clinical practice), and part of the plan quality could depend on this decision.

The beam energy in particular, and the choice of the flattened or unflattened beam (whenever available), more than the specific dosimetric evaluation in terms of target coverage and dose homogeneity, and OARs sparing, could improve the long term patient sequela, including a different risk of second cancer induction due to neutron production or radiation scattering.

For those reasons, solid understanding of the rationale behind the specific choices made in the treatment planning process is fundamental for treatment quality. How to deal with the CT dataset artifacts, which are the best settings for reducing the interplay effect, the level of fluence modulation generating a safely deliverable plan, and, ultimately, maintaining knowledge of the dose to be applied in the overlapping region when large targets require a multiple isocentric setting, have here been viewed.

It is important today, at a time when the intensity-modulated era is becoming ever more automated as regards the whole sequential process, so as to embrace the adaptive concept, that we consciously maintain our knowledge of the possible uncertainties that could occur in practical situations, in order to be able to critically evaluate the treatment planning results in relation to the planning aspect, even in the presence of inverse planning and *a fortiori* in the event of an adaptive process frame.

References

[1] Bortfeld T and Schlegel W 1993 Optimization of beam orientations in radiation therapy: some theoretical considerations *Phys. Med. Biol.* **38** 291–304

[2] Pirzkall A, Carol M P and Pickett B *et al* 2002 The effect of beam energy and number of fields on photon-based IMRT for deep-seated targets *Int. J. Radiat. Oncol. Biol. Phys.* **53** 434–42

[3] Benedict S H, Yenice K M, Followill D, Galvin J M, Hinson W and Kavanagh B *et al* 2010 Stereotactic body radiation therapy: the report of AAPM Task Group 101 *Med. Phys.* **37** 4078–101

[4] Hoppe B S, Laser B, Kowalski A V, Fontenla S C, Pena-Greenberg E and Yorke E D *et al* 2008 Acute skin toxicity following stereotactic body radiation therapy for stage I non-small-cell lung cancer: who's at risk? *Int. J. Radiat. Oncol. Biol. Phys.* **72** 1283–6

[5] Pugachev A B, Boyer A L and Xing L 2000 Beam orientation optimization in intensity-modulated radiation treatment planning *Med. Phys.* **27** 1238–45

[6] Djajaputra D, Wu Q, Wu Y and Mohan R 2003 Algorithm and performance of a clinical IMRT beam-angle optimization system *Phys. Med. Biol.* **48** 3191–212

[7] Gaede S and Wong E 2004 An algorithm for systematic selection of beam directions for IMRT *Med. Phys.* **31** 376–88

[8] Lee E K, Fox T and Crocker I 2006 Simultaneous beam geometry and intensity map optimization in intensity-modulated radiation therapy *Int. J. Radiat. Oncol. Biol. Phys.* **64** 301–20

[9] Srivastava S P, Das I J, Kumar A and Johnstone P A S 2011 Dosimetric comparison of manual and beam angle optimization of gantry angles in IMRT *Med. Dosim.* **36** 313–6

[10] Grosshans D, Boehling N S, Palmer M, Spicer C, Erice R and Cox J D *et al* 2012 Improving cardiac dosimetry: alternative beam arrangements for intensity modulated radiation therapy planning in patients with carcinoma of distal esophagus *Pract. Rad. Onc.* **2** 41–5

[11] Yirmibesoglu E, Fried D V, Kostich M, Rosenman J, Shockley W and Weissler M *et al* 2013 Dosimetric evaluation of an ipsilateral intensity modulated radiotherapy beam arrangement for parotid malignancies *Radiol. Oncol.* **47** 411–8

[12] Shukla A K, Kumar S, Sandhu I S, Oinam A S, Sing R and Kapoor R 2016 Dosimetric study of beam angle optimization in intensity-modulated radiation therapy planning *J. Cancer Res. Therap.* **12** 1045–9

[13] Ishii K, Okada W, Ogino R, Kubo K, Kishimoto S and Nakahara R *et al* 2016 A treatment-planning comparison of three beam arrangement strategies for stereotactic body radiation therapy for centrally located lung tumors using volumetric-modulated arc therapy *J. Rad. Res.* **57** 273–9

[14] Fu Y, Deng M, Zhou X, Lin Q, Du B and Tian X *et al* 2017 Dosimetric effect of beam arrangement for intentisy-modulated radiation therapy in the treatment of upper thoracic esophageal carcinoma *Med. Dos.* **42** 47–52

[15] Tian Q, Zhang F, Wang Y and Qu W 2014 Impact of different beam directions on intensity-modulated radiation therapy dose delivered to functioning lung tissue identified using single-photon emission computed tomography *Contemp. Oncol. (Pozn.)* **18** 436–41

[16] Mancosu P, Cozzi L, Fogliata A, Lattuada P, Reggiori G and Cantone M C *et al* 2010 Collimator angle influence on dose distribution optimization for vertebral metastases using volumentric modulated arc therapy *Med. Phys.* **37** 4133–7

[17] Kim J I, Ahn B S, Choi C H, Park J M and Park S Y 2018 Optimal collimator rotation based on the outline of multiple brain targets in VMAT *Radiat. Oncol.* **13** 88

[18] Ohira S, Sagawa T, Ueda Y, Inui S, Masaoka A and Akino Y *et al* 2019 Effect of collimator angle on HyperArc stereotactic radiosurgery planning for single and multiple brain metastases *Med. Dosim.*

[19] Li X, Wu J, Palta M, Zhang Y, Sheng Y and Zhang J *et al* 2019 A collimator setting optimization algorithm for dual-arc volumetric modulated arc therapy in pancreas stereotactic body radiation therapy *Technol. Cancer Res. Treat.* **18** 1–9

[20] Isa M, Rehman J, Afzal M and Chow J C L 2014 Dosimetric dependence on the collimator angle in prostate volumetric modulated arc therapy *Int. J. Cancer Ther. Oncol.* **2** 020419

[21] Tas B, Bilge H and Ozturk S T 2016 An investigation of the dose distribution effect related with collimator angle in volumetric arc therapy of prostate cancer *J. Med. Phys.* **41** 100–5

[22] Li M H, Huang S F, Chang C C, Lin J C and Tsai J T 2018 Variations in dosimetric distribution and plan complexity with collimator angles in hypofractionated volumetric arc radiotherapy for treating prostate cancer *Appl. J. Clin. Med. Phys.* **19** 93–102

[23] Sharma S, Manigandan D, Gyal S, Sahai P, Subramani V and Chander S *et al* 2015 Influence of collimator rotation on dose distribution and delivery in intensity modulated radiation therapy for parotid cancer *Int. J. Cancer Ther. Oncol.* **3** 3212

[24] Ahn B S, Park S Y, Park J M, Choi C H, Chun M and Kim J I 2017 Dosimetric effects of sectional adjustments of collimator angles on volumetric modulated arc therapy for irregularly-shaped targets *PLoS One* **12** e0174924

[25] Kim Y H, Park H R, Kim W T, Kim D W and Ki Y *et al* 2015 Effect of the collimator angle on dosimetric verification of volumetric modulated arc therapy *J. Kor. Phys. Soc.* **67** 243–7

[26] Zhang P, Happersett L, Yang Y, Yamada Y, Mageras G and Hunt M 2010 Optimization of collimator trajectory in volumetric modulated arc therapy: development and evaluation for paraspinal SBRT *Int. J. Radiat. Oncol. Biol. Phys.* **77** 591–9

[27] Fix M K, Frei D, Volken W, Terribilini D and Manser P 2016 Volumetric modulated arc therapy optimization including dynamic collimator rotation *Radiother. Oncol.* **119** S763

[28] Lyu Q, O'Connor D, Ruan D, Yu V, Nguyen and Sheng K 2018 VMAT otpimization with dynamic collimator rotation *Med. Phys.* **45** 2399–410

[29] Smyth G, Evans P M, Bamber J C and Bedford J L 2019 Recent developments in non-coplanar radiotherapy *Br. J. Radiol.* **92** 20180908

[30] Dong P, Lee P, Ruan D, Long T, Romeijn E and Yang Y *et al* 2013 4π non-coplanar liver SBRT: a novel delivery technique *Int. J. Radiat. Oncol. Biol. Phys.* **85** 1360–6

[31] Dong P, Lee P, Ruan D, Long T, Romeijn E and Low D A *et al* 2013 4π noncoplanar stereotactic body radiation therapy for centrally located or larger lung tumors *Int. J. Radiat. Oncol. Biol. Phys.* **86** 407–13

[32] Nguyen D, Rwigema J C, Yu V Y, Kaprealian T, Kupelian P and Selch M *et al* 2014 Feasibility of extreme dose escalation for glioblastoma multiforme using 4π radiotherapy *Radiat. Oncol.* **9** 239

[33] Rwigema J C, Nguyen D, Heron D E, Chen A M, Lee P and Wang P C *et al* 2015 4π noncoplanar stereotactic body radiation therapy for head-and-neck cancer: potential to improve tumor control and late toxicity *Int. J. Radiat. Oncol. Biol. Phys.* **91** 401–9

[34] Dong P, Nguyen D, Ruan D, King C, Long T and Romeijn E *et al* 2014 Feasibility of prostate robotic radiation therapy on conventional C-arm linacs *Pract. Radiat. Oncol.* **4** 254–60

[35] Tran A, Zhang J, Woods K, Yu V, Nguyen D and Gustafson G *et al* 2017 Treatment planning comparison of IMPT, VMAT and 4π radiotherapy for prostate cases *Radiat. Oncol.* **12** 10

[36] Tran A, Woods K, Nguyen D, Yu V Y, Niu T and Cao M *et al* 2017 Predicting liver SBRT eligibility and plan quality for VMAT and 4π plans *Radiat. Oncol.* **12** 70

[37] Murzin V L, Woods K, Moiseenko V, Karunamuni R, Tringale K R and Seibert T M *et al* 2018 4π plan optimization for cortical-sparing brain radiotherapy *Radiother. Oncol.* **127** 128–35

[38] Yu V Y, Landers A, Woods K, Nguyen D, Cao M and Du D *et al* 2018 A prospective 4π radiation therapy clinical study in recurrent high grade glioma patients *Int. J. Radiat. Oncol. Biol. Phys.* **101** 144–51

[39] Chang D S, Bartlett G K, Das I J and Cardens H R 2013 Beam angle selection for intensity-modulated radiotherapy (IMRT) treatment of unresectable pancreatic cancer: are non-coplanar beam angles necessary? *Clin. Transl. Oncol.* **15** 720–4

[40] Orlandi E, Giandini T, Iannacone E, De Ponti E, Carrara M and Mongioj V *et al* 2014 Radiotherapy for unresectable sinonasal cancers: dosimetric comparison of intensity modulated radiation therapy with coplanar and non-coplanar volumetric modulated Arc therapy *Radiother. Oncol.* **113** 260–6

[41] Woods K, Nguyen D, Tran A, Yu V Y, Cao M and Niu T *et al* 2016 Viability of Non-Coplanar VMAT for liver SBRT as compared to coplanar VMAT and beam orientation optimized 4π IMRT *Adv. Radiat. Oncol.* **1** 67–75

[42] Wild E, Bangert M, Nill S and Oelfke U 2015 Noncoplanar VMAT for nasopharyngeal tumors: plan quality versus treatment time *Med. Phys.* **42** 2157–68

[43] Voet P W, Breedveld S, Dirkx M L, Levendag P C and Heijmen B J 2012 Integrated multicriterial optimization of beam angles and intensity profiles for coplanar and non-coplanar head and neck IMRT and implications for VMAT *Med. Phys.* **39** 4858–65

[44] Audet C, Poffenbarger B A, Chang P, Jackson P S, Lundahl R E and Ryu S I *et al* 2011 Evaluation of volumetric modulated arc therapy for cranial radiosurgery using multiple noncoplanar arcs *Med. Phys.* **38** 5863–72

[45] Clark G M, Popple R A, Prendergast B M, Spencer S A, Thomas E M and Stewart J G *et al* 2012 Plan quality and treatment planning technique for single isocenter cranial radio-surgery with volumetric modulated arc therapy *Pract. Radiat. Oncol.* **2** 306–13

[46] Thomas E M, Popple R A, Wu X, Clark G M, Markert J M and Guthrie B L *et al* 2014 Comparison of plan quality and delivery time between volumetric arc therapy (RapidArc) and gamma knife radiosurgery for multiple cranial metastases *Neurosurgery* **75** 409–18
[47] Lutz W, Winston K R and Maleki N 1988 A system for stereotactic radiosurgery with linear accelerator *Int. J. Radiat. Oncol. Biol. Phys.* **14** 373–81
[48] Panet-Raymond V, Ansbacher W, Zavgorodni S, Bendorffe B, Nichol A and Truong P T *et al* 2012 Coplanar versus noncoplanar intensity-modulated radiation therapy (IMRT) and volumetric-modulated arc therapy (VMAT) treatment planning for fronto-temporal high-grade glioma *J. Appl. Clin. Med. Phys.* **13** 44–53
[49] Uto M, Mizowaki T, Ogura K and Hiraoka M 2016 Non-coplanar volumetric-modulated arc therapy (VMAT) for craniopharyngiomas reduced radiation doses to the bilateral hippocampus: a planning study comparing dynamic conformal arc therapy, coplanar VMAT, and non-coplanar VMAT *Radiat. Oncol.* **11** 86
[50] Smyth G, Bamber J C, Evans P M and Bedford J L 2013 Trajectory optimization for dynamic couch rotation during volumetric modulated arc radiotherapy *Phys. Med. Biol.* **58** 8163–77
[51] Smyth G, Evans P M, Bamber J C, Mandeville H C, Welsh L C and Saran F H *et al* 2016 Non-coplanar trajectories to improve organ at risk sparing in volumetric modulated arc therapy for primary brain tumors *Radiother. Oncol.* **121** 124–31
[52] Smyth G, Evans P M, Bamber J C, Mandeville H C, Moore A R and Welsh L C *et al* 2019 Dosimetric accuracy of dynamic couch rotating during volumetric modulated arc therapy (DCR-VMAT) for primary brain tumours *Phys. Med. Biol.* **64** 08NT01
[53] Fix M K, Frei D, Volken W, Terribilini D, Mueller S and Elicin O *et al* 2018 Part 1: optimization and evaluation of dynamic trajectory radiotherapy *Med. Phys.* **45** 4201–12
[54] Reggiori G, Mancosu P, Castiglioni S, Alongi F, Pellegrini C and Lobefalo F *et al* 2012 Can volumetric modulated arc therapy with flattening filter free beams play a role in stereotactic body radiotherapy for liver lesions? A volume-based analysis *Med. Phys.* **39** 1112–8
[55] Chung J B, Kim J S, Eom K Y, Kim I A, Kang S W and Lee J W *et al* 2015 Comparison of VMAT-SABR treatment plans with flattening filter (FF) and flattening filter-free (FFF) beam for localized prostate cancer *J. Appl. Clin. Med. Phys.* **16** 302–13
[56] Ong *et al* 2012 arc delivery for stereotactic body radiotherapy of vertebral and lung tumors *Int. J. Radiat. Oncol. Biol. Phys.* **83** e137–43
[57] Liu H W, Olivotto I, Lau H, Nugent Z and Khan R 2016 Role of volumetric-modulated arc therapy with flattening filter free delivery in lung stereotactic body radiotherapy *J. Med. Imag. Rad. Sci.* **47** 155–9
[58] Lai Y, Chen S, Xu C, Shi L, Fu L and Ha H *et al* 2017 Dosimetric superiority of flattening filter free beams for single-fraction stereotactic radiosurgery in single brain metastasis *Oncotarget* **8** 35272–9
[59] Spruijt K H, Dahele M, Cuijpers J P, Jeulink M, Rietveld D and Slotman B J *et al* 2013 Flattening filter free vs flattened beams for breast irradiation *Int. J. Rad. Oncol. Biol. Phys.* **85** 506–13
[60] Koivumäki T, Heikkilä J, Koskela K, Sillanmäki S and Seppälä J 2016 Flattening filter free technique in breath-hold treatments of left-sided breast cancer: the effect on beam-on time and dose distribution *Radiother. Oncol.* **118** 194–8

[61] Jia F, Xu D, Yue H, Wu H and Li G 2018 Comparison of flattening filter and flattening filter-free volumetric modulated arc radiotherapy in patients with locally advanced nasopharyngeal carcinoma *Med. Sci. Monit.* **24** 8500–5

[62] Vassiliev O N, Kry S F, Kuban K A, Salehpour M, Mohan R and Titt U 2007 Treatment-planning study of prostate cancer intensity-modulated radiotherapy with a Varian Clinac operater without a flattening filter *Int. J. Radiat. Oncol. Biol. Phys.* **68** 1567–71

[63] Zwahlen D R, Lang S, Hrbacek J, Glanzmann C, Kloeck S and Najafi Y *et al* 2012 The use of photon beams of a flattening filter-free linear accelerator for hypofractionated volumetric modulated arc therapy in localized prostate cancer *Int. J. Radiat. Oncol. Biol. Phys.* **83** 1655–60

[64] Nicolini G, Ghosh-Laskar S, Shrivastava S K, Banerjee S, Chaudhary S and Agarwal J P *et al* 2012 Volumetric modulation arc radiotherapy with flattening filter-free beams compared with static gantry IMRT and 3D conformal radiotherapy for advanced esophageal cancer: a feasibility study *Int. J. Radiat. Oncol. Biol. Phys.* **84** 553–60

[65] Subramanian S, Thirumalaiswamy S, Srinivas C, Gandhi G A, Kathirvel M and Kumar K K *et al* 2012 Chest wall radiotherapy with volumetric modulated arcs and the potential role of flattening filter free photon beams *Strahlenther. Onkol.* **188** 484–91

[66] Kragl G, Baier F, Lutz S, Albrich D, Dalaryd M and Kroupa B *et al* 2011 Flattening filter free beams in SBRT and IMRT: dosimetric assessment of peripheral doses *Z. Med. Phys.* **21** 91–101

[67] Stathakis S, Esquivel C, Gutierrez A, Buckey C R and Papanikolau N 2009 Treatment planning and delivery of IMRT using 6 and 18 MV phtotn beams without flattening filter *Appl. Rad. Isot.* **67** 1629–37

[68] Cashmore J, Ramtohul M and Ford D 2011 Lowering whole-body radiation doses in pediatric intensity-modulated radiotherapy through the use of unflattened photon beams *Int. J. Radiat. Oncol. Biol. Phys.* **80** 1220–7

[69] Mohan R, Arnfield M, Tong S, Wu Q and Siebers J 2000 The impact of fluctuations in intensity patterns on the number of monitor units and the quality and accuracy of intensity modulated radiotherapy *Med. Phys.* **27** 1226–37

[70] Llacer J, Solberg T D and Promberger C 2001 Comparative behaviour of the dynamically penalized likelihood algorithm in inverse radiation therapy planning *Phys. Med. Biol.* **46** 2637–63

[71] Webb S 2001 A simple method to control aspects of fluence modulation in IMRT planning *Phys. Med. Biol.* **46** N187–95

[72] Webb S 2003 The physical basis of IMRT and inverse planning *Br. J. Radiol.* **76** 678–89

[73] Nicolini G, Fogliata A, Vanetti E, Clivio A, Ammazzalorso F and Cozzi L 2007 What is an acceptably smoothed fluence? Dosimetric and delivery considerations for dynamic sliding window IMRT *Radiat. Oncol.* **2** 42

[74] Park J M, Park S Y, Kim H, Kim J H, Carlson J and Ye S J 2014 Modulation indices for volumetric modulated arc therapy *Phys. Med. Biol.* **59** 7315–40

[75] Park J M, Park S Y and Kim H 2015 Modulation index for VMAT considering both mechanical and dose calculation uncertainties *Phys. Med. Biol.* **60** 7101–25

[76] McNiven A L, Sharpe M B and Purdie T G 2010 A new metric for assessing IMRT modulation complexity and plan deliverability *Med. Phys.* **37** 505–15

[77] Masi L, Doro R, Favuzza V, Cipressi S and Livi L 2013 Impact of plan parameters on the dosimetric accuracy of volumetric modulated arc therapy *Med. Phys.* **40** 071817

[78] McGarry C K, Agnew C E, Hussein M, Tsang Y, McWilliam A and Hounsell A R *et al* 2016 The role of complexity metrics in a multi-institutional dosimetry audit of VMAT *Br. J. Radiol.* **89** 20150445

[79] Karin T, Crowe S B, Kenny J, Knight R T and Trapp J V 2014 Predicting the likelihood of QA failure using treatment plan accuracy metrics *J. Phys. Conf. Ser.* **489** 012051

[80] Du W, Cho S H, Zhang X, Hoffman K E and Kudchadker R J 2014 Quantification of beam complexity in intensity-modulated radiation therapy treatment plans *Med. Phys.* **41** 021716

[81] Crowe S B, Kairn T, Middlebrook N, Sutherland B, Hill B and Kenny J *et al* 2015 Examination of the properties of IMRT and VMAT beams and evaluation against pre-treatment quality assurance results *Phys. Med. Biol.* **60** 2587–601

[82] Park S Y, Kim J I, Chun M, Ahn H and Park J M 2018 Assessment of the modulation degrees of intensity-modulated radiation therapy plans *Radiat. Oncol.* **13** 244

[83] Park S Y, Kim J I, Oh D H and Park J M 2019 Evaluation of the plan delivery accuracy of intensity-modulated therapy by texture analysis using fluence maps *Phys. Med.* **59** 64–74

[84] Antoine M, Ralite F, Soustiel C, Marsac T, Sargos P and Cugny A *et al* 2019 Use of metrics to quantify IMRT and VMAT treatment plan complexity: a systematic review and perspectives *Phys. Med.* **64** 98–108

[85] Cheng C W, Das I J and Chen D J 1994 Dosimetry in the moving gap region in craniospinal irradiation *Br. J. Radiol.* **67** 1017–22

[86] Wu Q, Arnfield M, Tong S, Wu Y and Mohan R 2000 Dynamic splitting of large intensity-modulated fields *Phys. Med. Biol.* **45** 1731–40

[87] Malhotra H K, Raina S, Avadhani J S, deBoer S and Podgorsak M B 2006 Technical and dosimetric consideration in IMRT treatment planning for large target volumes *J. Appl. Clin. Med. Phys.* **6** 77–87

[88] Srivastava S P, Das I J, Kumar A and Johnstone P A S 2011 Dosimetric comparison of split field and fixed jaw techniques for large IMRT target volumes in the head and neck *Med. Dosim.* **36** 6–9

[89] Yom S S, Frija E D, Mahajan A, Chang E, Klein K and Shiu A *et al* 2007 Field-in-field technique with intrafractionally modulated junction shifts for craniospinal irradiation *Int. J. Radiat. Oncol. Biol. Phys.* **69** 1193–8

[90] South M, Chiu J K, The B S, Bloch C, Schroeder T M and Paulino A C 2008 Supine craniospinal irradiation using intrafractional junction shifts and field-in-field dose shaping: early experience at Methodist Hospital *Int. J. Radiat. Oncol. Biol. Phys.* **71** 477–83

[91] Wilkinson J M, Lewis J, Lawrence G P, Lucraft H H and Murphy E 2007 Craniospinal irradiation using a forward planned segmented field technique *Br. J. Radiol.* **80** 209–15

[92] Sharma D S, Gupta T, Jalali R, Master Z, Phurailatpam R D and Sarin R 2009 High-precision radiotherapy for craniospinal irradiation: evaluation of three-dimensional conformal radiotherapy, intensity-modulated radiation therapy and helical TomoTherapy *Br. J. Radiol.* **82** 1000–9

[93] Clair W H St., Adams J A, Bues M, Fullerton B C, La Shell S and Kooy H M *et al* 2004 Advantage of protons compared to conventional x-ray or IMRT in the treatment of a pediatric patient with medulloblastoma *Int. J. Radiat. Oncol. Biol. Phys.* **58** 727–34

[94] Pai Panandiker A, Ning H, Likhacheva A, Ullman K, Arora B and Ondos J *et al* 2007 Craniospinal irradiation with spinal IMRT to improve target homogeneity *Int. J. Radiat. Oncol. Biol. Phys.* **68** 1402–9

[95] Zeng G G, Heaton R K, Catton C N, Chung P W, O'Sullivan B and Lau M *et al* 2007 A two isocenter IMRT technique with a controlled junction dose for long volume targets *Phys. Med. Biol.* **52** 4541–52

[96] Cao F, Ramaseshan R, Corns R, Harrop S, Nuraney N and Steiner P *et al* 2012 A three-isocenter jagged-junction IMRT approach for craniospinal irradiation without beam edge matching for field junctions *Int. J. Radiat. Oncol. Biol. Phys.* **84** 648–54

[97] Hadley A and Ding G X 2014 A single-gradient junction technique to replace multiple-junction shifts for craniospinal irradiation treatment *Med. Dosim.* **39** 314–9

[98] Seppälä J, Kulmala J, Lindholm P and Minn H 2010 A method to improve target dose homogeneity of craniospinal irradiation using dynamic split field IMRT *Radiother. Oncol.* **96** 209–15

[99] Fogliata A, Bergström S, Cafaro I, Clivio A, Cozzi L and Dipasquale G *et al* 2011 Craniospinal irradiation with volumetric modulated arc therapy: a multi-institutional treatment experience *Radiother. Oncol.* **99** 79–85

[100] Chen J, Chen C, Atwood T F, Gibbs I C and Soltys S G *et al* 2012 Volumetric modulated arc therapy planning method for supine craniospinal irradiation *J. Radiat. Oncol.* **1** 291–7

[101] Lee Y K, Brooks C J, Bedford J L, Warrington A P and Saran F H 2012 Development and evaluation of multiple isocentric volumetric modulated arc therapy technique for craniospinal axis radiotherapy planning *Int. J. Radiat. Oncol. Biol. Phys.* **82** 1006–12

[102] Myers P, Stathakis S, Mavroidis P, Esquivel C and Papanikolaou N 2013 Evaluation of localization errors for craniospinal axis irradiation delivery using volume modulated arc therapy and proposal of a technique to minimize such errors *Radiother. Oncol.* **108** 107–13

[103] Strojnik A, Méndez I and Peterlin P 2016 Reducing the dosimetric impact of positional errors in field junctions for craniospinal irradiation using VMAT *Rep. Pract. Oncol. Radiother.* **21** 232–9

[104] Hsieh J 1995 Image artifacts, causes, and correction *Medical CT and Ultrasound, Current Technology and Application* ed L W Goldman and J B Fowlkers (Madison, WI: Advanced Medical Publishing) p 487–518

[105] Reft C, Alecu R, Das I J, Gerbi B J, Keall P and Lief E *et al* 2003 Dosimetric considerations for patients whit hip prostheses undergoing pelvic irradiation. Report of the AAPM Radiation Therapy Committee Task Group 63 *Med. Phys.* **30** 1162–82

[106] Wei J, Sandison G A, His W C, Ringor M and Lu X 2006 Dosimetric impact of a CT metal artefact suppression algorithm for proton, electron and photon therapies *Phys. Med. Biol.* **51** 5183–97

[107] Bazalova M, Baulieu L, Palefsky S and Verhaegen F 2007 Correction of CT artifacts and its influence on Monte Carlo dose calculations *Med. Phys.* **34** 2119–32

[108] Ezzell G A, Galvin J M, Low D, Palta J R, Rosen I and Sharpe M B *et al* 2003 Guidance document on delivery, treatment planning, and clinical implementation of IMRT: report of the IMRT subcommittee of the AAPM radiation therapy committee *Med. Phys.* **30** 2089–115

[109] Kim Y, Tomé W A, Bal M, McNutt T R and Spies L 2006 The impact of dental metal artifacts on head and neck IMRT dose distributions *Radiother. Oncol.* **79** 198–202

[110] Kim Y and Tomé W A 2007 On the radiobiological impact of metal artifact in head-and-neck IMRT in terms of tumor control probability (TCP) and normal tissue complication probability (NTCP) *Med. Bio. Eng. Comput.* **45** 1045–51

[111] Webster G J, Rowbottom C G and Mackay R I 2009 Evaluation of the impact of dental artefacts on intensity-modulated radiotherapy planning for the head and neck *Radiother. Oncol.* **93** 553–8
[112] Lin M H, Li J, Price R A Jr, Wang L, Lee C C and Ma C M 2013 The dosimetric impact of dental implants on head-and-neck volumetric modulated arc therapy *Phys. Med. Biol.* **58** 1027–40
[113] Giantsoudi D, De Man B, Verburg J, Trofimov A, Jin Y and Wang G *et al* 2017 Metal artifacts in computed tomography for radiation therapy planning: dosimetric effects and impact of metal artifact reduction *Phys. Med. Biol.* **62** R49–80
[114] Maerz M, Koelbl O and Dobler B 2015 Influence of metallic dental implants and metal artefacts on dose calculation accuracy *Strahlenther. Onkol.* **191** 234–41
[115] Spadea M F, Verburg J, Baroni G and Seco J 2013 Dosimetric assessment of a novel metal artifact reduction method in CT images *J. Appl. Clin. Med. Phys.* **14** 299–304
[116] Spadea M F, Verburg J M, Baroni G and Seco J 2014 The impact of low-Z and high-Z metal implants in IMRT: a Monte Carlo study of dose inaccuracies in commercial dose algorithms *Med. Phys.* **41** 011702
[117] Lin C I, Feng Y, Jiang W and Huang Z 2018 Quantification of dosimetric effects of dental metallic implant on volumetric-modulated arc therapy plans *Int. J. Cancer Clin. Res.* **5** 092
[118] Bär E, Schwahofer A, Kuchenbecker S and Häring P 2015 Improving radiotherapy planning in patients with metallic implants using the iterative metal artifact reduction (iMAR) algorithm *Biomed. Phys. Eng. Express* **1** 025206
[119] Ziemann C, Stille M, Cremers F, Buzug T M and Rades D 2018 Improvement of dose calculation in radiation therapy due to metal artifact correction using the augmented likelihood image reconstruction *J. Appl. Clin. Med. Phys.* **19** 227–33
[120] Yu C X, Jaffray D A and Wong J W 1998 The effects of intra-fraction organ motion on the delivery of dynamic intensity modulation *Phys. Med. Biol.* **43** 91–104
[121] Yang J N, Mackie T R, Reckwerdt P, Deasy J O and Thomadsen B R 1997 An investigation of tomotherapy beam delivery *Med. Phys.* **24** 425–36
[122] Bortfeld T, Jokivarsi K, Goitein M, Kung J and Jiang S B 2002 Effects of intra-fraction motion on IMRT dose delivery: statistical analysis and simulation *Phys. Med. Biol.* **47** 2203–20
[123] Court L E, Wagar M, Ionascu D, Berbeco R and Chin L 2008 Management of the interplay effect when using dynamic MLC sequences to treat moving targets *Med. Phys.* **35** 1926–31
[124] Court L, Wagar M, Berbeco R, Reisner A, Winey B and Allen A M *et al* 2010 Evaluation of the interplay effect when using RapidArc to treat targets moving in the craniocaudal or right-left direction *Med. Phys.* **37** 4–11
[125] Ong C L, Verbakel W F A R, Cuijpers J P, Slotman B J and Senan S 2011 Dosimetric impact of interplay effect on RapidArc lung stereotactic treatment delivery *Int. J. Radiat. Oncol. Biol. Phys.* **79** 305–11
[126] Rao M, Wu J, Cao D, Wong T, Mehta V and Shepard D *et al* 2012 Dosimetric impact of breathing motion in lung stereotactic body radiotherapy treatment using image-modulated radiotherapy and volumetric modulated arc therapy *Int. J. Radiat. Oncol. Biol. Phys.* **83** e251–6
[127] Ong C L, Dahele M, Slotman B J and Verbakel W F A R 2013 Dosimetric impact of the interplay effect during stereotactic lung radiation therapy delivery using flattening filter-free beams and volumetric modulated arc therapy *Int. J. Radiat. Oncol. Biol. Phys.* **86** 743–8

[128] Zou W, Yin L, Shen J, Corradetti M N, Kirk M and Munbodh R *et al* 2014 Dynamic simulation of motion effects in IMAT lung SBRT *Radiat. Oncol.* **9** 225

[129] Tyler M K 2016 Quantification of interplay and gradient effects for lung stereotactic ablative radiotherapy (SABR) treatments *J. Appl. Clin. Med. Phys.* **17** 158–66

[130] Mukhlisin P S A 2016 Dosimetric impact of interplay effect in lung IMRT and VMAT treatment using in-house dynamic thorax phantom *J. Phys. Conf. Ser.* **694** 012009

[131] Kuno K, Monzen H, Tamura M, Hirata M, Ishii K and Okada W *et al* 2018 Minimizing dose variation from the interplay effect in stereotactic radiation therapy using volumetric modulated arc therapy for lung cancer *J. Appl. Clin. Med. Phys.* **19** 121–7

[132] Hubley E and Pierce G 2017 The influence of plan modulation on the interplay effect in VMAT liver SBRT treatments *Phys. Med.* **40** 115–21

[133] Ecclestone G and Pierce G 2015 The role of VMAT interplay effect for liver stereotactic body radiation therapy *Proceedings of the World Congress on Medical Physics and Biomedical Engineering, June 7-12 Toronto, IFMBE* ed D Jaffray vol 51 (Cham: Springer)

[134] Sasaki M, Nakamura M, Mukumoto N, Goto Y, Ishihara Y and Nakata M *et al* 2019 Variation in accumulated dose of volumetric-modulated arc therapy for pancreatic cancer due to different beam starting phases *J. Appl. Clin. Med. Phys.* **20** 118–26

[135] Netherton T, Li Y, Nitsch P, Shaitelman S, Balter P and Gao S *et al* 2018 Interplay effect on a 6-MV flattening-filter-free linear accelerator with high dose rate and fast multi-leaf collimator motion treating breast and lung phantoms *Med. Phys.* **45** 2369–76

[136] Wakai N, Zhou P, Das I, Takashina M, Koizumi M and Ogawa K *et al* 2013 Impact of motion interplay effect on step and shoot IMRT *Int. J. Radiat. Oncol. Biol. Phys.* **87** S701

[137] Gauer T, Sothmann T, Blanck O, Petersen C and Werner R 2018 Under-reported dosimetry errors due to interplay effects during VMAT dose delivery in extreme hypo-fractionated stereotactic radiotherapy *Strahlenther. Onkol.* **194** 570–9

[138] Edvardsson A, Nordström F, Ceberg C and Ceberg S 2018 Motion induced interplay effects for VMAT radiotherapy *Phys. Med. Biol.* **63** 085012

[139] Edvardsson A 2018 *Dosimetric Effects of Breathing Motion in Radiotherapy* (Lund: Lund University, Faculty of Science, Department of Medical Radiation Physics)

[140] Das I J and Kase K R 1992 Higher energy: is it necessary, is it worth the cost of radiation oncology? *Med. Phys.* **19** 917–25

[141] Söderström S, Eklöf A and Brahme A 1999 Aspects on the optimal photon beam energy for radiation therapy *Acta Oncol.* **38** 179–87

[142] Laughlin J S, Mohan R and Kutcher G J 1986 Choice of optimum megavoltage for accelerators for photon beam treatment *Int. J. Radiat. Oncol. Biol. Phys.* **12** 1551–7

[143] Welsh J S, Mackie T R and Limmer J P 2007 High-energy photons in IMRT: uncertainties and risks for questionable gain *Technol. Cancer Res. Treat.* **6** 147–9

[144] deBoer S F, Kumek Y, Jaggernauth W and Podgorsak M B 2007 The effect of beam energy on the quality of IMRT plans for the prostate conformal radiotherapy *Technol. Cancer Res. Treat.* **6** 139–46

[145] Followill D, Geis P and Boyer A 1997 Estimates of whole-body dose equivalent produced by beam intensity modulated conformal therapy *Int. J. Radiat. Oncol. Biol. Phys.* **38** 667–72

[146] Chibani O and Ma C M C 2003 Photonuclear dose calculations for high-energy photon beams from Siemens and Varian linacs *Med. Phys.* **30** 1990–2000

[147] Hall E J and Wuu C S 2003 Radiation-induced second cancers: the impact or 3D-CRT and IMRT *Int. J. Radiat. Oncol. Biol. Phys.* **56** 83–8

[148] Kry S F, Salehpour M, Followill D, Stovall M, Kuban D A and White A *et al* 2005 The calculated risk of fatal secondary malignancies from intensity-modulated radiation therapy *Int. J. Radiat. Oncol. Biol. Phys.* **62** 1195–203
[149] Rawlinson J A, Islam M K and Galbraith D M 2002 Dose to radiation therapists from activation at high-energy accelerators used for conventional and intensity-modulated radiation therapy *Med. Phys.* **29** 598–608
[150] Perrin B, Walker A and Mackay R 2003 A model to calculate the induced dose rate around an 18 MV Elekta linear accelerator *Phys. Med. Biol.* **48** N75–81
[151] Zanini A, Durisi E, Fasolo F, Ongaro C, Visca L and Nastasi U *et al* 2004 Monte Carlo simulation of the photoneutron field in linac radiotherapy treatments with different collimation systems *Phys. Med. Biol.* **49** 571–82
[152] Howell R M, Ferenci M S, Hertel N E, Fullerton G D, Fox T and Davis L W 2005 Measurements of secondary neutron dose from 15 MV and 18 MV IMRT *Radiat. Prot. Dosim.* **115** 508–12
[153] Howell R M, Kry S F, Burgett E, Hertel N E and Followill D S 2009 Secondary neutron spectra from modern Varian, Siemens, and Elekta linacs with multileaf collimators *Med. Phys.* **36** 4027–38
[154] Naseri A and Mesbahi A 2010 A review of photoneutrons characteristics in radiation therapy with high-energy photon beams *Rep. Pract. Oncol. Radiother.* **15** 138–44
[155] Takam R, Bezak E, Marcu L G and Yeoh E 2011 Out-of-field neutron and leakage photon exposures and the associated risk of second cancers in high-energy photon radiotherapy: current status *Radiat. Res.* **176** 508–20
[156] Patil B J, Chavan S T, Pethe S N, Krishnan R, Bhoraskar V N and Dhole S D 2011 Estimation of neutron production from accelerator head assembly of 15 MV medical linac using FLUKA simulations *Nucl. Instr. Meth. Phys. Res.* B **269** 3261–5
[157] Israngkul-Na-Ayuthaya I, Suriyapee S and Pengvanich P 2015 Evaluation of equivalent dose from neutrons and activation products from a 15-MV x-ray linac *J. Radiat. Res.* **56** 919–26
[158] Yücel H, Çobanbaş İ, Kolbaşi A, Yüksel A Ö and Kaya V 2016 Measurement of photo-neutron dose from an 18-MV medical linac using a foil activation method in view of radiation protection of patients *Nucl. Eng. Technol.* **48** 525–32
[159] Horst F, Fehrenbacher G and Zink K 2017 On the neutron radiation field and air activation around a medical electron linac *Radiat. Prot. Dosim.* **174** 147–58
[160] Weiss E, Siebers J V and Keall P J 2007 An analysis of 6-MV versus 18-MV photon energy plans for intensity-modulated radiation therapy (IMRT) of lung cancer *Radiother. Oncol.* **82** 55–62
[161] Solaiappan G, Singaravelu G, Prakasarao A, Rabbani B and Supe S S 2009 Influence of photon beam energy on IMRT plan quality for radiotherapy of prostate cancer *Rep. Pract. Oncol. Radiother.* **14** 18–31
[162] Tyagi A, Supe S S, Sandeep and Sing M P 2010 A dosimetric analysis of 6 MV versus 15 MV photon energy plans for intensity modulated radiation therapy (IMRT) of carcinoma of cervix *Rep. Pract. Oncol. Radiother.* **15** 125–31
[163] Sung W, Park J M, Choi C H, Ha S W and Ye S J 2012 The effect of photon energy on intensity-modulated radiation therapy (IMRT) plans for prostate cancer *Radiat. Oncol. J.* **30** 27–35

[164] Kumar L, Yadav G, Raman K, Bhushan M and Pal M 2015 The dosimetric impact of different photon beam energy on RapidArc radiotherapy planning for cervix carcinoma *J. Med. Phys.* **40** 207–13

[165] Hälg R A, Besserer J, Boschung M, Mayer S and Schneider U 2012 Monitor units are not predictive of neutron dose for high-energy IMRT *Radiat. Oncol.* **7** 138

[166] Li D, Deng X, Xue Y, Lou Z, Zhang Y and Guo W *et al* 2017 Neutron dose distribution in the treatment room for an accelerator in the flattening filter-free mode *Prec. Radiat. Oncol.* **1** 13–9

[167] Dawn S, Pal R, Bakashi A K, Kinhikar R A, Joshi K and Jamema S V *et al* 2018 Evaluation of in-field neutron production for medical linacs with and without flattening filter for various beam parameters—Experimental and Monte Carlo simulation *Radiat. Meas.* **118** 98–107

IOP Publishing

Intensity Modulated Radiation Therapy
A clinical overview
Indra J Das, Nicholas J Sanfilippo, Antonella Fogliata and Luca Cozzi

Chapter 9

Optimization

The optimization processes can determine the optimal solution of different requests. It could be, in the IMRT or VMAT flow, the optimization of the gantry angles of the fixed beams or the arc span for the arc therapy, or the optimization of the number of fields/arcs, or the optimization of the collimator rotation, or the optimization of the fluence maps, or other parameters. In this chapter, only the fluence map optimization is described, which is relevent to this book.

9.1 The inverse planning concept

To understand the need of the optimization algorithm to solve the inverse planning process, we have to look at the origin of the intensity modulation, that could be dated to 1982 with the seminal work of Brahme [1]. In their work, the authors intended to determine the dose profile needed to deliver a high dose to a ring shape target of inner radius r_0 and outer radius r, while maximally sparing the OAR with a circular shape of radius r_0 (where to deliver no primary fluence) located inside the target, as shown in figure 9.1.

They showed how to obtain the mathematical solution to this problem, giving the fundaments for the inverse planning concept. Interesting to note is that, at the time of the paper, the MLC was not yet available (the beam modulation was done in terms of different thicknesses for blocks), and the delivery was supposed to be through a rotating source (arc). In this archetypal problem of intensity modulation, in a simplified vision, during the rotation, a homogeneous beam could irradiate the target, and a block can shield the OAR. The points lying in the target and close to the OAR will result more blocked than those in the target and close to its external periphery. To obtain a homogeneous dose in the target, more dose is needed to be delivered in the region of the target close to the OAR, resulting in an inhomogeneous delivered fluence (shown as different block thickness in figure 9.1). This established the concept of the planning as an inverse problem: knowing the goal of homogeneous dose in the target with maximal sparing of the OAR, the solution of the

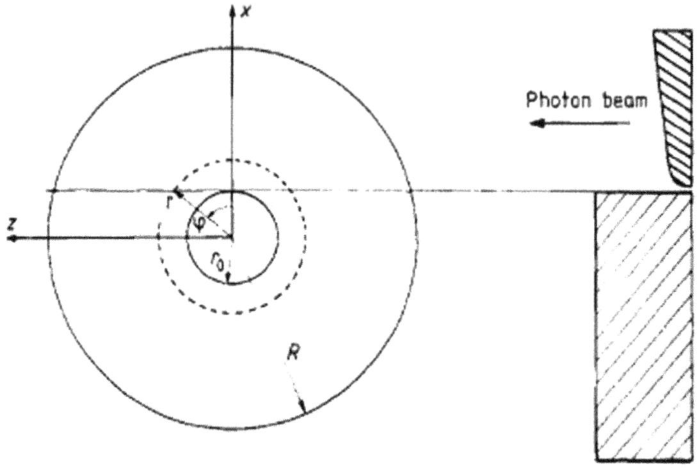

Figure 9.1. The 'Brahme's problem': a geometry with an inner circle to block and an annulus just outside to homogenously irradiate. From Brahme *et al* [1], reproduced with permission. Copyright IOP Publishing Ltd. All rights reserved.

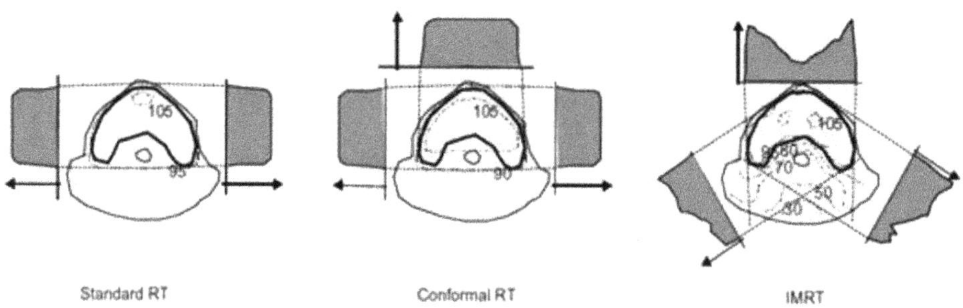

Figure 9.2. Uniform beams or arcs can deliver only concave treatment volumes. Non-uniform beams can also deliver convex treatment volumes. [2], reprinted by permission of Taylor & Francis Ltd.

problem is the shape of the fluence (or the varying thickness of the block). In 1988 Brahme [3] proposed the new inverse approach for beam optimization. The method derived the optimum incident beam dose distribution for the desired dose distribution in the target volume. He determined that the optimum shape of the incident beam for each gantry angle can be obtained by inverse back-projection of the point irradiation density on the position of the radiation source for that incident beam. In his work, Brahme proved that, as shown in figure 9.2, aiming to irradiate concave target volumes, uniform beams cannot produce concave treatment volumes (isodoses). It is only with the non-uniform beam irradiation, i.e., when the fluence is modulated across the fields, that the treatment volume can conform around the target volume following the specific shape.

The inverse planning problem is similar to the back-projection used in the CT reconstruction imaging, as then described by Bortfeld in 1990 [4]. In the CT image reconstruction problem, given the measured radiation projection along a large number of incident angles, the density distribution is to be computed. In a mirrored way, given the desired dose distribution, the beam profile from a large number of beam entrances is to be calculated. These concepts have been discussed in chapter 4 of this book.

The problem of the inverse planning resides in the fact that the ideal solution, in some part of the beam, gives a negative dose that is not physically realizable. Considering the archetypal Brahme problem in figure 9.1, the ideal dose distribution is the prescription dose in the ring-shaped target, and zero dose in the OAR embedded in the target. Although no direct dose is delivered to the OAR, an amount of scattered dose is delivered anyhow, and this is physically unavoidable. A mathematical optimization process, under the limit of zero dose to the OAR, would propose a negative dose to compensate for the scatter. To solve this problem, two methods were introduced. With the first approach, all the negative dose voxels were reset to zero [5]. The second method [6] required adding, to each entrance, a uniform beam sufficient to keep the non-negative intensity. The results won't be the ideal solution which is impossible to deliver, and this is one of the reasons why the optimal solution derived from the optimization process is not necessarily the best. A strategy needs to be defined to find the *best* possible plan physically realisable, and this can be attempted only when the problem is clearly defined.

9.2 The goals and the cost function

The way to thoroughly define the problem for the inverse planning is ideally strictly linked to the clinical results related to the dose levels to deliver to each target and OAR. However, the dose–volume effects, the various tissue radiosensitivities are not known, and the clinical importance of the physical dose homogeneity in the target volume is pretty undetermined. A biological approach (described later in this chapter) would be desirable, but the physical one is more robust.

The physical parameters that we could correlate to the clinical results have the advantage, in contrast to the biological parameters, of being **well-defined** and **measurable**: the physical absorbed dose and the volume of a structure are well-defined, computable, and quantifiable with reasonable accuracy.

Let us now suppose we know which is the desirable physical dose distribution in each beam element (bixel), $D^d(x,y,z)$, i.e., we have a conceptually well-defined problem to solve [7]. Consider an iterative optimization process that, at each iteration, generates a plan with dose distribution $D^o(x,y,z)$ in each bixel (x,y,z) of a volume, accounting for an importance factor $P(x,y,z)$ which can include the clinical trade-offs between target coverage and OAR sparing, or different OAR sparing levels. A cost function can be generated:

$$\text{cost} = \sum_{(x,y,z)\epsilon \text{Volume}} P(x, y, z)[D^o(x, y, z) - D^d(x, y, z)]^2 \tag{9.1}$$

The optimized dose distribution D^o which better approximates the desired one D^d and better respects the required importance P, is that which minimizes the cost. The problem is hence translated in the minimization, through an iterative process, of a *cost function*, often called also *objective function.*

The dose distribution can be expressed as:

$$\mathbf{D} = A \cdot \mathbf{b} \tag{9.2}$$

where **D** is the 3D dose distribution, **b** is the intensity parameter to optimize per each bixel, A is the matrix linking each dose-space element to the corresponding beam-space element, and represents the elemental dose in the specific bixels. The solution of (9.2) is:

$$\mathbf{b} = A^{-1} \cdot \mathbf{D} \tag{9.3}$$

which gives the intensity modulation required to deliver the dose **D**.

The desired dose distribution $D^d(x,y,z)$ cannot be practically given as such, and the physical dose and dose–volume parameters have to be addressed to feed the cost function and possibly find the optimal dose by the minimization of the cost. Those parameters are the *optimization objectives.*

In practice, we need to feed the optimization process with such knowledge, which is a 3D dose distribution on the patient anatomy based on the CT dataset. The anatomy (target and OAR), is based on the contours from the CT, affected by the uncertainties arising from contouring, image quality, eventual image co-registration. Additionally, the structure delineation cannot discriminate the radiosensitivity and the functionality of the structures and sub-structures of the different organs. Onto this simplified anatomy, the desired dose distribution needs to be simplified, since it is impracticable to describe a 3D dose distribution. The first step is the use of the DVH, which is a summary of a dose distribution inside each structure: the spatial information is lost, and for complex structures, this could be a piece of important information missing. From the DVH we can imagine extracting some physical dose–volume parameters which correlate with clinical results, also considering the knowledge from the clinical studies, where only a few physical parameters are given as tolerance dose (or dose–volume) levels. In this way, the dose distribution is reduced from a 3D distribution to a few parameters (scalars) per structure, the *optimization objectives*, oversimplifying the requests (that are imprecise and not well known).

9.3 The optimization objectives

The optimization objectives should be derived from the clinical experience, in the sense that they should be obtained from studies analyzing the correlation between accurately computed dose distribution and clinical observations.

For target structures, since a homogeneous dose distribution is generally desired, two dose objectives, or *constraints* can be set, in terms of minimum and maximum doses: D_{min} and D_{max}. With these constraints, the wish is to have, in all the bixels located inside the structure delineated as the target, a dose between D_{min} and D_{max}.

For the OAR, simple maximum dose constraints can work only for serial organs, like the spinal cord. However, the vast majority of the critical structures are not purely serial and present more or less significant volume effects. In those cases, the maximum dose constraints are generally not sufficient, and it is more appropriate to use the *DVH constraints*, or *dose–volume constraints*, which to a certain extent account for the volume dependence response. They are formulated in a way that no more than a certain amount of the structure volume *V* should receive more than a certain amount of dose *D*. In figure 9.3, this is shown on a hypothetical DVH. To an initial DVH (green), the dose–volume (D-V) constraint is applied, generating a region in the DVH where the cumulative DVH cannot reside. The resulting DVH (blue), after the optimization, has to lie below the forbidden zone.

With the DVH constraint, the spatial information is lost, and there is an infinite number of plans fulfilling the constraint criteria, producing the *degeneracy problem*. The inverse planning process cannot decide which is the best solution since the infinite solutions are acceptable. The decision can then be transferred back to the planner, who can add further dose–volume or even technical constraints that could drive the optimization toward a clinically and technically better solution.

An example of a technical constraint could be the smoothness of the intensity map. It has been proven that high fluence gradients that have no clinical need should be avoided to improve the accuracy in the dose delivery. This is achievable with a technical constraint to add to the cost function able to smooth the final fluence.

It could happen that different dose–volume constraints on different structures would conflict, and a solution fulfilling all the requests is impossible to find. An *importance factor* that can also be called a *penalty factor*, can be used in the cost function, allowing some permeability toward the forbidden region of the DVH, and can be interpreted as the price to pay for violating the dose–volume constraint. For example, with a small penalty, some overdose inside the forbidden region is allowed since its clinical consequence is only of a mild and acceptable complication. In contrast, a strong penalty would reduce the constraint permeability, hence not allowing the constraint overcoming since it may have a too severe clinical consequence and must be prevented. Although these are physical and not biological criteria, it appears evident that the importance of the translation of the constraints and penalties from the clinical knowledge into the mathematical language.

With all the points above described, it is possible to generate the cost function, as the sum of the contributions for all the structures, are they target or OAR, that

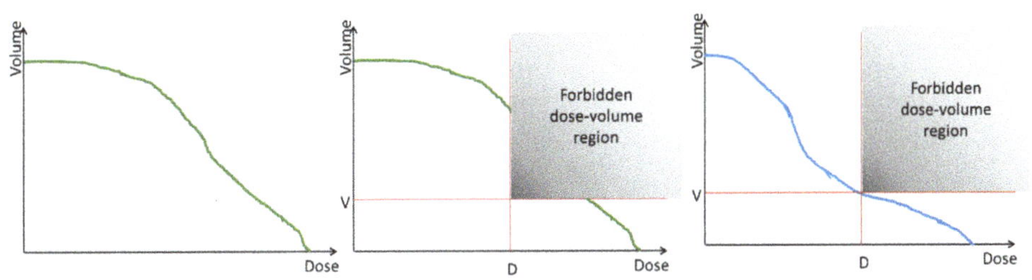

Figure 9.3. dose–volume constraint: initial DVH (on the left), application of the D-V constraint with the forbidden DVH region, resulting DVH after the optimization having applied the D-V constraint (on the right).

violate the dose–volume objectives. The bixels not violating the objectives won't contribute to the cost through the Heaviside function $H(x)$:

$$\text{Cost}(k) = \sum_{i=1}^{\text{Total } N \text{ bixel}} P_k \cdot \left(D_i^o - D_k^d\right)^2 \cdot H\left(D_k^d - D_i^o\right) \tag{9.4}$$

where k is the structure, P is the penalty, D^o is the optimizing dose, D^d is the desired dose, H is the Heaviside function, where $H(x) = 0$ for $x < 0$ and $H(x) = 1$ for $x > 0$. The penalty has different names in the clinical practice: penalty, priority, weight, importance. The global cost function will be combined, by summing up the cost of all the involved structures, be they targets or OARs:

$$\text{Total Cost} = \sum_{\text{PTVs}} \text{Cost(PTV)} + \sum_{\text{OARs}} \text{Cost(OAR)} \tag{9.5}$$

The optimization dose is changed along with a high number of iterations in the optimization process, and the changing variable is the fluence intensity per bixel. The optimization algorithms (the mathematical solution) to minimize the cost function are described in the next paragraph.

To visualize with an example of what happens during the optimization iterations, a simplification is shown in figure 9.4. A target structure is presented in the BEV in red, together with the beam divided into several pencil beams (the circles). The fluence intensity of each pencil is changed during each iteration, according to the optimization algorithm. The dose distribution is computed, the cost evaluated at each iteration, that will ideally continue until the cost cannot be further reduced (the minimum of the cost function is achieved). The final result will be the map of the pencil beam intensities over each field which minimized the cost function.

This example shows a simple approximation of pencils. However, an important parameter to adjust for the optimization is the size of the bixel, which translates into the optimization resolution. Bortfeld *et al* [8] determined that the optimal sampling should be related to the penumbra width, and should be about 1.5–2 mm. Attention on this point has to be paid to the risk of over-modulation when the optimization resolution is too fine, as described in chapter 8 on treatment planning, discussing the modulation degree and the delivery accuracy.

The continuously updated cost function during the optimization is shown in figure 9.5, where a case of a modification of a dose–volume constraint is also presented. These cost functions are cumulative of the whole plan. However,

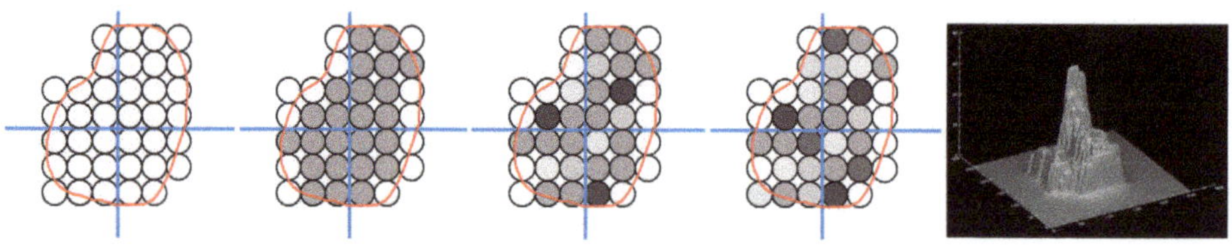

Figure 9.4. Example of intensity pixel changes at four iterations. On the right, the optimal fluence at the end of the optimization.

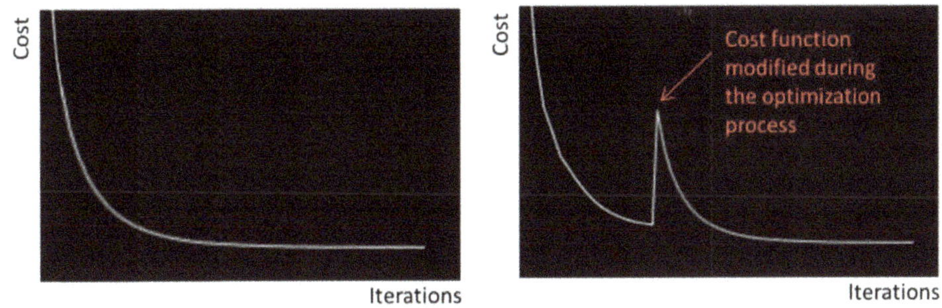

Figure 9.5. Cost function during its minimization process (plan optimization), decreasing to a plateau. On the left: no interactions during the optimization: the cost continuously decreases until the plateau, where no further reduction is possible with the given dose–volume constraints and beam geometry. On the right: during the optimization the cost is varied by a modification of the dose–volume constraints (the desired dose) or the importance factor (priority) or the calculation conditions (multiple resolution levels for VMAT optimization).

structure-specific cost functions can also be evaluated during the optimization process.

9.4 The optimization algorithms

The initial clinical problem is being translated into a computational problem, and over the years, many approaches have been explored aiming to solve the radiotherapy planning. The algorithms proposed are, as said, almost all iterative processes. From a starting point of fluence intensity (that could be 0 or given by an initial guess), at each iteration, the optimization algorithm will determine a new fluence distribution, for which a dose distribution is computed. This is evaluated relative to the clinical objectives included in the cost function. When the convergence is achieved, i.e., the minimum of the cost function is determined, the optimal plan is obtained (figure 9.6).

Two main classes of optimization algorithm exist: the deterministic and the stochastic algorithms. Of the former category, the most common is the *gradient technique*, of the latter, the *simulated annealing*. In the following, a brief description of the concept of each of them is given. This can also be seen in the figure 2.5 animation of this book.

9.4.1 The deterministic algorithms

In the deterministic algorithms, the intensity fluence modifications follow deterministic rules, i.e., no random steps are involved. Those mostly applied, refer to the *gradient technique* discussed below as well as shown in figure 2.5 of this book.

The gradient technique [4, 9–11]. To visualize the technique, let us consider the cost function, as shown in figure 9.7, and the initial guess x_0 determined on the right of the plot. At the point x_0, the gradient of the cost function is positive. At the first iteration the variable modification rule will determine x_1 by subtracting to x_0 an amount proportional to the gradient of the cost function in x_0 (according to a factor α):

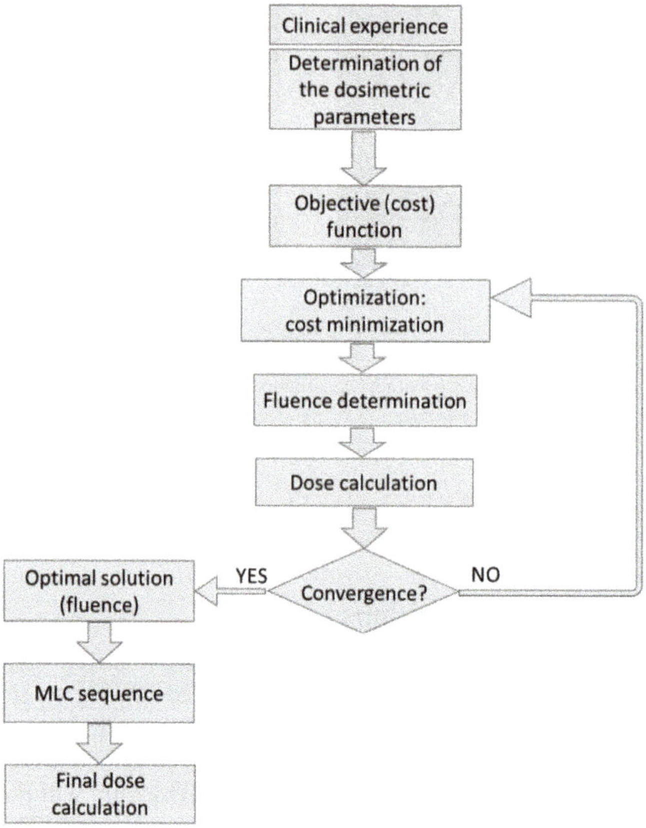

Figure 9.6. Flow of the plan optimization process.

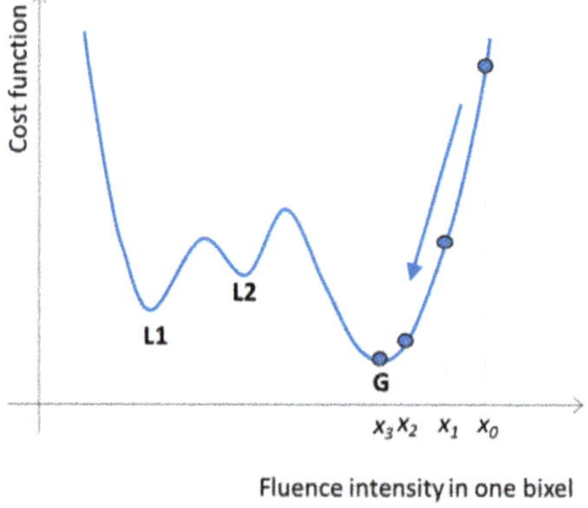

Figure 9.7. The concept of gradient technique optimization. The minimum of the cost function is determined running downhill through a descent gradient from the position x_0 to x_3, where the global minimum G is found. The cost, in this case, also presents two local minima L1 and L2.

$$x_{i+1} = x_i - \alpha \cdot \nabla \mathrm{Cost}(x_i) \quad (9.6)$$

Until the gradient remains positive, the next x_{i+1} points will similarly run downhill, with step sizes that are larger for steeper slopes. In the point having a gradient equal to 0 (and by consequence, in the iterative process, a 0 step size), the minimum of the cost is reached, and the solution x is found. During the optimization, whenever the intensity becomes negative, it is set to 0 to allow a physically realisable solution.

This method has the advantage of being fast, but it could easily be trapped in a local instead of the global minimum if the cost function presents more minima. Let us consider the cost function in figure 9.7 again: if the initial condition x_0 is set on the left side of the plot, instead of the right, with the descent gradient, the solution would be trapped in the local minimum L1, with no possibility to escape from it since the gradient there is zero.

For convex cost functions, only one minimum exists, and the gradient technique is an excellent approach, quickly finding the unique solution. However, in practice, the cost functions are generally not convex: dose–volume constraints would, in principle, add local minima, and this is done in the actual planning process.

The gradient techniques have been refined with some different mathematical approaches. From the original *steepest descent* approach, the *Newton's method* (or *quasi-Newton*) modified the factor α using the inverse Hessian operator, or an approximation of it. Another approach, named the *conjugated gradient*, starting from an initial point, the cost is evaluated following the direction along the line presenting the steepest descent gradient.

As seen, the disadvantage of the gradient approach to the cost function minimization is the possibility to remain trapped in a local minimum. In contrast, theoretically, the global minimum is the desirable goal. Moreover, relevant in the clinical practice, the higher the number of dose–volume constraints, the higher the number of local minima, and the possibility to be stuck there. However, studies have been conducted to estimate, which is the relevance of achieving the global instead of a local minimum of the cost [12, 13]. Bortfeld [11] listed three possible reasons why, in contrast to the theoretical expectations, the local minima trap seems not to be a problem. Firstly, if we can use simple cost functions, with only minimum and maximum dose constraints, there are no local minima in the function. Second, the starting point selection in a position not too far from the global minimum, allows the optimization not to be trapped in a local minimum, and analytical methods to find the best initial guess can be used. Lastly, the values of the cost function at the local minima are often not too different from the value in the global minimum, leading to similar results.

9.4.2 The stochastic algorithms

The stochastic algorithms do not use deterministic rules for modifying the fluence to explore the cost function, while each position in the search space has a random component. The most used stochastic approach is the *simulated annealing*, and it was also historically introduced by Webb [14] as one of the first methods to solve the intensity-modulated radiotherapy planning problem. The origin of this method (as

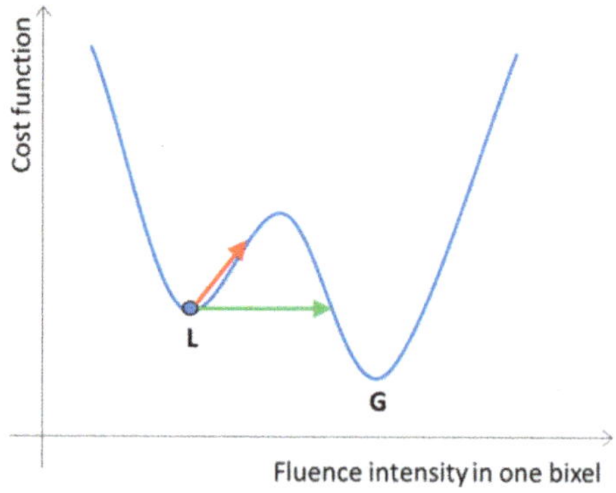

Figure 9.8. Simulated annealing: how to escape from a local minimum L, through tunneling (green arrow) or hill-climbing (red arrow).

also suggested by the name) has been already explained in chapter 2 and comes from the solid-state physics. With the annealing process, a material is rapidly heated to very high temperatures and then cooled down slowly to allow the material to reach the optimal crystal state with the minimization of the internal energy of the solid.

The simulated annealing [15–18]. It is not a pure downhill technique as the deterministic one, the intensity fluence modification along the iterations has a random component, and for that reason, it is possible to escape from local minima. There are mainly two ways of escaping: the first is called *hill-climbing*, the second *tunneling*, as depicted in figure 9.8: from a local minimum the optimizer can follow the red arrow (hill-climbing) or the green arrow (tunneling) jumping out of the local minimum position.

The simulated annealing, different from the gradient technique, does not reject fluence intensity solutions leading to an increase of the cost function. At the same time, they are accepted with a probability that depends on the temperature (annealing). The temperature determines the average size of the random steps to jump in the search space, which is the amount of the fluence intensity variation: the higher the temperature, the higher the probability of acceptance and of searching in the space. In these phases, tunneling is heavily used, allowing significant changes. With the progress of the iterations, the temperature is gradually reduced, and toward the end of the process, the optimization will be in the valley of the global minimum. Only the downhill changes will be accepted, bringing to the global minimum solution.

The advantages and disadvantages of the simulated annealing are the opposite of those of the gradient method: it does not get trapped in local minima, but it is slow since it has to widely explore the solution space with an enormous increase of the number of iterations.

9.5 The direct aperture optimization

The two optimization approaches so far described are both beamlet-based inverse planning methods: the beams are discretized in a large number of beamlets, as depicted in figure 9.4. The algorithms, driven by a set of dose and dose–volume constraints on targets and OARs, determine the fluence intensity maps that minimize the cost function.

Once the optimal fluence is determined, the MLC sequencer generates the MLC positions that would deliver a fluence (as similar as possible to the optimal fluence) accounting for the collimating device limitations (figure 9.5). The deliverable fluence could generate a plan with a deteriorated quality.

Moreover, the number of MU able to deliver those fluences is often quite high. This is ultimately associated with increased treatment time, a more considerable leakage through the MLC, an increase of the total body dose with the consequence of raising the risk of second cancer induction. It is hence clear that attempts to find ways of reducing MU without compromising the plan quality have been taken [19]. One of the main objectives was to reduce complexity. In this frame, the *direct aperture optimization* had its fundamental role, following the planner concept of the field-in-field technique seen as a forward IMRT. This, contrary to the *beamlet-based optimization*, can be defined as *aperture-based optimization*, DAO [20–22].

With DAO, weights and shapes of apertures are simultaneously optimized according to a user-specified number *n* of apertures per beam (the higher the *n*, the higher the complexity). The optimization of the aperture shapes is a concave problem, and a *simulated annealing* approach is then used. The DAO method can reduce the number of MU significantly relative to the other techniques [20], which has been found a natural application to the intensity-modulated arc therapy [22]. The VMAT dose-optimization proposed by Otto [23] employs a similar aperture-based method by incorporating MLC leaf positions and MU weights as optimization parameters. The optimization accounts for all the delivery constraints (MLC limitations), and no additional sequencing steps are then required.

The problem of the conversion algorithms from optimal to actual fluence determined by the realisable leaf sequence has been the subject of investigations since it could easily reduce the plan quality that can significantly deviate from the optimal plan [24–26]. The DAO approach can account for the delivery constraints (machine and MLC related technical limitations) in the optimization phase. This has the advantage of not requiring the sequencing step after the optimal fluence determination, making the DAO a robust optimization method, resulting in the final actual fluences with no translation from the optimal fluences.

9.6 The biological optimization

In the previous section, the inverse plan optimization through physical objectives was guided by the need to use measurable and well-defined parameters, and it was clear that only the physical parameters (dose and volumes) have those characteristics. However, it is not the physics, but the biologic mechanisms, that are responsible for the radiation-induced damage. There is an impressive number of different factors that guide the response of the organs and the tumor to the radiation. At a very superficial approach, we can identify some of those factors that can modify the radiation response: the volume effect, the different radiation sensitivity in the population, the variation in radiation sensitivity inside the tumor, the different clonogenic cell density inside the tumor, the direct impact of other treatment modalities that could be part of the patient care (as the chemotherapy, the hormonal therapy, the surgery), the patient characteristics. All this provides evidence of the difficulty to unambiguously define biological parameters to use in the optimization of the planning process.

We should start from the assumption that the final goal of radiotherapy is the patient cure rather than the delivery of a specified dose to a particular region.

The physical dose–volume criteria can fix a constraint to prevent the DVH of an OAR to enter the forbidden dose–volume region depicted in figure 9.3. Let us now consider the DVHs in figure 9.9: all the curves in the left-hand side plot fulfill the dose–volume criterion of no more than *V'* volume receiving *D'* dose or more, but it is evident at a glance that the DVH which possibly induces less toxicity is the lowest one. On the right-hand side of the same figure, the two DVHs, both meeting the criterion, can produce different responses; the red DVH will be better for a more serial organ, while for a more parallel organ the blue one should be preferred. Additionally, we should also consider the physiological interaction between different organs (as described in chapter 7 of this book). With this simple example, it is clear that limiting to only physical dose–volume constraints, we miss the biological characteristics of the organs and their specific response to the radiation, resulting in optimal plans not clinically optimized, and possibly deviating from the patient cure goal.

All this clarifies the interest of the community in developing quantitative models able to predict the biological response of the specific human tissues to a particular radiation dose distribution.

Beforehand we need the radiobiological models, and then the inverse treatment planning should develop a suitable way to include in the cost function clinical and biological criteria based on those models, aiming to obtain plans fulfilling the biological and clinical, more than physical, endpoints.

9.6.1 The radiobiological models for TCP, NTCP, EUD

It was in the 1980s and 1990s when the development of radiobiological models to estimate the probability of locally controlling the tumor (TCP) and of inducing

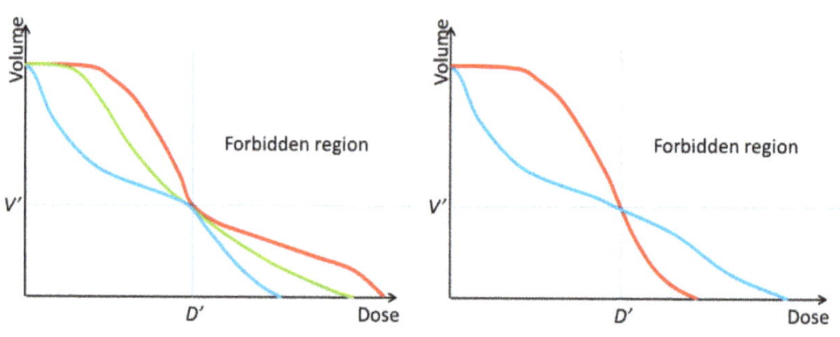

Figure 9.9. DVHs of a critical structure.

complications on normal tissues (NTCP) after radiation treatment was of primary scientific interest [27] The TCP and NTCP models have been mainly used to evaluate plans and to compare rival plans. A considerable number of studies aimed to determine the best parameters correlating clinical to dosimetric data. A summary and a lot of meta-analysis work have been done within the QUANTEC project for what concerns the NTCP for all the OAR. However, the resulting parameters present large uncertainties, in part deriving from the model, but mainly from the way the data were reported, due also to the intrinsic nature of the radiation treatment that does not produce deterministic effects on the human being (the dose criteria meeting does not guarantee the absence of complications) [28].

The current radiobiological models are mainly the TCP model (from the works of Nahum) [29–31] for the tumor response modeling, the Relative Seriality model [32] and the Lyman–Kutcher–Burman model [33–35] for the NTCP modeling. However, also in cases where dosimetric metrics as EUD and gEUD (for tumors and OAR) [36–38] are closely correlated with TCP and NTCP, they can be used as radiobiological models.

Nahum [27] classified the biological optimization, i.e., the use of the radiobiological models for plan optimization, in four different levels, from a pure individualization of the prescription dose based on isotoxic effects (level I) to an optimization based on individual patient biology, as could be the case of genomic (level V). Level III concerns the use of radiobiological functions (TCP, NTCP, EUD) in the inverse planning algorithms.

The potential of a biological-based optimization is shown in figure 9.10 [27]: the two prescription doses indicated by the arrows (50 and 72 Gy) are associated with the same NTCP level (isotoxic) in the two cases where large and small volumes, respectively, are irradiated to high dose levels, as could be the case of 3DCRT or

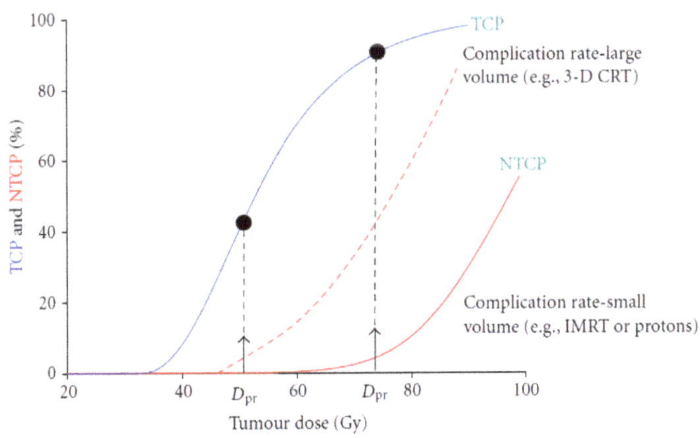

Figure 9.10. Potential of biological-based optimization. From Nahum *et al* [27], reproduced with permission. Copyright 2012 A E Nahum and J Uzan. Open access CC BY 4.0.

IMRT treatments. Those two isotoxic dose prescriptions would result in a TCP improvement (e.g., IMRT treatment to 72 Gy) from ~45% to ~90%.

In this way, the focus moves from the physical dose concept to the biological and clinical effect of that dose.

In level III of the biological optimization, the optimizer can find solutions by reducing the target dose adjacent to a critical structure, while boosting other parts of the target volumes (this would be better exploited in level IV, where the inverse planning optimization is also based on functional imaging). This approach would result in a target dose, which is no longer uniform, but with the effect that the hot and cold spots in the target are taken into account in the TCP estimation [39].

A method to optimally balance the TCP maximization and NTCP minimization is the P_+ approach of maximizing the *uncomplicated tumor local control probability* [40–42]:

$$P_+ = P(B) - P(I) \tag{9.7}$$

where P_+ is the probability for uncomplicated tumor control, $P(B)$ is the probability for tumor control, $P(I)$ is the probability of inducing radiation-related injury. The inclusion of the biological engines in the cost function, due to the non-convex nature of the TCP and NTCP functions, suffers from the same physical optimization of solutions trapped in local minima.

As pointed out in the Task Group 166 of the AAMP [43] on the biological models for treatment planning, the potential of the biological models is to provide an inherent prioritization of the multiple dose–volume constraints in a single figure of merit. The report was mostly looking at the EUD/gEUD concept, which are the biological indices more commonly available in the inverse planning systems:

$$\text{gEUD} = \left(\sum_i v_i D_i^{a}\right)^{1/a} \tag{9.8}$$

were v_i is the fractional volume receiving a dose D_i of the ith pixel in the structure. The parameter a is tissue-specific and describes the volume effect: high values of a indicate a serial organ, low values (for $a = 1$ EUD equals the mean dose) are for parallel tissue. With the gEUD, large volumes receiving low–medium dose levels are allowed while keeping low the high dose for high a values; hot spots are allowed while attempting to reduce the volume receiving the low dose levels for low a values.

The gEUD inclusion in the cost function for what relates the serial responding organs do not give rise to local minima of the optimization problem since, for $a \geqslant 1$, the problem is convex [44]. For parallel responses, gEUD, as well as TCP and NTCP, could create local minima in the cost function (the function is no longer convex); however, this risk is less than for the case of using dose–volume objectives [45]. A challenging balance between the clinical and the mathematical criticalities should drive to the right choice of the cost function, aiming to take advantage of using the biological concept [46].

9.7 Benefit and deficiencies in biological optimization

The main objection in using biological optimization engines remains the high uncertainty of the used parameters associated with the available model, which are still too simplistic (although continually refined) and are based on weak clinical grounds for such a variate patient population. Their clinical use as the unique index of judging and prescribing a treatment is hence open to criticism. What is in this view possible and safe today is to combine the biological optimization with physical dose–volume constraints, which are today still more reliable in predicting clinical outcomes and are more consistent with the whole radiotherapy experience.

On the possible clinical implementation of the biological models in radiotherapy (and the objectives in the inverse planning is the first step), it is interesting to read today, 15 years after publication, the debate published in 2005, attempting to have a future vision of the next decade (now over) on the biological treatment plan optimization [47]. The opponents were debating whether the biological response coming from the molecular technologies would have replaced the traditional dose-optimization approaches based on surrogate measures as the maximization and uniformity in the target and dose limits to the normal tissues. They agreed substantially on the compelling need for biological-based treatment planning, as well as on the major issues related to the biological model implementation in the clinical practice. The current models relating the dose distribution to treatment outcomes are highly non-linear: small variations in physical or biological factors could significantly impact on the biologic response estimation, which is tissue and patient-specific. On the physical parameter side, as we have seen in the paragraphs above, we can rely on well-defined and reliable quantities (the volume and the dose). This is not the case of the biological parameters. For example, the clonogenic cell density and radiosensitivity distribution are not constant throughout the PTV, leading to the used assumption that a uniform dose distribution maximizes the tumor control is incorrect. Notwithstanding decades of experience and a lot of studies and efforts, the knowledge on the radiation response of the tumors and the OAR is still unreliable and not well documented. Despite the developments on the models, the clinical outcome and toxicity prediction are poor due to the significant uncertainty in the biological parameters, to add to the other sources of uncertainty (patient- and treatment-related) which contribute to the low knowledge about the complications. All this, still today, makes the biological model not mature enough in my opinion, and a great deal of caution has to be used for clinical application in a decision-making process.

Summarizing, no big changes in the radiotherapy community have been made in the last 15 years to make the biological optimization robust enough to be clinically used, and the conclusions of the debate are still valid. Prospective clinical trials to evaluate the clinical impact of biologically-based planning strategies are still lacking, and the demonstration of the potential clinical benefit with respect to physically-based planning is missing.

At a 20-year distance, the opinion expressed by Bortfeld in 1999 [11] could be seen as a visionary concept we should maybe turn to today: perhaps we should better understand which planning criteria are clinically relevant or not, rather than use or not the biological models in the optimization process. The actual knowledge is based on physically-based optimization criteria with clinical relevance, and maybe we should not give this concept up without solid and cogent foundations.

The TCP and NTCP models, however, summarizing the biological and clinical knowledge, remain fundamental in the plan evaluation, although more work has to be done to make them a reliable tool for plan optimization; especially the biological parameters α and β that are not very well understood for all tumor types, histology and grade.

9.8 Robust optimization

The optimization processes so far described do not account for intra-fraction organ and patient motion during the delivery. This uncertainty was traditionally (before the advent of intensity modulation) taken into account by adding internal and set-up margins from CTV to PTV, and this is the actual common approach in almost all the radiotherapy photon treatments, also intensity-modulation based.

A different concept, commonly named *robust optimization*, aimed to incorporate the motion and related uncertainties into the plan optimization process, making the PTV approach out-of-date. This has been recently applied to IMPT (intensity-modulated proton therapy), and these methods are now introduced in the photon beam in the IMRT planning. A comprehensive topical review on the robust optimization subject was published in 2018 by Unkelbach *et al* [48], presenting the concept and main applications in radiotherapy. In the remaining paragraphs of this section, a summary is given for what concerns the first approaches and the photon IMRT implementations.

In the typical inverse planning process, a dose distribution d is a linear function of the incident fluence x: $d = Dx$, and D denotes the dose-influence matrix collecting the dose contributions of all beamlets to each voxel. The uncertainty in the matrix D models the geometric uncertainty as to the set-up errors and the organ motion. The geometric uncertainty is the most studied in the robust optimization frame.

Each scenario generating geometric uncertainty is indexed by k, and each error scenario gives a different dose distribution due to a different dose-influence matrix: $d^k = D^k x$. The robust optimization concept, instead of considering a fixed dose-influence matrix D, evaluates the possibility that the delivered dose distribution is one of the d^k, depending on the delivery scenario. Hence, an optimal and robust optimization would generate a plan with dose distribution d^k which is useful for (possibly) all the error scenarios that may occur. Mathematically, two approaches have been followed: the *stochastic programming* approach, which optimizes the expected plan quality, and the *minimax* approach, which optimizes the plan quality for the worst-case scenario and has been mainly investigated for IMPT planning [49]. The *stochastic programming* has been applied on both IMRT and IMPT [50–54]. In this approach, each error scenario is associated with an importance weight p_k (that could be considered the probability that the scenario k occurs). The cost function to minimize becomes:

$$\text{cost} = \sum_k p_k f(d^k(x)) \tag{9.9}$$

The uncertainties to handle as inter-fraction motions have systematic and random components (as shown in chapter 7). As a first approximation, the inter-fraction motion is often modeled as a set-up error. This can be a translation (plus a rotation), or, with a more accurate approach including deformations of the tumor and the surrounding tissues, using the principal component analysis (PCA), as approached by different groups on different anatomical sites [55–58]. A schematic view of the *stochastic programming* is shown in figure 9.11 [48], where two cases of 1 single fraction and 30 fractions are shown in a hypothetical 1D simplified example, where the probability of a maximum shift of 10 mm is described by a Gaussian distribution with 3 mm standard deviation, which would model the penumbra. The single fraction on the left shows the incorporation of the uncertainty induces the nominal dose (the blue profile), which yields the expected dose (the red profile) to adequately cover the CTV (the gray region of 6 cm). The effect is to extend the irradiated region around the CTV without defining geometrically and explicitly the PTV. When a large number of fractions are considered, the nominal dose will present horns at the target edges. This feature is the result of the fact that the tumor may be underdosed in some fractions in the region close to the normal tissue; the horns serve to compensate for the fractions and location of the target underdose [50, 59].

The horns are the mechanism allowing the delivery of a steeper dose gradient at the edges of the target; however, they can be questionable, especially in the frame of IGRT treatment, where the errors are minimized.

Refinements of the robust optimization methods were studied. Interesting is the concept of Baum *et al* [60]: the sum of all the probabilities p_k of a scenario k where the voxel i is in a given structure, corresponds to the probability that the voxel i belongs to that structure, and is called the *coverage probability*, which enters in the cost function as a penalty. The concept can be applied to the target and the OAR.

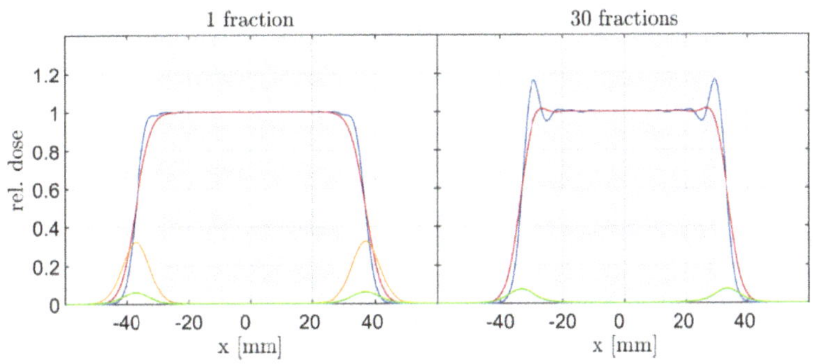

Figure 9.11. Schematic representation of the stochastic programming in the single and 30 fractions cases. The blue profiles represent the nominal dose, the red profiles the expected dose according to the probability of set-up errors. Adapted from Unkelbach *et al* [48], reproduced with permission. Copyright 2018 Institute of Physics and Engineering in Medicine. All rights reserved.

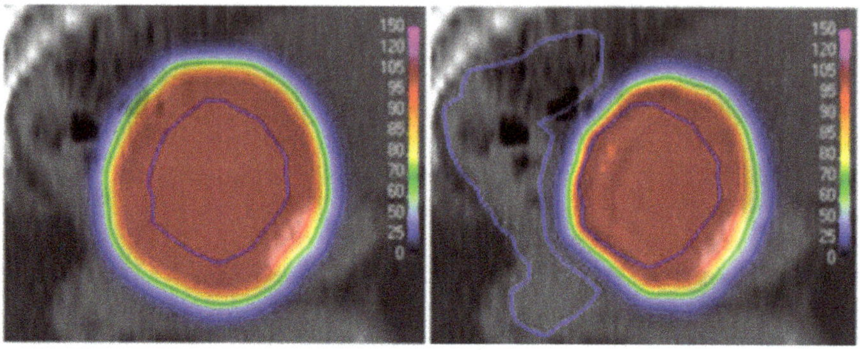

Figure 9.12. Example of robust optimization in a prostate case. On the left: uncompromised target coverage. On the right: a conflict between target coverage and OAR sparing. Adapted from Unkelbach *et al* [48], reproduced with permission. Copyright 2018 Institute of Physics and Engineering in Medicine. All rights reserved.

A clinical example is shown in figure 9.12 [49] for the *stochastic programming* method. Here, a prostate treatment is optimized: the first sagittal slice shows the dose distribution with no compromise to the target coverage, and no close OAR to spare: the dose expanded outside the CTV accounts for the possible set-up errors, without using the PTV concept. The second dose distribution presents the case where the OAR (the rectum) needs to be spared: the conflict is solved with a higher dose gradient in the direction of the rectum, and a higher dose at the edge of the CTV to compensate for the possible underdosing during more posterior target position.

The robust optimization concept is still far from being the standard in photon IMRT plan optimization (today only the planning system from RaySearch has the photon robust optimization clinically available). However, its importance, more than simply overcoming the PTV concept, would allow delivering the dose distribution to the patient more consistently with what planned, and this should be the main aim of the entire planning and delivery processes. For this reason, it would be desirable to see in the next future all the planning system moving toward the adoption of this approach.

References

[1] Brahme A, Roos J E and Lax I 1982 Solution of an integral equation encountered in rotation therapy *Phys. Med. Biol.* **27** 1221–9

[2] Cozzi L and Fogliata A 2014 IMRT in the treatment of head and neck cancer: is the present already the future? *Expert Rev. Anticancer Ther.* **2** 297–308

[3] Brahme A 1988 Optimization of stationary and moving beam radiation therapy techniques *Radiother. Oncol.* **12** 129–40

[4] Bortfeld T, Bürkelbach J, Boesecke R and Schlegel W 1990 Methods of image reconstruction from projections applied to conformation radiotherapy *Phys. Med. Biol.* **35** 1423–34

[5] Barth N 1990 An inverse problem in radiation therapy *Int. J. Radiat. Oncol. Biol. Phys.* **18** 425–31

[6] Cormack A 1987 A problem in rotation therapy with x-rays *Int. J. Radiat. Oncol. Biol. Phys.* **13** 623–30

[7] Webb S 2003 The physical basis of IMRT and inverse planning *Br. J. Radiol.* **76** 678–89

[8] Bortfeld T, Oelfke U and Nill S 2000 What is the optimum leaf width of a multileaf collimator? *Med. Phys.* **27** 2494–502

[9] Spirou S V and Chui C S 1998 A gradient inverse planning algorithm with dose–volume constraints *Med. Phys.* **25** 321–33

[10] Gustafsson A, Lind B K and Brahme A 1994 A generalized pencil beam algorithm for optimization of radiation therapy *Med. Phys.* **21** 343–56

[11] Bortfeld T 1999 Optimized planning using physical objectives and constraints *Semin. Radiat. Oncol.* **9** 20–34

[12] Llacer J, Deasy J O, Bortfeld T R, Solberg T D and Promberger C 2003 Absence of multiple local minima effects in intensity modulated optimization with dose–volume constraints *Phys. Med. Biol.* **48** 183–210

[13] Wu Q and Mohan R 2002 Multiple local minima in IMRT optimization based on dose–volume criteria *Med. Phys.* **29** 1514–27

[14] Webb S 1989 Optimisation of conformal radiotherapy dose distributions by simulated annealing *Phys. Med. Biol.* **34** 1349–70

[15] Webb S 1991 Optimization by simulated annealing of three-dimensional conformal treatment planning for radiation fields defined by a multileaf collimator *Phys. Med. Biol.* **36** 1201–26

[16] Webb S 1992 Optimization by simulated annealing of three-dimensional, conformal treatment planning for radiation fields defined by a multileaf collimator: II. Inclusion of the two-dimensional modulation of the x-ray intensity *Phys. Med. Biol.* **37** 1689–704

[17] Morrill S M, Lane R G, Jacobson G and Rosen I I 1991 Treatment planning optimization using constrained simulated annealing *Phys. Med. Biol.* **36** 1341–61

[18] Mageras G S and Mohan R 1993 Application of fast simulated annealing to optimization of conformal radiation treatments *Med. Phys.* **20** 639–47

[19] Broderick M, Leech M and Coffey M 2009 Direct aperture optimization as a means of reducing the complexity of intensity modulated radiation therapy plans *Radiat. Oncol.* **4** 8

[20] Shepard D M, Earl M A, Li X A, Naqvi S and Yu C 2002 Direct aperture optimization: a turnkey solution for step-and-shoot IMRT *Med. Phys.* **29** 1007–18

[21] De Gersem W, Claus F, de Wagter C, Van Duyse B and De Neve W 2001 Leaf position optimization for step-and-shoot IMRT *Int. J. Radiat. Oncol. Biol. Phys.* **51** 1371–88

[22] Earl M A, Shepard D M, Naqvi S, Li X A and Yu C X 2003 Inverse planning for intensity-modulated arc therapy using direct aperture optimization *Phys. Med. Biol.* **48** 1075–89

[23] Otto K 2008 Volumetric modulated arc therapy: IMRT in a single gantry arc *Med. Phys.* **35** 310–7

[24] Siebers J V, Lauterbach M, Keall P J and Mohan R 2002 Incorporating multi-leaf collimator leaf sequencing into iterative IMRT optimization *Med. Phys.* **29** 952–9

[25] Alber M and Nüsslin F 2001 Optimization of intensity modulated radiotherapy under constraints for static and dynamic MLC delivery *Phys. Med. Biol.* **46** 3229–39

[26] Litzenberg D W, Moran J M and Fraass B A 2002 Incorporating of realistic delivery limitations into dynamic MLC treatment delivery *Med. Phys.* **29** 810–20

[27] Nahum A E and Uzan J 2012 (Radio)Biological optimization of external-beam radiotherapy *Comput. Math. Method Med.* **2012** 329214

[28] Jackson A, Marks L B, Bentzen S M, Eisbruch A, Yorke E D and Ten Haken R K *et al* 2010 The lessons of QUANTEC: reccomendations for reporting and gathering data on dose–volume dependencies of treatment outcome *Int. J. Radiat. Oncol. Biol. Phys.* **76** S155–60

[29] Nahum A R and Tait D M 1993 Maximizing local control by customized dose prescription for pelvic tumours *Tumor Response Monitoring and Treatment planning* ed A Breit *et al* (Heidelberg: Springer) pp 425–31

[30] Webb S and Nahum A E 1993 A model for calculating tumour control probability in radiotherapy including the effects of inhomogeneous distributions of dose and clonogenic cell density *Phys. Med. Biol.* **38** 653–66

[31] Nahum A E and Sanchez-Nieto B 2001 Tumour control probability modelling: basic principles and applications in treatment planning *Phys. Med.* **17** 13–23

[32] Källman P, Ågren A and Brahme A 1992 Tumour and normal tissue responses to fractionated non-uniform dose delivery *Int. J. Radiat. Biol.* **62** 249–62

[33] Lyman J T 1985 Complication probabilities as assessed from dose–volume histograms *Radiat. Res.* **104** S13–9

[34] Kutcher G J and Burman C 1989 Calculation of complication probability factors for non uniform normal tissue irradiation: the effective volume method *Int. J. Radiat. Oncol. Biol. Phys.* **16** 1623–30

[35] Kutcher G J, Burman C, Brewster L, Goitein M and Mohan R 1991 Histogram reduction method for calculating complication probabilities for three-dimensional treatment planning evaluations *Int. J. Radiat. Oncol. Biol. Phys.* **21** 137–46

[36] Niemierko A 1997 Reporting and analysing dose distributions: a concept of equivalent uniform dose *Med. Phys.* **24** 103–10

[37] Ebert M A 2000 Viability of the EUD and TCP concepts as reliable dose indicators *Phys. Med. Biol.* **45** 441–57

[38] Niemierko A 1999 A generalized concept of equivalent uniform dose (EUD) *Med. Phys.* **26** 1101

[39] De Gersem W R, Derycke S, Colle C O, De Wagter C and De Neve W J 1999 Inhomogeneous target-dose distributions: a dimension more for optimization? *Int. J. Radiat. Oncol. Biol. Phys.* **44** 461–8

[40] Ågren A, Brahme A and Turesson I 1990 Optimization of uncomplicated control for head and neck tumors *Int. J. Radiat. Oncol. Biol. Phys.* **19** 1077–85

[41] Brahme A 2001 Individualizing cancer treatment: biological optimization models in treatment and planning *Int. J. Radiat. Oncol. Biol. Phys.* **49** 327–37

[42] Peñagarícano J A, Papanikolaou N, Wu C and Yan Y 2005 An assessment of Biologically-based Optimization (BORT) in the IMRT era *Med. Dosim.* **30** 12–9

[43] Li X A, Alber M, Deasy J O, Jackson A, Lee K W K and Marks L B *et al* 2012 The use and QA of biologically related models for treatment planning: short report of the TG-166 of the therapy physics committee of the AAPM *Med. Phys.* **39** 1386–409

[44] Choi B and Deasy J O 2002 The generalized equivalent uniform dose function as a basis for intensity-modulated treatment planning *Phys. Med. Biol.* **47** 3579–89

[45] Romeijn H E, Dempsey J F and Li J G 2004 A unifying framework for multi-criteria fluence map optimization models *Phys. Med. Biol.* **49** 1991–2013

[46] Wu Q, Mohan R, Niemierko A and Schmidt-Ullrich R 2002 Optimization of intensity-modulated radiotherapy plans based on the equivalent uniform dose *Int. J. Radiat. Oncol. Biol. Phys.* **52** 224–35

[47] Ling C C and Li X A 2005 Over the next decade the success of radiation treatment planning will be judged by the immediate biological response of tumor cells rather than by surrogate measures such as dose maximization and uniformity *Med. Phys.* **32** 2189–92

[48] Unkelbach J, Alber M, Bangert M, Bokrantz R, Chan T C Y and Deasy J O *et al* 2018 Robust radiotherapy planning *Phys. Med. Biol.* **63** 22TR02

[49] Fredriksson A, Forsgren A and Hårdemark B 2011 Minimax optimization for handling range and set-up uncertainties in proton therapy *Med. Phys.* **38** 1672–84

[50] Unkelbach J and Oelfke U 2005 Incorporating organ movements in IMRT treatment planning for prostate cancer: minimizing uncertainties in the inverse planning process *Med. Phys.* **32** 2471–83

[51] Witte M G, van der Geer J, Schneider C, Lebesque J V, Alber M and van Herk M 2007 IMRT optimization including random and systematic geometric errors based on the expectation of TCP and NTCP *Med. Phys.* **34** 3544–55

[52] Heath E, Unkelbach J and Oelfke U 2009 Incorporating uncertainties in respiratory motion into 4D treatment plan optimization *Med. Phys.* **36** 3059–71

[53] Bohoslavsky R, Witte M G, Janssen T M and Van Herk M 2013 Probabilistic objective functions for margin-less IMRT planning *Phys. Med. Biol.* **58** 3563

[54] Fontanarosa D, van der Laan H P, Witte M, Shakirin G, Roelofs E and Langendijk J A *et al* 2013 An in silico comparison between margin-based and probabilistic target-planning approaches in head and neck cancer patients *Radiother. Oncol.* **109** 430–6

[55] Price G J and Moore C J 2007 A method to calculate coverage probability from uncertainties in radiotherapy via a statistical shape model *Phys. Med. Biol.* **52** 1947

[56] Zhang Q, Pevsner A, Hertanto A, Hu Y C, Rosenzweig K E, Ling C C and Mageras G S 2007 A patient-specific respiratory model of anatomical motion for radiation treatment planning *Med. Phys.* **34** 4772–81

[57] Thörnqvist S, Hysing L B, Zolnay A G, Söhn M, Hoogeman M S, Muren L P and Heijmen B J 2013 Adaptive radiotherapy in locally advanced prostate cancer using a statistical deformable motion model *Acta Oncol.* **52** 1423–9

[58] Xu H, Vile D J, Sharma M, Gordon J J and Siebers J V 2014 Coverage-based treatment planning to accommodate deformable organ variations in prostate cancer treatment *Med. Phys.* **41** 101705

[59] Unkelbach J and Oelfke U 2004 Inverse planning incorporating organ movements via probability distributions of voxel locations *Radiother. Oncol.* **73** S347

[60] Baum C, Alber M, Birkner M and Nüsslin F 2006 Robust treatment planning for intensity modulated radiotherapy of prostate cancer based on coverage probabilities *Radiother. Oncol.* **78** 27–35

Chapter 10

Dose calculation

In this chapter, the importance of accuracy in the dose calculation process in intensity modulation treatment is overviewed. Since IMRT requires optimization based on dose, it is critical that a proper understanding of the dose calculation and related accuracy required in radiotherapy is known. A summary of the various algorithms that have become available over the decades is given. It is of fundamental importance, in the clinical practice, to understand the limitations and the areas of applicability of the calculation process implemented in our clinical routine.

Then, several particular situations are evaluated, where the overall treatment accuracy might be influenced by the dose calculation algorithm.

10.1 Required accuracy in dose calculation

The level of accuracy required in the estimation of the dose distribution of radiotherapy treatments has to be related to the clinical aspects and is linked to the dose-effect curves, be they describing the target or a critical structure, and in particular to their slope (figure 10.1). The sigmoidal curves of the tumor control probability (TCP) and normal tissue complication probability (NTCP) for a specific endpoint as a function of the tumor or organ delivered dose are characterized by mainly two parameters. The first, D_{50}, is the dose that yields a tumor or organ response in 50% of the patient population; the second, γ, is the normalized dose gradient of the curve [1]. It is only the proper estimation of the dose delivered with a specific treatment plan that includes the dose distribution in the patient tissue as well as the computation of the MU needed to achieve the desired dose level, which allows knowledge about the complication-free tumor control to be improved.

The 'proper estimation' of the *delivered* dose is the result of the achievable accuracy of the dose distribution that is a complex concept and is related to two kinds of uncertainties: random and systematic. The random errors are more related to the delivery, while the systematic ones could be mostly ascribed to the dose determination chain and the machine adjustment. Since the accuracy of the dose

doi:10.1088/978-0-7503-1335-3ch10

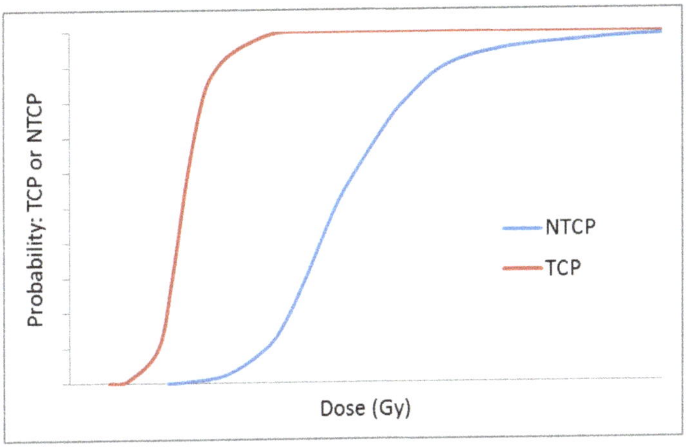

Figure 10.1. Sigmoidal dose–response curves of tumor control probability (TCP) and normal tissue complication probability (NTCP).

calculation is a systematic error, it cannot be compensated by other factors as the fractionated treatment, and for this reason, has to be kept as small as possible.

The requirements for the dose variations dated a long time ago, starting in 1976 with the ICRU Report 24 recommendations [2], then investigated by Brahme [1, 3], by Van Dyk [4], to the ICRU 50 [5], and more specifically for intensity-modulated treatment by ICRU 83 [6]. However, the early estimates are still valid and applicable, notwithstanding the technological improvements, which moved, over the years, from a 1D approach to the actual 4D. The TCP and NTCP curves remain the starting point for the accuracy requirements. In the steepest region of the dose–response curve, a 5% dose variation can lead to 10%–20% and 20%–30% in TCP and NTCP change, respectively [7]. The probability variation as a function of the dose depends on the point where the sigmoid curve is used since the gradient is not a constant value. However, a generally accepted threshold for accuracy requirement, valid for most situations, has to be defined, and the case of the highest gradient should, for safety reasons, be considered. The ICRU 24 recommended an accuracy in the delivered dose to the target volume of ±5%, estimated on the highest gradient. This can translate into a dose calculation accuracy requirement of 3%. However, in particular critical conditions, the needed accuracy could be more stringent. It could be the case for certain types of tumors, where a variation of a maximum 3.5% of the dose should be delivered [1, 8], that translated into a dose calculation accuracy need of 2%. Boyer and Schultheiss [9] estimated that an overall 1% increased accuracy can result in a 2% improvement of cure, determined as complication-free tumor control.

In general, an overall required delivery accuracy in the dose distribution should be in the range 3%–5%, and commonly a 2% dose calculation accuracy is considered the recommendable objective. Noteworthy in the advanced technologies are the increasing sources of dose delivery uncertainty. To cite just some of those sources: the volume definition and delineation accuracy, associated with the imaging modality (together with distortion, resolution, contrast issues) and co-registration;

the anatomy changes during the treatment course, like a possible (and clinically desirable) shrinkage of the tumor, or some radiation-induced variations during the treatment (as discussed in chapter 7); the organ and patient motion during the treatment session delivery, coming from breathing, heart beating, which also add the interplay effect for the intensity-modulated techniques. All these additional uncertainties would increase the need for accurate dose calculation algorithms. This is particularly relevant today since the accuracy of the dose relative to the prescription should determine the clinical outcome, for both TCP and NTCP variables, in a complication-free tumor control concept [10].

Moreover, the increased complexity of the treatment fields as the intensity-modulated beams and arcs in place of the standard static beams increases the sources of uncertainty. This makes the dose calculation process a fundamental but challenging part for the success of the high precision planning and delivery of radiotherapy treatments.

10.2 Dose calculation algorithms and classification

The importance of the dose calculation accuracy for treatment planning purposes has been, over the years, of primary interest for the medical physics community.

A fascinating historical review on the developments of radiotherapy, starting from the very first approaches in the late 19th century was published in 1995 by Fraass [11]. It was only in the 1950s, with the advent of computer technology, that the dose calculation started to be available, by using some empirical methods. The patient's anatomy was determined by simple body outline contouring in a single slice through a pantograph, and the patient information was, of course, ignored. The distance and depth were the essential parameters allowing the dose estimation. Later, in the 1970s, the CT scanner technology was introduced in the medical field, and the radiotherapy had the opportunity to know and use the patient and organ anatomy, and, more important, the density information as the fundamental concept in the absorbed dose calculation process. Initially, the computation used empirical methods, but they had quite limited accuracy. The evolution of the CT scanners also allowed the introduction of a dose computation approach based on voxel considerations, and not on purely empirical data. The physics foundation, in terms of the interaction of the radiation with the medium, the cross-sections, the transport equations, was well known. It required technological advances in terms of computational science to be able to calculate the dose distribution inside the patient anatomy with enough accuracy in a practically reasonable time, using semi-analytical or analytical methods, and Monte Carlo simulations.

Excellent review works, over the years, described the evolution of the dose calculation systems. Among these reviews, we can cite the works of Ahnesjö and Aspradakis in 1999 [12], Papanikolaou and Stathakis in 2009 [10], and Knöös in 2017 regarding 3D dose computation [13]. They have provided interesting overviews on this subject from different perspectives. Additionally, the Report 85 of the AAPM (American Association of Physics in Medicine) [14] on the heterogeneity

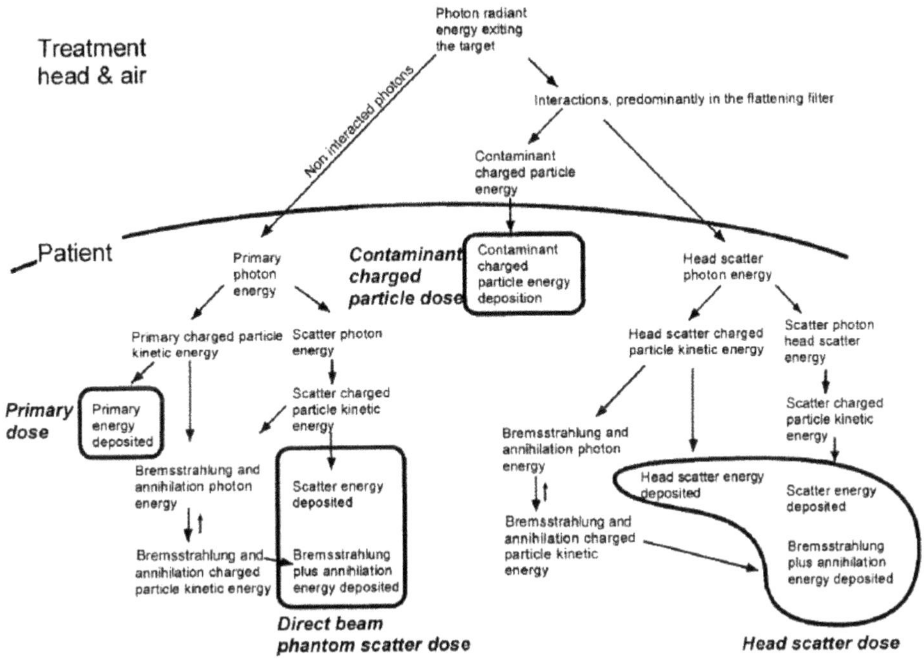

Figure 10.2. Interaction history of the main components of the dose deposition and referred to in the dose calculation: primary dose, phantom scatter dose, contaminant charged particle dose, head scatter dose. From Ahnesjö *et al* [12], reproduced with permission. Copyright IOP Publishing Ltd. All rights reserved.

correction in the dose calculation has also provided a summary pointing to tissue inhomogeneities handling over the years.

The complexity of the radiation beam and the multiplicity of the interactions occurring in the patient (medium) and also in the treatment machine are very high. This is well summarized in figure 10.2, from the Ahnesjö and Aspradakis paper [12], presenting the various components involved in the dose deposition.

The absorbed dose deposited by the primary photon beam can be calculated explicitly. The management of the scattered dose is more demanding, particularly in the presence of tissue heterogeneities.

In the following, a brief description of the dose calculation algorithms over the years is given, starting from the early empirical algorithms with corrections to account for scattering and inhomogeneity, continuing with the model-based algorithms, and to those fully including the radiation transport, according to a general classification described in the IAEA document TRS-430 [15].

In the next section, the current classification in type 'a', 'b' as initially suggested by Knöös in 2006, and then extended to type 'c' will be summarized [16].

10.2.1 The empirical models

The very early dose computations (the 1950s) were purely empirical, based on broad beam data, measured in water. Data were depth dose curves (PDD), tissue–phantom ratio (TPR), tissue–air ratio (TAR), output factors (OF). The algorithms, basically, reproduced at their best the input data entered in the system but mainly in water.

The *TAR method* [17] combined the two effects of beam attenuation (the primary beam handling) and the scattered radiation. By reducing the cross-sectional area toward zero, the remaining radiation approximates the primary beam only. This method allows the scatter to be separated from the primary component solely with a difference between TARs.

Another purely empirical approach is discussed by the ESTRO formalism for monitor unit (MU) calculation in high energy photon beams [18, 19], where the measured TPR, output factors and volume scatter ratio (similar to the tissue–air ratio) were the key elements of the calculation. It was in this frame, for the volume scatter ratio measurements, that the mini-phantom concept was introduced. In those methods the scatter radiation was empirically included.

The inclusion of the scattering and the density information from the CT scan allowed a step forward to more sophisticated models.

10.2.2 The semi-empirical, correction-based algorithms

The correction-based algorithms started with the fundamental papers of 1972 by Cunningham [20, 21]. The empirical solution of separating the primary and scatter radiation components by using the scatter air ratio, as in the *TAR method* was combined with the *Clarkson sector integration* [22] concepts. This yielded to the *IREEG* program code for dose calculation.

The following methods also included the 3D patient information, available from the patient CT scan.

The *TAR model* thus evolved into the *ETAR method* (equivalent tissue–air ratio), from the Sontag and Cunningham works [23, 24], based on the O'Connor rectilinear density scaling algorithm for scattering integration [25] to account for different body densities. The O'Connor method evaluated the dose in two media of different density but the same atomic composition, postulating that the ratio of secondary scattered and primary photon fluences are constant in the two media when the geometric distances are scaled inversely to the distance. The inherent assumption of this theory leads to limited applications to heterogeneous tissues, where both density and atomic composition change simultaneously. However, this theorem has been widely used, also in the further evolution of the dose calculation algorithms.

Other approaches modeled the scattered particle transport and the inhomogeneities through correction factors. Among those, the *differential scatter air ratio model dSAR* [26], where the scatter contribution was determined by a scatter–air ratio table that was numerically differentiated.

The *dSAR* method was later improved, by combining a primary and an analytical first scatter calculation with an empirically determined residual scatter component, proposing the *Delta Volume DVOL method* [27]. However, the high computation demand (at that time) did not allow the implementation of those last two methods in clinical practice.

Particularly regarding the heterogeneity handling, noteworthy are the linear attenuation method, the equivalent path length (EPL), the Batho power-law method, all based on a 1D description of the density changes (along the ray path). The first, the *Linear attenuation method*, is straightforward and adjusted the dose with tabulated per cent per cm correction factors according to the tissue and the beam energy. A step forward has been made with the *EPL method*, where the correction factor was expressed as the exponential of the effective attenuation coefficient multiplied by the difference between the physical and radiological depth. Then, the *Power-law method* initially proposed by Batho [28, 29] was generalized by Sontag and Cunningham [30], by using the ratio of TAR powered with the relative electron densities of the tissue as the correction factor.

Interesting to note, as also underlined by the AAPM Report 85 [14], is the use of the correction factors related to the required dose estimation accuracy. In the case of a calculation method which includes a first step of dose calculation in a homogeneous medium, and a second step, independent from the first, taking into account the inhomogeneity by a correction factor, the required total uncertainty has to be divided into the two phases. Let us assume a simplified case where an overall accuracy of 2% is required. Let us also assume an even weight is assigned to the uncertainty from the two steps. All these conditions would then imply that the uncertainty in each step should not exceed 1.4%. The consequence is that the dose calculation in water needs to be more accurate than the global dose calculation requirements.

10.2.3 The kernel-based algorithms: pencil beam, AAA, collapsed cone

It was in the mid-1980s when the energy deposition kernel concept started to be used in the radiotherapy dose calculation. The kernel (or point spread function) is the response of a system to a point source and can describe the scatter (response) generated by the energy fluence in a point (the point source) that crosses the medium. The TERMA (total energy released per mass) is the energy fluence, differential in energy, multiplied by the mass attenuation coefficient in the primary photons, thus describing energy released by the primary photons. A point kernel can be determined (using, for example, Monte Carlo simulations, but also an analytical method can be applied) to describe the transport of energy by the electrons released in the first interaction and the scattered photons. The absorbed dose in a point can be thus calculated by a convolution of the TERMA with the point kernel (figure 10.3):

$$D(\boldsymbol{r}) = \int\int \frac{\mu_E}{\rho} \Psi_E(\boldsymbol{r}) \cdot K_E(\boldsymbol{r} - \boldsymbol{r}')d\boldsymbol{r}\, dE \tag{10.1}$$

In some cases, the integral over the energy is performed before the convolution, and it can be quickly solved by using the Fourier transform, as in the Boyer approach using the Fast Fourier Transform (FFT) [31, 32], assuming the approximation of an invariant kernel. However, the point spread kernel is not spatially invariant due to energy variations, divergence, and the varying density and composition of the

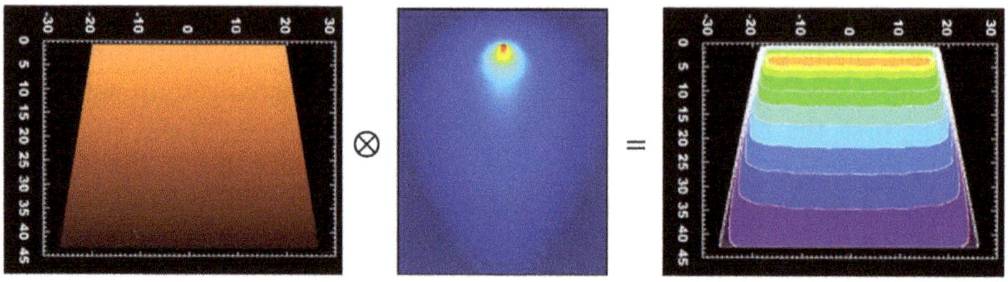

Figure 10.3. Schematic of the absorbed dose distribution as a convolution between TERMA and dose kernel. Adapted from Knöös [13], reproduced with permission. Copyright IOP Publishing Ltd. Open access CC BY 3.0.

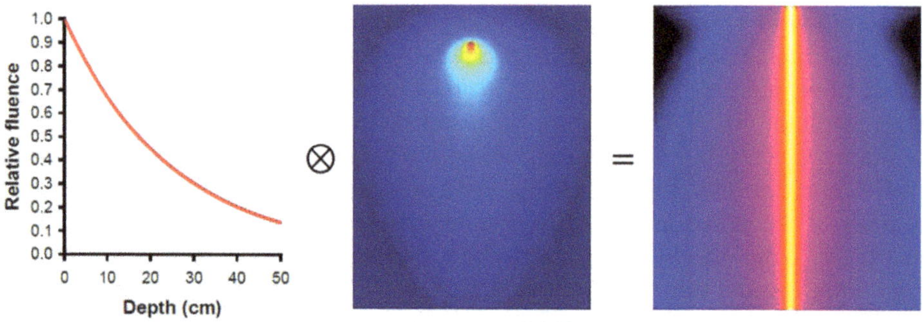

Figure 10.4. The pencil beam principle: convolution of the TERMA along a ray line with the point spread kernel describing the energy transport and absorption. From Knöös [13], reproduced with permission. Copyright IOP Publishing Ltd. Open access CC BY 3.0.

patient tissue. A superposition is hence needed to account for those variations, yielding to a more accurate dose estimation at the cost of a very time-consuming calculation process.

Two methods allowed increasing the calculation speed, namely the pencil beam and the collapsed cone. The *pencil beam* approach reduces the calculation problem from a 3D to a 2D convolution, by the integration of the point kernel along the depth line, as shown in figure 10.4. Here the pencil beam is determined as a convolution of the TERMA along a ray line with the point spread kernel describing the energy transport and absorption.

The dose is then computed applying the pencil beam convolution (and shown in figure 10.5):

$$D(x, y, z) = \iint \frac{\mu_E}{\rho} \cdot \Psi_E(x', y') \cdot P(x - x', y - y', z)dx'dy' \tag{10.2}$$

where z is the water equivalent depth, i.e., the radiological depth that considers the density of the voxel along the pencil.

In equation (10.2), the pencil beams are pre-calculated (analytically or via Monte Carlo simulations), and they are spatially invariant, and a fast calculation with a fast Fourier transform is possible. However, the pencil beams are not spatially invariant

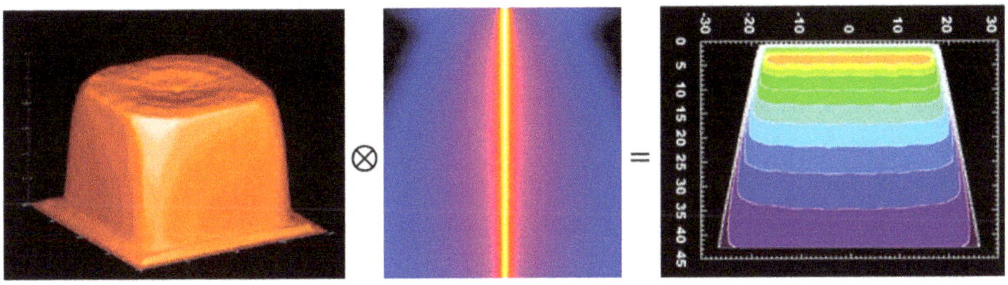

Figure 10.5. Dose distribution obtained by convolution of the 2D energy fluence with the pencil beam. Adapted from Knöös [13], reproduced with permission. Copyright IOP Publishing Ltd. Open access CC BY 3.0.

due to the off-axis variation of the energy spectrum due, for flattened beams, to the presence of the flattening filter making the beam softer going away from the central axis, or also due to the inhomogeneities. When the kernels are considered energy-dependent, the simple convolution does not hold, and a *superposition* approach should be applied, for which the FFT can no longer be adopted.

The pencil beam approach scales for inhomogeneity only in the forward direction, i.e., no scaling is done in directions different from that of propagation. The missing lateral density scaling has effects also on the penumbra. For example, the field edge passing through the lung tissue is not correctly modeled by the pencil beam, and this effect needs to be carefully considered when multiple overlapping fields (or segments of a step and shoot intensity-modulated field) have to be computed by summation. The pencil beam algorithm has been implemented in most of the treatment planning systems and used clinically for many years and as we will see is not ideal for dose calculation in IMRT.

The *anisotropic analytical algorithm* (AAA) realized a step forward in accounting for the lateral electron transport in the presence of inhomogeneities. The AAA was implemented for clinical use only in the Varian Eclipse treatment planning system [33–36].

The lateral transport is modeled along with the four main lateral directions (figure 10.6). Here, the pencil beam is a sum of three terms, one approximating the primary electrons set in motion along the pencil beam, the others describing scattered photons. The density scaling, also in the lateral directions, uses the radiological distance to the calculation points.

The other approach to account for lateral electron transport while increasing computation speed is the *collapsed cone convolution* algorithm, first proposed by Ahnesjö in 1989 [38]. The secondary radiation kernel is, in this model, angularly discretized into a finite number of directions. The polyenergetic point kernels are parametrized and described as a sum of two exponentials [39]. Each discretization direction represents a cone, where the total energy therein released is transported (collapsed) along its central axis. A lattice of collapsed cone lines is built to cover the irradiated volume in many directions (figure 10.7) entirely. The use of density scaling along each collapsed cone direction gives a better detailed, 3-dimensional correction for heterogeneities. However, voxels falling between the collapsed cone lines would

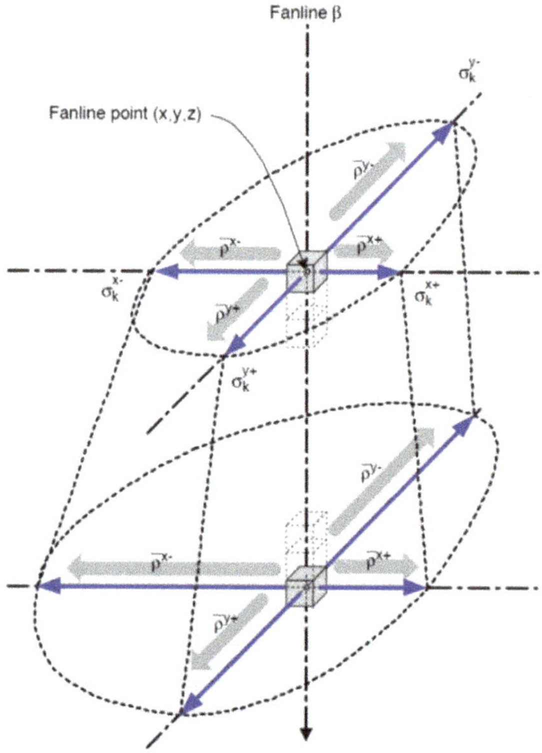

Figure 10.6. Density scaling for the photon scatter kernels in the AAA algorithm. From Sievinen *et al* Varian white paper [37].

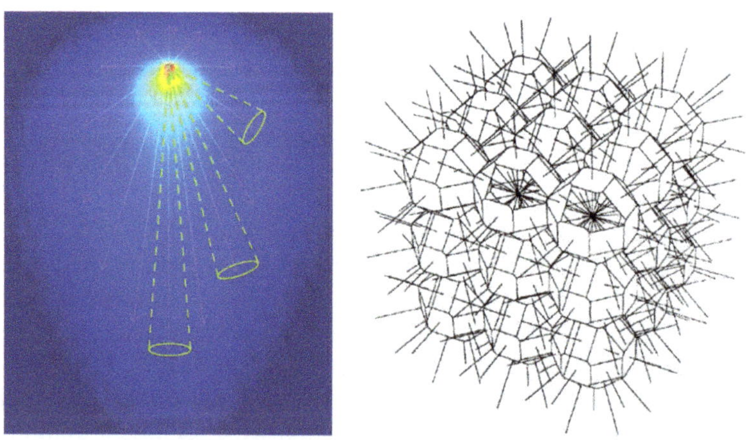

Figure 10.7. On the left: the kernel with the angular discretization and the schematic representation of the cones. On the right: example of a lattice of cone axes. From Ahnesjö [12], reproduced with permission.

receive no energy; for this reason, a large number of cone directions (~100) is needed in the kernel discretization to achieve enough accuracy at all distances.

The collapsed cone convolution algorithm has been implemented in some treatment planning systems, like Pinnacle (Philips), RayStation (RaySearch Laboratories), and used clinically with better dose calculation.

The model-based algorithms (non-empirical) are based on two main components: the modeling of the radiation source, and the in-patient dose calculation. The first component describes the beam source model, determining the fundamental physical parameters required for the dose calculation in the medium for any field geometry and patient anatomy. The second component is the dose calculation algorithm core, which calculates the dose deposition in the patient (medium) using the fundamental physical parameters determined in the first component.

10.2.4 The electron transport explicit algorithms: Monte Carlo, LBTE solvers

The evolution of the photon dose calculation algorithms briefly described in the previous paragraphs yielded to continuous improvement in the accuracy of the estimation of the dose delivered to the patient. With the convolution and superposition models, some pre-determined Monte Carlo simulations results were used, as the kernel computation, to cite an example. The full use of the Monte Carlo dose calculation in the treatment planning systems is in this view the natural, logical further step, also considering the enormously improved computing power. Today's computations allow simulations of detailed 3D geometries both for the treatment unit generating the beam, and the patient anatomy using the CT scan data. The Monte Carlo simulations have been considered the gold standard for dose calculation: the inclusion of the 'true physics' should overcome the limitations of the analytical models.

The physics of the ionizing particles traveling through a medium and interacting with the matter is macroscopically summarized by the linear Boltzmann transport equations (LBTE) [40]:

$$\hat{\Omega} \cdot \vec{\nabla}\Phi^{\gamma} + \sigma_t^{\gamma}\Phi^{\gamma} = q^{\gamma\gamma} + q^{\gamma} \tag{10.3}$$

$$\hat{\Omega} \cdot \vec{\nabla}\Phi^{e} + \sigma_t^{e}\Phi^{e} - \frac{\partial}{\partial E}(S_R\Phi^{e}) = q^{ee} + q^{\gamma e} + q^{e} \tag{10.4}$$

where $\hat{\Omega}$ is the unit direction vector; Φ^{γ} is the photon angular fluence, Φ^{e} is the electron angular fluence, and are a function of the position, the energy, and the direction; $q^{\gamma\gamma}$ is the photon source resulting from photon interactions (photon to photon scattering source), q^{ee} is the electron source resulting from electron interactions (electron to electron scattering source), $q^{\gamma e}$ is the electron source resulting from photon interactions (photon to electron scattering source), and are a function of the position, the energy, and the direction; q^{γ} is the external photon source and represents the photons coming from the linac, q^{e} is the external electron source and represents the electrons coming from the linac, both are a function of the energy and the direction; σ_t^{γ} and σ_t^{e} are the macroscopic total cross-sections for photons and electrons, respectively; S_R is the restricted collisional plus radiative stopping power.

There are two practical approaches to solve the LBTE: a stochastic and a deterministic method.

The *Monte Carlo method* is the stochastic approach that utilizes random sampling for obtaining numerical solutions. It predicts the particle transport across the medium by tracking a statistically significant number of particles through successive random interactions.

Similar to the model-based algorithms, the beam modelization is separate from the patient dose calculation. Three steps are mainly used for Monte Carlo dose distribution calculations in the radiotherapy planning (figure 10.8). Firstly, a phase space summarizing the radiation beam at a position downstream to the beam generation after the primary collimation in the linac head, that is machine-specific, but not patient-specific. Then, a second phase space is generally computed positioned after the secondary collimation (jaws and MLC). The third step is the simulation of the patient-specific geometry, where the dose distribution is calculated.

The simulation of the accelerator linac heads (the first and second steps) was pioneered by Petti [41] and Mohan [42], and today the most used code for this purpose is the EGSnrc-based BEAM code [43]. In the phase space generation, some parameters have to be tuned (for example the initial electron energy and spread, the

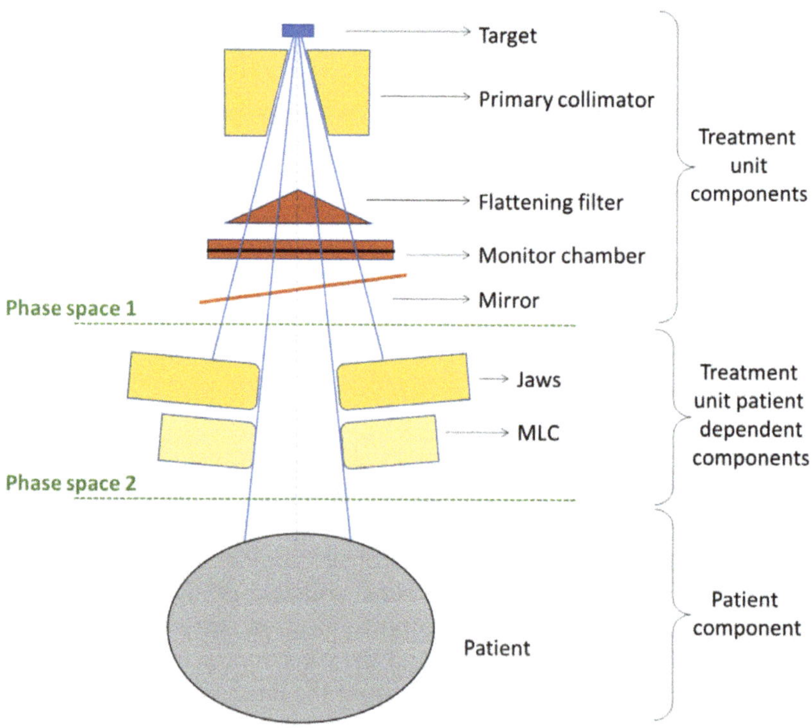

Figure 10.8. Treatment unit and patient-related components for Monte Carlo simulation (not to scale).

focal spot) and a validation process has to confirm that the phase space is in accordance with measured data of the clinical beam. Moreover, to achieve sufficient accuracy, variance-reduction techniques have to be applied to increase the statistical efficiency of the simulation. Being subject to stochastic errors, an insufficient number of histories give unacceptable uncertainty.

Regarding the in-patient part of the simulation process, the resulting dose calculation is more accurate than any other analytical-based algorithm, where rather crude approximations are adopted, especially concerning inhomogeneity handling. However, the Monte Carlo planning systems also have uncertainties in this view: the material of which a specific tissue is composed is translated from the CT number to a particular human tissue. The human tissues are limited to only a few compositions as lung, adipose, muscle, cartilage, and bone. Their elemental compositions are based on ICRP or ICRU reports [44–46]. These provide the average values based on a limited set of human body samples in contrast with the ICRU Report 44 request to always take into account the variability of the body-tissue compositions (that are not physical constants and cannot be considered at the same standing) [45].

All these aspects suggest that no Monte Carlo calculation should be considered free of errors, and, particularly in treatment planning, the uncertainties involved remain ‘uncertain’ [47].

Interesting reviews of the Monte Carlo usage in the treatment planning system were published in 2007 by Reynaert and colleagues [48], and more recently, in 2018, Andreo [47].

Over time, different Monte Carlo codes have been developed over the years, specifically optimized for radiotherapy dose calculation [49], such as XVMC [50], VMC++ [51], DPM [52], allowing the implementation in some clinical treatment planning systems. Among those: Monaco (Elekta), RayStation (RaySearch), iPlan (BrainLab). Other full Monte Carlo solutions are also available on the web, such as PRIMO, which is a free system usable for research purposes [53].

The LBTE equations can also be solved through *deterministic methods*, which simulate the effect of an infinite number of particles by discretizing the phase space variables. An analytical solution of the LBTE is not feasible, and the deterministic methods use numerical solutions. One of those is the grid-based solver (or discrete ordinate method) [40, 54–56].

The energy fluence is generated by a different model and summarized in a phase space. Once the radiation enters the patient, the discrete ordinates are applied, giving photon and electron sources in each voxel. The photon and electron energies are discretized in directions, space and angle, and energy. Once all the fluences are determined according to the discretization, the final dose is obtained by integrating the fluences in energy and angular direction. On the usage of LBTE solvers in the dose calculation for radiotherapy planning, a recent and comprehensive review by Bedford [57] has been published.

Based on the work of Vassiliev *et al* [40], Varian Eclipse treatment planning system has implemented an LBTE solver in the clinical practice which is called Acuros-XB dose calculation algorithm.

Noteworthy is that both approaches to the LBTE solutions, whether Monte Carlo or a deterministic method, have inherent errors, the first in terms of stochastic uncertainties, the second, in the form of the discrete ordinate solvers, in terms of uncertainty produced by the discretization process. The uncertainty reduction may be improved by increasing the number of histories in the Monte Carlo case, or by using a finer discretization in the deterministic solver.

Similarly to the model-based algorithms, that are based on the modeling of the radiation source and the in-patient dose calculation, also the LBTE based algorithms, here briefly described, have the same structure (figure 10.8). The beam characteristics are derived in a phase space generated separately from the process involving the dose calculation in the patient anatomy, where the Monte Carlo or LBTE solver simulates or computes the energy deposition. The phase space can be fully simulated via Monte Carlo (and then verified against measurements), once the linac head geometry is known, or with multiple-source models [58]. Just to give a couple of examples, PRIMO, that is a Monte Carlo based system, generates fully simulated phase space (or can use pre-calculated phase spaces). In contrast, Acuros, is a deterministic method for which the photon beam source model is adopted, similar to the AAA algorithm [59].

10.3 Type 'a', 'b', 'c' algorithm classification

The photon dose calculation algorithms have been classified by Knöös in 2006 [16]. In this first paper, several algorithms implemented in different commercial TPS were compared, and variations on simple clinical situations were assessed. The cases selected included a two tangential breast field treatment, a 3D conformal box for prostate, two lateral fields in head and neck, and lung boost treatment with five fields. Using conformal plans, the authors focused their attention on the clinical impact of only the dose calculation algorithm.

The algorithms were initially classified into two groups, aiming, in essence, to isolate and differentiate only the heterogeneity and the scatter volume handling:

- *Type 'a'* models: are the algorithms primarily based on equivalent path length scaling for inhomogeneity corrections. The changes in lateral electron transport are not modeled. To this type belong all the empirical models and the pencil beam which handles the inhomogeneity along the fan line with one-dimensional path length.
- *Type 'b'* models: are the algorithms that consider approximately the changes in lateral transport of electrons. Here the electron modeling is not explicitly performed, while approximate modeling is included. To this type belong, as paradigmatic examples, the collapsed cones (implemented in Pinnacle, RaySearch, and other systems) with the energy transported along the cones mimicking a 3D transport, and being probably the most accurate among this category of algorithms. The anisotropic analytical algorithm AAA (on the Varian Eclipse system) also belongs to this group, by including the lateral density scaling in six directions; the multigrid superposition algorithm (on the XiO planning system) is also part of this category of models.

The third category of algorithms has been later introduced extending the Knöös classification, as *type 'c'* models (initially introduced as such by Ojala [60]). Type 'c' models are properly the Monte Carlo based systems and the algorithms presenting the same degree of accuracy in dose estimation, as the linear Boltzmann transport equation solvers, like the Acuros algorithm. In those systems, the physics generating the dose absorption process is fully included. By using appropriate approximations, *type 'c'* algorithms are certainly the most accurate descriptors of the absorbed dose distribution in the medium (patient) and should be the choice in IMRT.

Knöös *et al* [16], comparing some *type 'a'* and *type 'b'* algorithms, concluded that in many situations, the differences are small and possibly not clinically relevant. This could be the case of the prostate and pelvic region. Regarding the head and neck, where there are a number of small inhomogeneities, the use of more sophisticated models should be preferred. Significant differences have been found in the tangential breast setting, with the missing lateral scattering and the low-density lung on one side. The most complicated situation of the lung, with large low-density volumes, showed variations, especially for higher energy photon beams, of possible clinical relevance, and *type 'a'* algorithms should be avoided.

The characteristics of the three model categories in the most complex clinical case of stereotactic lung treatment was published in 2017 [61]. The increased complexity is due to the small fields to deliver dose in low-density volumes. This particular situation makes the electronic equilibrium and volume scatter a challenging task. Figure 10.9 reports an example of rather small fields with lung inhomogeneity for the three model categories. A pencil beam convolution algorithm for the *type 'a'*, the anisotropic analytical algorithm AAA as the *type 'b'* and the Acuros-XB algorithms

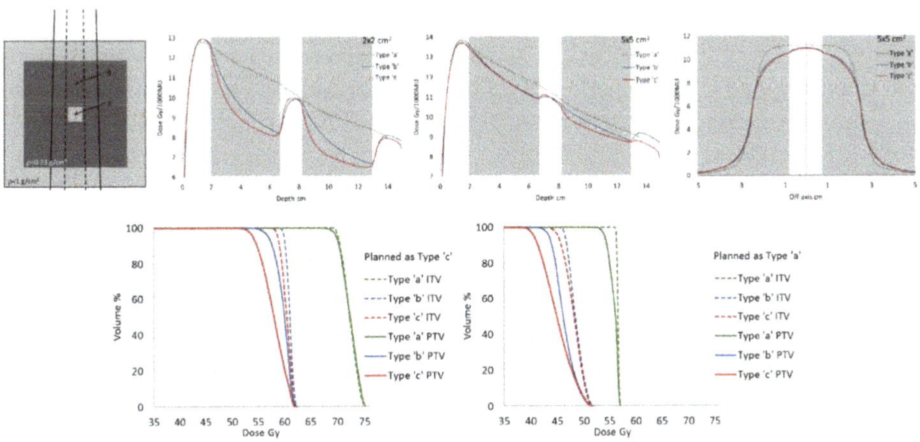

Figure 10.9. First row: phantom setting with single 2 × 2 and 5 × 5 cm^2 field; depth doses along the central beam axis for the 2 × 2 cm^2 and the 5 × 5 cm^2; lateral profile for the 5 × 5 cm^2 across the mid-phantom. Second row: the lung SBRT example: ITV and PTV DVHs of a clinical IMRT case planned with type 'c' (left) and type 'a' (right) algorithms, using in each plot settings the same number of MU. Adapted from Fogliata *et al* [61], reproduced with permission from Associazione Italiana di Fisica Medica.

type 'c' (all from the Eclipse planning system). Here the difference in estimating the dose in the lung region is shown. Another critical effect of clinical relevance is the MU calculation in the lung SBRT case, as shown in the second part of figure 10.9. In this case a 7-field, six MV IMRT treatment was planned to deliver 54 Gy in three fractions as 95% PTV coverage: in the first case by using the *type 'c'* (assumed to be the most accurate), in the second by using the *type 'a'* (with the least accuracy) algorithms. The plans were then recomputed with the three algorithms, using the same MU as the original plan (Acuros and pencil beam in the first and second cases, respectively). The PTV and ITV DVH are reported, showing a dramatic dose overestimation when the *type 'a'* algorithm is used, and a non-negligible overestimation of the target coverage for the *type 'b'* model. A similar observation has also been noted by Jones *et al* [62].

The lung SBRT is probably the clinical case where the dose calculation algorithm has the highest impact. The imperfect calculation is part of the prior clinical knowledge: the predictions of a vast number of studies were based on *type 'a'* algorithms, and most of the clinical data we today refer to, come from the results of those studies.

The example of the RTOG trials on lung SBRT is quite impressive. The RTOG-0236 (phase II trial of SBRT in medically inoperable stage I/II NSCLC, activated in 2004 and closed in 2006) and the RTOG-0618 (phase II trial of SBRT inoperable stage I/II NSCLC, activated in 2007 and closed in 2010), in the protocol guidelines, cited that 'for purposes of dose planning and calculation of monitor units for actual treatment, all tissues within the body, including lung, will be assumed to have unit (water) density (no correction for tissue heterogeneity)'. In those cases hence the clinical results correlating with dosimetric data were affected by a rather gross error.

More recent trials such as the RTOG-0813 (phase I/II study of SBRT for early-stage centrally located medically inoperable NSCLC, activated in 2009), and the RTOG-0915 (randomized phase II of SBRT for medically inoperable stage I NSCLC, activated in 2009), in the protocol guidelines, cited that 'for purposes of dose planning and calculation of monitor units for actual treatment, this protocol will require tissue density heterogeneity corrections'. In particular, this last protocol, the SBRT treatment approach requires the use of the superposition/convolution or Monte Carlo based dose calculation algorithms. This protocol allows using a *type 'c'* algorithm for MU calculation and dose distribution that, in SBRT cases, would give dosimetric values significantly different from a *type 'b'* algorithm, or the missing inclusion of inhomogeneity correction (as in the previous trials). This fact shows that consistent use of the dose calculation algorithms in the clinical trials is not yet fully achieved, possibly lowering the strength of the accuracy of the dosimetric results emerging from those fundamental clinical studies.

This issue was pointed out by Timmermann *et al* [63] in their description of the RTOG-0236 trial results. They confirmed that, related to the 60 Gy prescribed at the edge of the PTV in three fractions, a later analysis with an appropriate inhomogeneity handling, showed that the RTOG-0236 trial overpredicted the actual PTV dose, and the delivered dose was closer to 54 Gy [64], thus reporting an inaccuracy of about 10% which is also shown by Akino *et al* [65].

10.4 Dose-to-medium or dose-to-water?

The Monte Carlo based dose calculations (or, similarly, through the LBTE solvers), by their intrinsic nature, compute the dose in the actual medium (tissue) crossed by the radiation beam. At the same time, it is generally not the case for most of the kernel-based algorithms. Indeed, for the latter, the kernels are commonly determined in water; the radiological scaling does not change the elemental composition of the medium, that remains water. Those algorithms hence compute the dose 'in-water' with different densities. The case of the Monte Carlo models is different, where the energy transport, in general, uses the physical properties of the (assigned) tissue of each voxel, and the dose can be thus computed 'in-medium'. Most of the Monte Carlo methods allow the reporting of the dose-to-water, although intrinsically calculated as dose-to-medium, by applying to each voxel a correction, given by the ratio of the mass stopping powers S/ρ between water and medium, correction based on the application of the Bragg–Gray cavity theory [66]. In principle, the dose-to-water intended to be the dose as if the crossed medium is water with different density

$$D_w = D_m(S/\rho)_m^w \tag{10.5}$$

In their paper, Siebers and coauthors reported the stopping power ratios to apply to the simulated dose-to-medium to report the dose-to-water for some human tissues under the most common radiotherapy photon beams. This issue has been recently elaborated in the AAPM TG-329 [67]. The correction values are rather closer to unity, except for the air and the cortical bone, where they are higher than 10%, this value represents the difference between dose-to-medium and dose-to-water reporting for the same deposited energy in the medium. This implies that, for the majority of the tissues, the dosimetric impact is not too significant, and the question of which is the procedure to follow in dose reporting seems to be not too urgent to solve. The dose handling with bone tissue remains an issue.

Reynaert and colleagues [68] studied the specific bone problem, and proposed, instead of correcting using the stopping power ratios, to use in its place the ratio of the mass-energy absorption coefficients in the regions of electronic equilibrium, since the electron range in the bone is short, and the voxels can be considered large cavities in the Bragg–Gray theory, and by consequence the mass-energy absorption coefficients $\overline{\mu_{en}}/\rho$ should be applied instead of the stopping power

$$D_w = D_m(\overline{\mu_{en}}/\rho)_m^w \tag{10.6}$$

This would suggest a correction of 5%–6% to bone in place of the 10%–11% of the Siebers method.

Andreo [47], in 2018, when discussing the Monte Carlo based treatment planning dose calculation, showed that the Siebers correction with the stopping power ratio is incorrect, since it assumes the same electron fluence in case of tissue or water crossed by the radiation, while it is not the case. For this reason, Andreo proposed an additional correction, the *fluence correction factor* accounting for this difference:

$$D_w = D_m(S/\rho)^w_m k_\phi \tag{10.7}$$

All these more recent proposals have been analyzed by Delbaere *et al* in 2019 [69], where the authors also compared calculations against measurements in bone-like slabs, considering measuring with acceptable approximations the dose-to-water. The interesting results showed a good agreement among measurements (as a dose-to-water expression), and the dose-to-water estimated by correcting the Monte Carlo simulated dose-to-medium according to the Reynaert formula with the ratio of the mass-energy absorption coefficient or the dose-to-water according to the Andreo formula with the stopping power ratio and the additional fluence correction factor. In the same study, the authors showed that the native Monte Carlo dose-to-water, using the Siebers correction with stopping power ratio, overestimated the measured dose by 4%. In comparison, the dose-to-medium was lower by about 6% with respect to the measurements acquired as in-water. This work also suggests the impossibility of comparing, for human tissues, measurements against dose-to-medium calculations, making it hard to commission, for clinical use, the dose calculation algorithms based on this inherent computation modality.

In a very interesting work published in 2010, Walters and colleagues [70] detailed the dose (to-medium and to-water). The authors suggested more precise modeling of the different types of bone tissues in the human body: the radiosensitive red bone marrow consisting of hematopoietic stem cells and bone surface osteogenic cells (hard or cortical bone), embedded in the spongious bone (spongy soft bone, light and porous). By using a well detailed virtual phantom that accounted for all those differences, they aimed to determine whether dose-to-medium or dose-to-water better estimated the dose received by the more sensitive tissues (red bone marrow and bone surface cells) inside the spongious structure. The amount of these tissues is different for bones in different location of the human skeleton, value expressed as trabecular bone volume fraction (TBVF), from the 10% of the ribs (with a density of 1.10 g cm^{-3}) to the 15% of the long bones, to the 20% of the pelvic bones, to the 55% of the mandible and cranium (with a density of 1.51 g cm^{-3}). A difference in the dose estimation reporting was expected for different bone locations. They found that with decreasing TBVF the difference between dose-to-medium and dose-to-water is less significant. However, for the cranium and mandible, the dose-to-medium significantly underestimated the absorbed dose by at least 5%. The authors suggested specifying the dose-to-water in Monte Carlo planning in the head and neck region since it provides a better estimate of dose to sensitive tissue in bone. However, this suggestion is not valid for the surrounding spongious bone, which is the predominant volume.

All the above discussion is valid for most of the Monte Carlo dose estimations. However, the dose-to-water conversion from dose-to-medium inherently computed can be applied differently. This is the case, for example with Acuros-XB implementation, where the dose-to-water is not calculated as a simple correction of the dose-to-medium. In this case, once the electron fluence Φ^e is determined, the dose is computed as:

$$D_i = \int_0^\infty dE \int_{4\pi} d\hat{\Omega} \frac{\sigma_{\mathrm{ED}}^e(\vec{r}, E)}{\rho(\vec{r})} \Phi^e(\vec{r}, E, \hat{\Omega}) \tag{10.8}$$

where D_i is the dose in the voxel I, σ_{ED}^e is the macroscopic electron energy deposition cross-section, ρ is the material density. When dose-to-medium is calculated, σ_{ED}^e and ρ are based on the specific material properties of the voxel. When the dose-to-water is instead computed, σ_{ED}^e and ρ are based on water. However, the energy-dependent electron fluence Φ^e is in both cases based on the properties of the materials of the patient in each voxel [40]

Delbaere [69] compared the Andreo and Reynaert corrections with the native Acuros conversion just described. They found that the Acuros dose-to-water was higher than the measured and Andreo or Reynaert corrected dose, by about 10%, presenting the same problems pointed out with the Siebers correction.

The dose-to-water obtained by Monte Carlo or Acuros is not the same dose-to-water that was intended with the analytical algorithms (which did not account for the elemental composition of the crossed medium) since in the dose calculation, or at least in the electron fluence estimation, the physical properties of the assumed medium are adopted.

In the absence of a clear indication or recommendation of what should be clinically used (which arrived only very recently with the AAPM TG-329 [67]), the community investigated the clinical practice on the differences between the two dose reporting methods, as shown in many papers published in the last decade, assessing its possible clinical impact. In 2006, Dogan *et al* [71] used a full Monte Carlo (EGS4) for calculating the dose of head and neck and prostate IMRT plans, finding a difference in the target dose coverage of 2.9% and 3.5% for the head and neck and prostate cases, respectively, and an overall range of differences from 0% to 8%, that can be considered as systematic dose errors. Later, when the commercial planning systems using Monte Carlo or LBTE solvers started to be available, the interest allowed an increase of publications, mainly on the Elekta Monaco Monte Carlo, and the Varian Acuros.

Radojčić [72] evaluated the dose-to-medium and dose-to-water reporting differences using the Elekta Monaco Monte Carlo planning system on nasopharyngeal cancer patients. They found that for the majority of the target and most of the organs at risk, the dosimetric parameter differences were not significant, while it was for the bony structures such as the mandible and the cochlea, where the dose-to-water was higher by almost 10% than the dose-to-medium estimation, concluding that this might have clinical consequences.

Muñoz-Montplet [73] assessed the dosimetric impact in using Acuros with dose-to-medium or dose-to-water reporting, comparing with AAA (dose-to-water in water) dose calculations for head and neck tumor planning with VMAT. They found that no systematic trend was observed between AAA and dose-to-water Acuros computations, with absolute dose differences ranging between −5.3 Gy (−7.3% for the maximum dose to the manidble) and 0.6 Gy (2.4% for a parotid mean dose). Conversely, the dose-to-water dose-volume parameters were significantly higher than dose-to-medium reporting, with absolute dose difference in a range of 0.1 Gy (1.8% for the mean brain dose) and 6.6 Gy (10% for the maximum dose to the mandible), with the largest absolute differences presented for the maximum doses to cochleae and the mandible (14% and 10%), that is in line, as a trend, with the discussions above, and especially the Walters concept of bone composition in the mandible.

Other authors reported on similar comparisons with Monaco Monte Carlo [74] or Acuros-XB [75, 76] for different anatomical sites such as head and neck, breast, lung, prostate, and pelvis, concluding that the most relevant difference is found in the bone, and in particular in the head and neck tumors.

It is clear, not only from the theory but also confirmed in the clinical field, that the most considerable relevance is in the regions where bones are involved. However, this is not the only tissue where the elemental composition plays a role, as pointed out by Fogliata *et al* [77, 78]. On Acuros and PRIMO Monte Carlo, it was found that the two main tissue components of the breast, the lobular and the adipose tissues receive up to 2% dose variation (more significant in the lobular than in the fat) due to their elemental composition more than the pure density difference. Although not clinically relevant, it is an indication of the unavoidable degrees of inaccuracy we have in our common clinical practice.

To summarize on the dose-to-medium and dose-to-water reporting, in the following an example of a head and neck VMAT plan with a simultaneous integrated boost to deliver 66 and 54 Gy in 30 fractions is presented with the support of the isodoses and the DVHs (figure 10.10), with the same plan initially optimized and calculated with Acuros and dose-to-medium reporting, then recomputed as dose-to-water as well as AAA, keeping identical MUs.

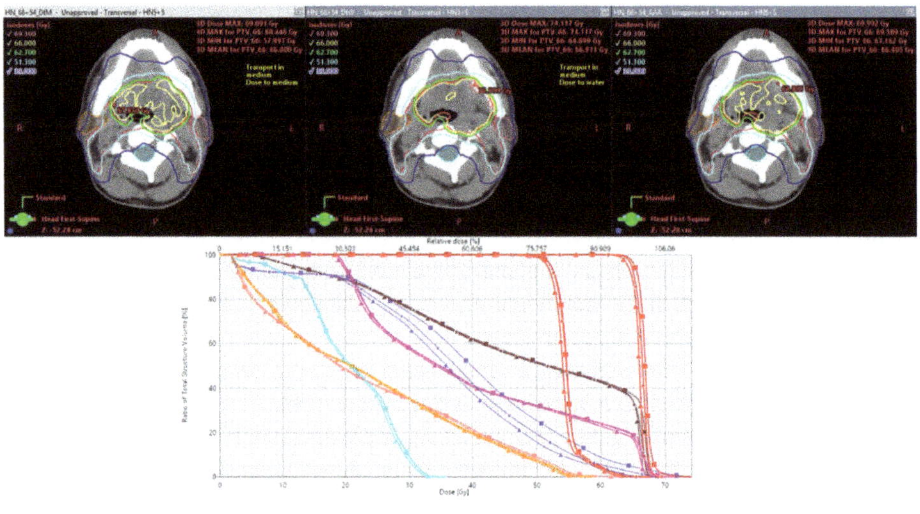

Figure 10.10. Head and neck VMAT example: isodoses and DVHs for targets and OARs of the same plan (same MUs) computed with Acuros dose-to-medium, Acuros dose-to-water, AAA. In the DVHs: Acuros dose-to-medium: triangles, Acuros dose-to-water: squares, AAA: dots.

In this exemplification, the mean doses to the 66 Gy and 54 Gy PTVs were 65.8 and 54.3 Gy in the dose-to-medium plan, while they were +1.2%, +1.0%, and +1.5%, +0.8% for the dose-to-water, AAA plans, respectively. The largest difference, as expected, was in the mandible, with $D_{10\%}$ of 53.6 Gy for dose-to-medium, and +10.0%, +3.5% for dose-to-water, AAA, respectively. The other OARs differences are not so large. These figures are similar to what was published by Dogan *et al* [71].

The same exercise on a prostate VMAT plan, conversely, did not show the significant variations pointed out for the head and neck case, supporting the concept expressed by Walters *et al* [70]. Here, in figure 10.11, a prostate case with urethra sparing with VMAT, in four fractions, indicating very high similarities.

Now, let us first assume that the Monte Carlo and LBTE solvers are more accurate than any analytical algorithm. However, the difference in the dose-to-water relative to the dose-to-medium (the inherent calculation) in some cases—the head and neck, for example—is not negligible. The difference could be close to the 2% that is required in the dose calculation accuracy, as shown in the first section of this chapter, suggesting the need of finding a solution to harmonize dose reporting to allow improving clinical knowledge.

Additionally, the absorbed dose estimation with Monte Carlo (or LBTE solver), naturally computed as dose-to-medium, assumes the knowledge of the elemental tissue composition as determined and reported in the ICRP and ICRU Reports [44–46], which also include some variability in the population. However, there are differences even in the elemental composition when used in two different systems. As an example, PRIMO with Monte Carlo and Eclipse with Acuros, have different tissue composition for nominally equal tissues, as shown in figure 10.12 [77]. This

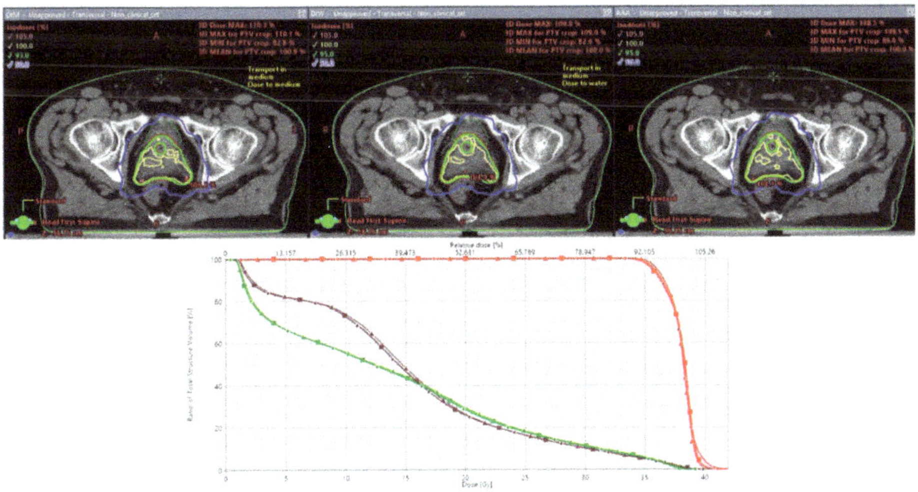

Figure 10.11. Prostate VMAT example: isodoses and DVHs for targets and OARs of the same plan (same MUs) computed with Acuros dose-to-medium, Acuros dose-to-water, AAA. In the DVHs: Acuros dose-to-medium: dots, Acuros dose-to-water: squares, AAA: triangles.

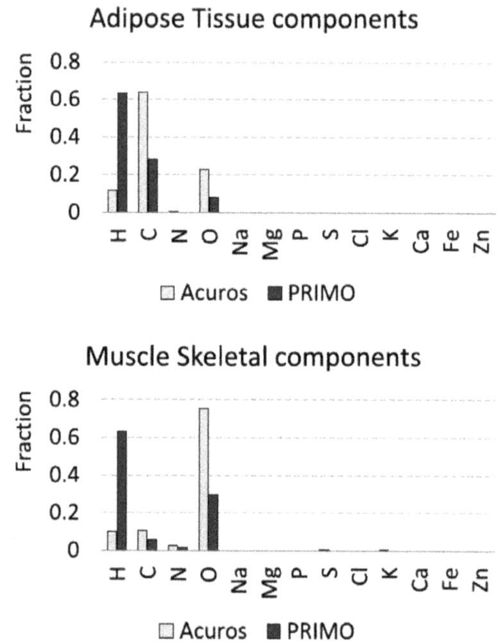

Figure 10.12. Default elemental component of adipose and muscle-skeletal tissues, as implemented in Eclipse, Acuros, and PRIMO, Monte Carlo. From Fogliata *et al* [77], reproduced with permission. Copyright the authors 2018. Open access CC BY 4.0.

difference, although defined as the same tissue, will produce different results in terms of absorbed dose.

Also, the range of the CT numbers to associate to each tissue is not uniquely defined, nor uniquely used. In general, Monte Carlo uses adjacent ranges to associate different tissues. This is not the case in the current Acuros implementation in Eclipse, where overlapping regions between two adjacent tissues are present, defining the tissue composition as a linear combination of the previous and next material. This is particularly interesting in the bone material, where the overlapping region between bone and the previous tissue, the cartilage, is rather large to minimize the discrepancies dosimetrically pointed out by Walters [70].

From these simple considerations, it is clear that the radiotherapy community needs to delineate, which is the road to follow in the next future in terms of dose-to-medium or dose-to-water. Moreover, better knowledge about the tissue assignment and elemental composition should be worth at the present status to improve the dose estimation accuracy. However, as per today, no consensus has yet been reached on the subject, the dilemma remains, and the community is still debating, since a couple of decades ago, about the dose reporting. There are reasons in favor of one or the other reporting methods, as summarized in the point/counterpoint debate a quite long time ago, in 2002, between Liu and Keall, the first in favor of dose-to-medium, the second of dose-to-water reporting [79], and then detailed in the Task Group No. 105 of the AAPM [80]. The discussion continued over the years, to more recent days, where Andreo [47, 81] in publications still discussed the same arguments.

The arguments *in favor of the dose-to-water* reporting are mainly three:

- first, the past clinical experience is based on the dose-to-water computation. With the exclusion of the most modern systems, the dose calculation algorithms adopted for a long time used measurements or calculations (the kernels) in water to describe the dose deposition in water-like tissue with different densities. Nothing different was possible, and hence the current experience (and trials) refers to clinical results in terms of therapeutic and normal tissue tolerance dose levels compliant with the dose-to-water (in water) computation, leaving to the community many dose criteria for TCP and NTCP that are dose-to-water, and not dose-to-medium criteria. What is generally not underlined at this point is the accuracy of the biological parameters currently in use, being much larger than the differences found between the dose-to-medium and dose-to-water.
- second, the beam calibration. The current dosimetry codes of practice determine the absorbed dose-*to-water*, which is the reference quantity in the clinics.
- third, the tumor cells embedded within a medium are more water-like than medium-like. This should also be related to the size of the cavity in the Bragg-Gray theory.

The arguments *in favor of the dose-to-medium* can be summarized:

- first, the chance to accurately and inherently compute the absorbed dose in the tissue is an advantageous feature. The dose-to-water calculation would bring back to the past when this accuracy level was not possible. With the dose-to-medium approach, new standards of practice should be established to reflect the achieved advantages of using Monte Carlo.
- second, the conversion from the inherently computed dose-to-medium to the dose-to-water requires corrections, as discussed above. As any new correction factor, this introduces additional and not negligible uncertainty in the dose-to-water estimation.
- third, the clinical impact is not expected to be significant for most of the tissues (the exception is the bone handling), giving thus no actual reason to correct back to dose-to-water, and the dose-to-medium reporting allows providing a closer relationship between the tissue response and the *actual* dose.

With no consensus on the dose reporting (till the very recent AAPM TG-329 [67]), there have been attempts over the years to drive the community toward one way, initially to dose-to-water reporting. In 2011 Ma *et al* [82], reassessing the findings for both the reportings, suggested the assignment of water material with variable electron density instead of the real biological tissue to be more compliant with the old calculations and to avoid additional corrections, thus inhibiting the advantages made available by the Monte Carlo dose estimation in the medium, in terms of both accuracy and knowledge advances. More recently, Andreo [47] suggested that the conversion from dose-to-medium to dose-to-water should be avoided due to the considerable uncertainty in the determination of the corrections, implicitly recommending the dose-to-medium reporting. Indeed, with the dose-to-medium approach, new standards of practice should be established to reflect the achieved advantages of using Monte Carlo. An effort on this road should be made by the community to review the biological parameters for TCP and NTCP estimations in light of the recent, more accurate dose estimation. This process could lead to a more robust knowledge of the relationships between dose and clinical outcomes.

An additional consideration, bringing the discussion in favor of the dose-to-medium reporting, concerns the interfaces between different materials. This is an unresolved problem in the dose-to-water conversion, as reported for example by Reynaert *et al*, and Andreo [47, 68], indicating the interfaces as regions where the dose conversion is not valid.

It is only very recently—the publication in *Medical Physics* dates to March 2020—that the AAPM (American Association of Physicists in Medicine) published the recommendations from the Task Group 329 on reference dose specifications for dose calculations as dose-to-water or dose-to-muscle, trying to put some order on one point of the whole debate on dose-to-medium versus dose-to-water reporting [67]. In the introduction, the authors started from the concept of beam calibration that is done in water according to the code of practice (AAPM TG-51 and IAEA RTS-398). However, historically in North America, the dose has been requested as dose-to-tissue (also called dose-to-muscle), this concept being more consistent with what was being delivered to the patient. But the big challenge of translating the linac calibration in water to the treatment planning reference dose remains open.

From Monte Carlo simulations the difference between water and muscle dose is estimated to be in the range of 0.7%–1.3%, giving the reason of a 1% correction that is (and has been) applied in most institutions to comply with some clinical trials requesting dose-to-muscle reporting. Considering the uncertainty of using or not this correction, this 1% (systematic) error represents a substantial portion of the total calculation uncertainty budget, which is required as ±2% to achieve an overall treatment accuracy of ±5% in the patient, as discussed at the beginning of this chapter. The Task Group document intended to clarify the link between the calibration dose measured in water and the calculated dose to soft tissue, without entering into the broader debate, nor in the accuracy of the different algorithm. However, this clarification could be the answer to the beam calibration, considered an issue in the dose reporting debate, and would weaken the dose-to-water reporting. The document finally recommends fundamentally that the linear accelerators should be calibrated in water and reported as dose-to-water, according to the current codes of practice (as AAPM TG-51 and IAEA RTS-398); for the systems and algorithms calculating dose-to-water, the dose should be manually corrected as dose-to-tissue by multiplying the dose by a correction factor equal to 0.99. They encourage the planning system vendors to evolve their algorithms to calculate and report dose-to-tissue.

Notwithstanding, the Task Group does not enter into the specific merit of the dose-to-medium or dose-to-water debate, the trend toward dose-to-medium is delineated.

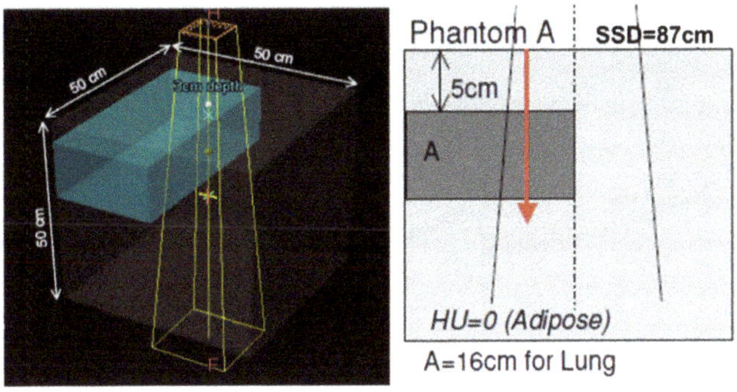

Figure 10.13. Geometrical layout of the phantom. Adapted from Fogliata *et al* [83], reproduced with permission. Copyright IOP Publishing Ltd. All rights reserved.

10.5 Dose calculation accuracy in various TPS implementations

A vast number of studies have been published over the years to assess the accuracy of the different dose calculation algorithms as implemented in the clinically released commercial treatment planning systems. Many compared the calculations against measurements in phantoms (homogeneous, with inhomogeneities, anthropomorphic) and others compared against Monte Carlo simulations, with validated Monte Carlo phase spaces of the linac head. Again, many others just compared different algorithms to each other. It was with the Knöös classification of the algorithms [16] that the salient differences and critical points were categorized, showing the significant differences between the different algorithm types according to this classification.

Just as an example of this plethora of literature, here is a summary of only a couple of studies summarizing many dose calculation algorithms together, under critical phantom conditions including heterogeneities, and compared against a validated full Monte Carlo simulation. However, similar results can be found for each algorithm implementation. Fogliata *et al* [83] presented data with different algorithms in different planning systems and compared with full Monte Carlo simulation. Although not recent, it gives a rather comprehensive overview of the main characteristics of each algorithm category. The study was based on a virtual phantom geometry, as in figure 10.13, with the insert mimicking the lung tissue with two different densities (0.20 g cm^{-3} or normal lung, and 0.035 g cm^{-3} or light lung), or bone. The different values for the two low densities intended on one side to evaluate the clinical aspect (normal lung), and on the other hand to highlight the potential problem in more extreme cases (light lung).

The algorithms analyzed were: pencil beam convolution (from Varian Eclipse and Nucletron Helax-TMS), fast Fourier Transform convolution (FFTC from CMS XiO) as *type 'a'* algorithms, multigrid superposition/convolution (MGS from CMS XiO), AAA (from Varian Eclipse), collapsed cone (from Nucletron Helax-TMS and Philips Pinnacle) as *type 'b'* algorithms. At that time, no commercial *type 'c'* algorithms were yet available. The results of that work are reported in figures 10.14, 10.15 as depth dose curves along the red arrow depicted in figure 10.13. In the

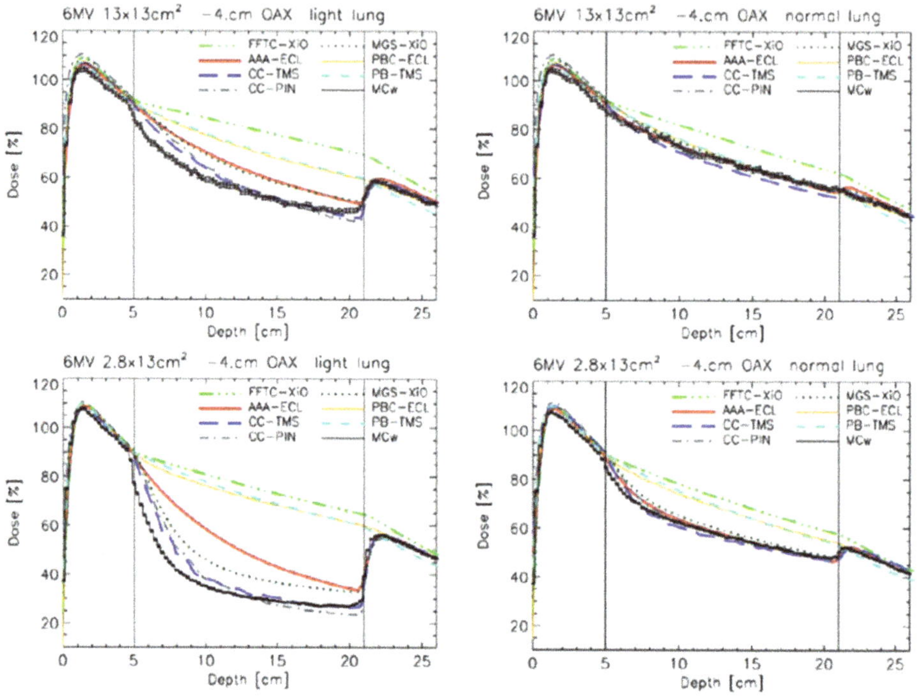

Figure 10.14. Depth dose curves for a 6 MV beam along the arrow in figure 10.13. Adapted from Fogliata *et al* [83], reproduced with permission.

figures (figures 10.14 and 10.15 for the 6 MV and 15 MV beam, respectively), the upper graphs refer to a square 13×13 cm^2 field, the bottom row to a 2.8×13 cm^2 (small in one direction); on the left, there are the plots estimated for the light lung phantom, on the right for the normal lung. The distinction between *type 'a'* algorithms is enhanced in the light lung for the smaller field, where the dose overestimation in the low-density region is evident, with the fast Fourier transform being the lower performing model. Different is the case of *type 'b'* algorithms, where a dose reduction in the lung is present. Among those, considering Monte Carlo as the benchmark, the collapsed cone is the model which better agrees with it even in the extreme conditions of the light lung, followed by the multigrid superposition, and then the AAA, which suffers more in the high energy case (figure 10.15).

The lateral profiles at isocentre at the half-thickness of the lung insert, to better understand the lateral scatterings which are reported in figure 10.16 for the 6 MV and 10.17 for the 15 MV. It shows the amount of dose in the lung insert (negative values of the off-axis position) reports the same as visualized in the depth dose curves; of interest in the lateral profile is the estimation of the beam penumbra in the low-density region, and the estimated behavior close to the interface between low and medium density (across the zero off-axis) (figure 10.17).

The inclusion of a *type 'c'* algorithms, Acuros-XB in the Eclipse planning system, was published by the same group in 2011 [78]. In figures 10.18 and 10.19, the depth

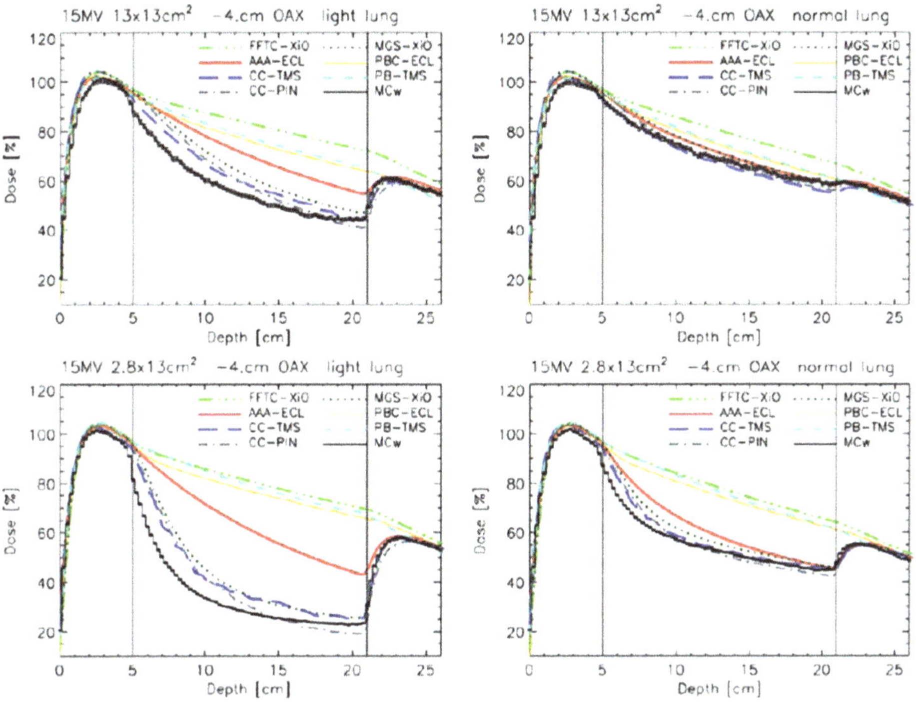

Figure 10.15. Depth dose curves for a 15 MV beam along the arrow in figure 10.13. Adapted from Fogliata *et al* [83], reproduced with permission. Copyright IOP Publishing Ltd. All rights reserved.

dose curves (analogous to figures 10.14 and 10.15) of that work are reported, showing a Monte Carlo as the benchmark (VMC++), the AAA as a *type 'b'* algorithm, which was the model mostly suffering from inaccuracy in the previous comparison and Acuros-XB as a *type 'c'* algorithm.

It is clear from these figures that advanced algorithms (possibly *type 'c'*) are most suited for dose calculations with heterogeneous medium in all possible clinical conditions.

10.6 Fluence to dose and MLC parameters: another source of uncertainty

The MLC dosimetric characteristics, mainly leaf transmission, interleaf leakage, tongue and groove effect, leaf end shapes play an important role in IMRT dose delivery. The inverse process of planning is conventionally divided into two steps: the fluence map is generated by the optimizer through the minimization of the cost function (as described in chapter 9 of this book), and then, at a second stage, this map is used to obtain the MLC sequence able to generate a fluence as similar as possible to the optimized fluence. Often, with this process, none of the mechanical limitations of the MLCs and dosimetric characteristics are included in the optimal fluence and have to be taken into account in the MLC sequencing process. Different is the case of the direct aperture optimization (DAO), where the second step of the

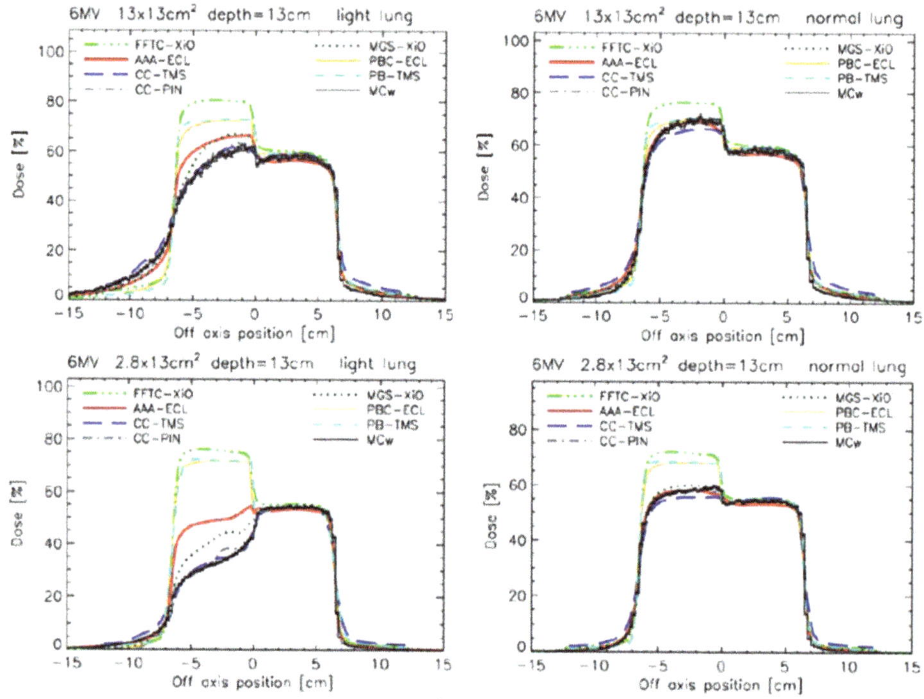

Figure 10.16. Lateral profile at mid-depth of the insert in figure 10.13 for 6 MV. Adapted from Fogliata *et al* [83], reproduced with permission. Copyright IOP Publishing Ltd. All rights reserved.

MLC sequencing step is not utilized, since the mechanical MLC constraints are included in the optimization process, generating a fluence that is directly deliverable [84].

Both the main optimization approaches need, for the dose computation, the estimation of the MLC parameters to be implemented in the clinical TPS. Those approximate estimations, as well as the good determination of those parameters used in the final dose calculation, generate additional uncertainties in the dose calculation of the dynamic, intensity-modulated deliveries.

Generally speaking, there are three main parameters to consider: the leaf transmission and interleaf leakage, the closed (or dosimetric) leaf gap and its offset, and the tongue and groove effect.

The first parameter, the leaf transmission, and its related interleaf leakage is the radiation transmitted through the leaves, and the interleaf leakage is the extra dose passing through two adjacent leaves. Simple point dose and profiles at pre-defined conditions can easily give an estimation of those parameters. Their setting could have an impact on the out-of-field dose estimation, as well as the OARs dose. These also impact, to some extent, the dose to the target in IMRT.

The second characteristic, the leaf gap (minimum, or closed, or dosimetric leaf gap) is generally defined as the minimum aperture (field) obtained by opposed closed leaves, that generates the transmission through the closed leaf gap modeling. This

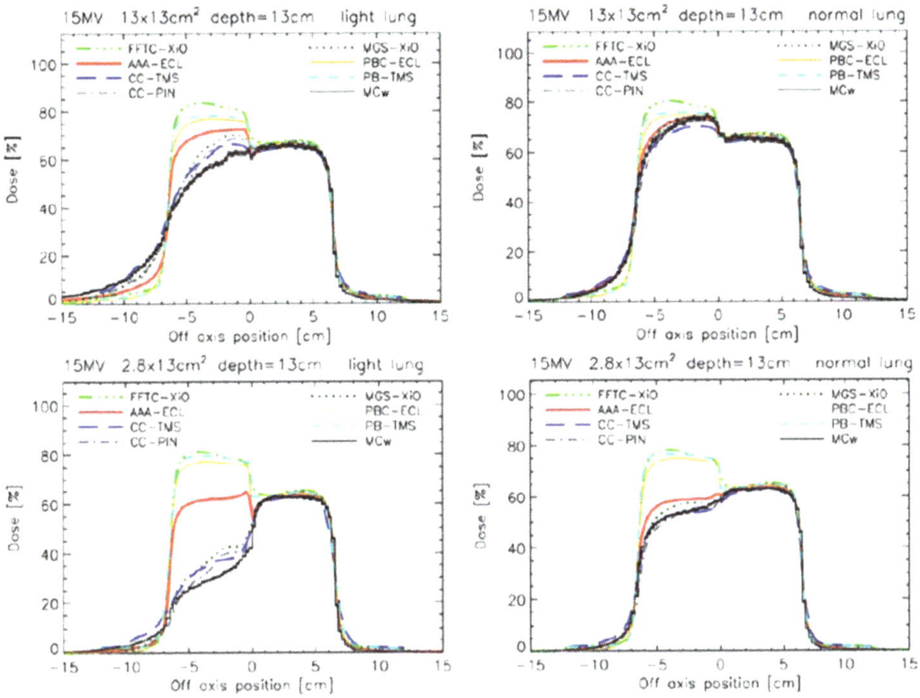

Figure 10.17. Lateral profile at mid-depth of the insert in figure 10.13 for 15 MV. Adapted from Fogliata *et al* [83], reproduced with permission. Copyright IOP Publishing Ltd. All rights reserved.

gap also describes the difference between the nominal field width defined by the MLC, and the dosimetric size determined by the profile (as full width half maximum in a flat beam) in the direction parallel to the leaf motion. Such a difference could be included in the planning system by offsetting the actual leaf position and the position that has to be planned to adjust the real, measured gap properly. This characteristic has an impact on the dose at the field edge, and, particularly important, for the small fields, in terms of size, penumbra and also MU calculation.

As the last characteristic, there is the tongue and groove effect. This effect describes the potential under-dosage in the interleaf region under dynamic leaf movement, related to some overlapping area between adjacent leaves according to the specific MLC design [85, 86]. The tongue and groove effect is hence opposite to the interleaf leakage and could be eliminated by synchronizing the movement of adjacent leaf pairs. This effect depends on the MLC profile design. In figure 10.20 different examples of MLC designs are shown [87], according to the strategies adopted by the three major linac vendors at the time of the Huq *et al* publication (2002). The Varian MLC presents a tongue and groove design, where a slot (the groove) cut along one leaf side houses a ridge (the tongue) on the side in front of the adjacent leaf aiming to minimize the interleaf transmission; this solution is currently used by the Varian Millennium and HDMLC (High Definition MLC). The Elekta MLC showed a combination of a partial tongue and groove design and a defocus of

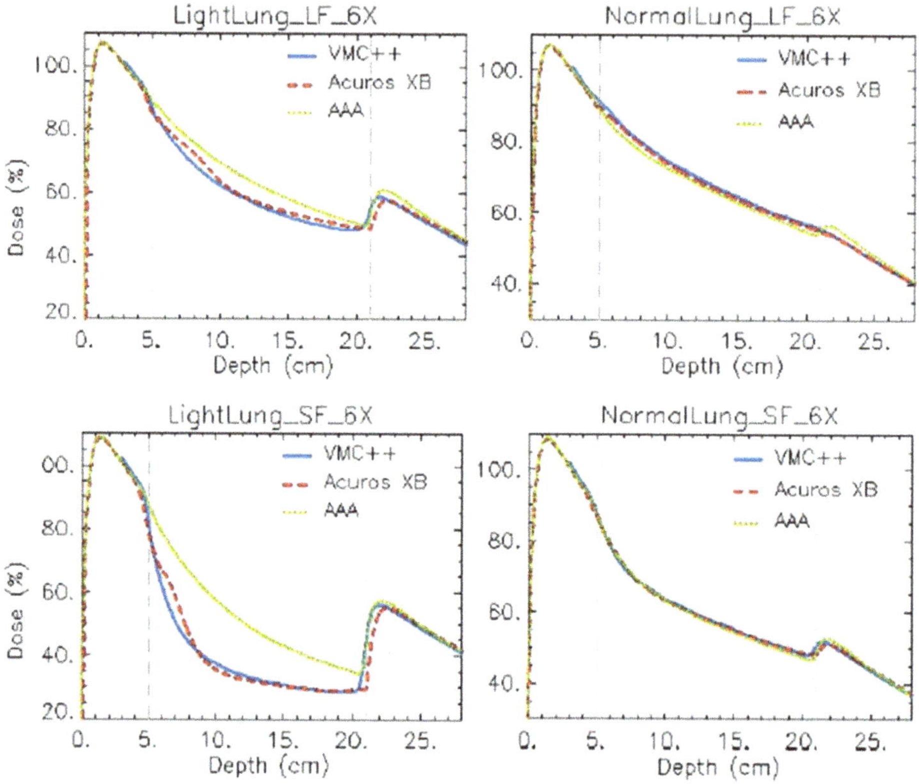

Figure 10.18. Depth dose curves for a 6 MV beam along the arrow in figure 10.13. LF = large field, 13 × 13 cm^2, SF = small field, 2.8 × 13 cm^2. Adapted from Fogliata *et al* [83], reproduced with permission. Copyright IOP Publishing Ltd. All rights reserved.

the MLC from the source, obtained by applying a leaf bank rotation. On the bottom part of figure 10.20, the concept of the design adopted for the current Elekta Agility MLC is shown, where the MLC interleaf gap is defocused with a leaf bank rotation, rather than purely using a tongue and groove design [88, 89].

The final dose calculation based on an optimized fluence has to include those MLC characteristics, modeled in the algorithm implementation (be it a *type 'a'*, *'b'* or *'c'*) using parameters able to describe the MLC design. The largest effect on the accuracy of them is on the small field calculations.

Several works have been published for different MLCs and different dose calculation algorithms, attempting to estimate the accuracy of the dose distribution and MU calculations and demonstrating the need for accurate tuning of the MLC parameters for improving dose calculation accuracy.

It is well known that patient-specific QA (PSQA) in IMRT/VMAT is heavily dependent on the MLC parameters [90–99]. Roche *et al* [100] using the Monaco Planning system showed that gamma passing rates were significantly proved (95% with 2%/2 mm) with a transmission probability filter optimization compared to the default setting with a pass rate of only 88% Additionally, Snyder *et al* [101] showed

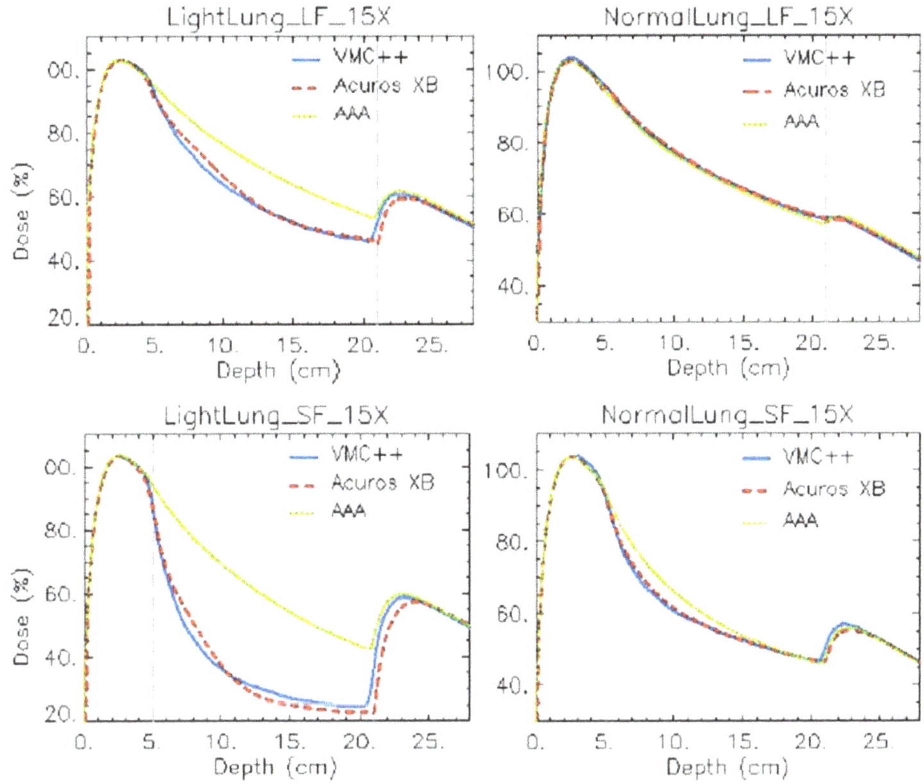

Figure 10.19. Depth dose curves for a 15 MV beam along the arrow in figure 10.13. LF = large field, 13 × 13 cm^2, SF = small field, 2.8 × 13 cm^2. Adapted from Fogliata *et al* [83], reproduced with permission. Copyright IOP Publishing Ltd. All rights reserved.

that the most accurate models were achievable by using a combination of vendor-provided and in-house procedures in Monaco Monte Carlo for the Agility MLC.

Gholampourkashi *et al* [102] using EGSnrc showed that the rotation of the leaf bank could be used for the defocusing to find the best tongue and groove parameter for the Monaco system. Attention has to be paid to the risk of over-modeling to obtain the best agreement on particular fields, which could lead to reduced accuracy of clinical dose distributions.

The MLC parameters were investigated by Bedford *et al* [103] in the Elekta Agility system based on data described by Starkschall *et al* [104] for the Pinnacle treatment planning system for the collapsed cone algorithm. The MLC parameters in Pinnacle on Varian MLCs were evaluated by Yao *et al* [99], for the mMLC on a BrainLab Novalis system by Feygelman *et al* [105], and on an Elekta beam modulator with a micro-MLC by Young *et al* [106].

Similarly, in the Varian environment, the dosimetric leaf gap and leaf transmission have been studied for both the AAA and Acuros-XB algorithms mostly for the Varian MLC, the Millennium 120-MLC and the high definition HDMLC [91, 107, 108]. The algorithms implemented in Eclipse, for the two dose calculation

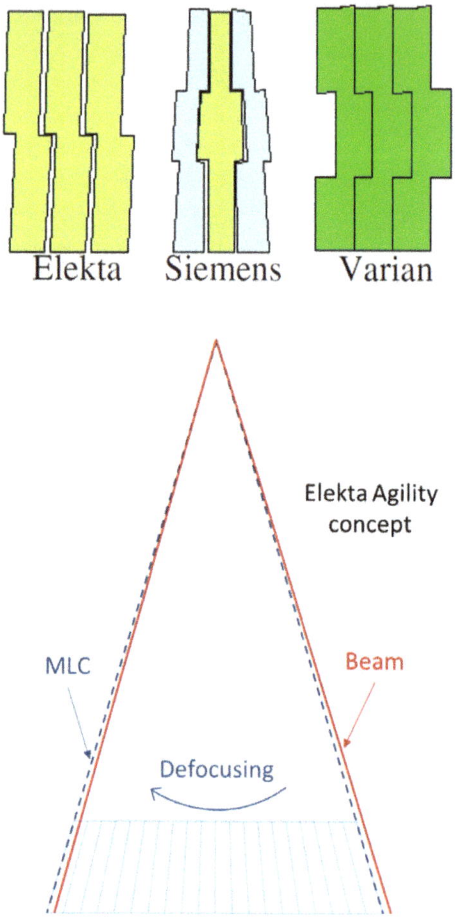

Figure 10.20. Interleaf and tongue and groove MLC design. On top: the end on view of various leaves from different manufacturers. Adapted from Huq *et al* [87], reproduced with permission. Copyright IOP Publishing Ltd. All rights reserved. On bottom: the MLC defocusing concept.

models, translate the user-defined MLC parameters into the fluence modeling. The rounded leaf end transmission is modeled by shifting the leaf tip positions in the actual fluence by moving back the leaves by half the value of the dosimetric leaf gap parameter. The tongue and groove effect also modifies the fluence, by blocking some of the radiation on the tongue side in the leaf overlapping region by using a parameter not modifiable by the user and depending on the MLC model.

An assessment for the MLC characteristics was also provided by Paganini *et al* [109] by assessing PRIMO Monte Carlo (Penelope) compared with measurements and the Eclipse Acuros which pointed out the suitability of an external Monte Carlo code as an independent dose calculation tool with reasonable accuracy. However, a check on all the possible sources of errors of any dose calculation system should be suggested.

It is obvious that the need for proper MLC parameters in each algorithm for each specific MLC type cannot be ignored. The overall accuracy of the dose calculation (analytical, deterministic, or stochastic) is not only dependent on a beam model (or full linac head simulation) but the MLC modeling in a planning system. Apart from the above, there is an additional source of uncertainty in the small fields that has to be taken in account, as described and reported in the recommendation documents from IAEA (TRS-483 on small fields [110]) and the upcoming AAPM TG-155 Report [111].

10.7 The out-of-field dose

Intensity-modulated techniques spill dose outside the treatment fields, thus it is critical to accurately estimate the out-of-field dose. Not only the OAR but also the targets are shielded by the MLC and the jaws (when present) during part of the treatment delivery in IMRT. The amount of shielding increases with increasing the number of fields to the limit of the rotational treatments as in VMAT. It is mostly in the last decade where a number of works dealing with the accuracy of the dose calculation algorithms in the region out of the primary beam started to appear in publications, when the potential increase of secondary cancer risk and its correlation with accurate doses delivered began to be considered a topic of concern.

Results from measurements [112] and Monte Carlo simulations [113–115] were reported regarding the doses at increasing distances from the radiation field edges. With Monte Carlo, the authors found local differences relative to measurements in an average of 16% (up to 50% at 50 cm). However, the doses at such large distances were down to 0.01% of the in-field dose, making the absolute dose difference of low clinical relevance. But this indicates that even the Monte Carlo calculations, considered the benchmark in all the situations, could suffer from the used approximations, mostly in terms of beam or linac head design simulation for out-of-field dose calculation. Taylor *et al* [116] published the need to reduce the out-of-field dose (photons and, not to forget, neutrons) to lower the secondary cancer risk and compared 3DCRT and IMRT. Monte Carlo simulations and measurements were also reported for FFF beams [117–120] and compared 3DCRT against IMRT [121], or evaluating multi-source models for the linac head [122].

Evaluations of the accuracy in the estimation of the out-of-field dose as computed by commercial treatment planning systems generally underestimate (30%–50%) the dose out of the primary beam, with differences increasing with the distance from the field border. Howell *et al* [123] found an underestimation of the AAA calculations of 40% (local) on average in a range of ~4–11 cm, a region clinically relevant not only for secondary cancer induction but also for the estimation of the OAR dose close to the target volume. Fogliata *et al* [124] also reported an overestimation of 44% with AAA and reduction to 30% with Acuros calculations at 10 cm distance to the field border. Quite similar results have been reported more recently for the same algorithms by Wang *et al* [125, 126], Alghamdi *et al* [127], Shine *et al* [128]. Not different are also the estimations of other algorithms implemented on other treatment planning systems, as the collapsed cone on Pinnacle [129], multigrid superposition on XiO [127], tomotherapy [130]. The case of the CyberKnife planning system has been shown to be different, underestimating the dose of up to 100% with Monte Carlo, and more than 250% with RayTracing (pencil beam) algorithm [131].

An interesting approach was followed by Schneider and colleagues [130] evaluating the tomotherapy and the CyberKnife out-of-field doses. Starting from an assumption of accepting a maximum error of 50% out of the primary beam (that is the accuracy achieved by other commercial treatment planning calculations as shown by Huang *et al* [129]) they quantified the dose value and the distance from the field border yielding to unsatisfactory accuracy. They found that tomotherapy calculation is acceptable for a dose level of 0.75 mGy per prescribed Gy at 35 cm distance. For CyberKnife, the acceptability was achieved for 10 mGy per prescribed Gy, corresponding to only 10 cm distance.

From various publications, it is clear that achievable accuracy in the low-dose regions is much lower than the in-field dose estimation accuracy. On one hand, we could argue that the out-of-field dose is at a very low dose level, and such accuracy could be acceptable. This is the case for locations very far from the treatment area, and the concern, in that region, is relative to the risk of secondary cancer induction, where the needed accuracy in estimating the risk is not too high. On the other hand, however, with the intensity-modulated fields (IMRT/VMAT) during the treatment delivery the leaves shield the OARs in the close vicinity of the target, and the critical structure requiring rather low doses relative to the dose prescription (as could be the example of the parotids in a head and neck treatment) would receive most of their dose as scattering or transmission. In any case, most of the dose can be considered as out-of-field. It could easily happen that about 10 Gy (or more) are computed by the planning system as out-of-field OAR dose. Considering the underestimation of about 50%, the actual dose to that OAR is probably 15 Gy. Such an inaccuracy could have a non-negligible clinical impact since the NTCP computations, and the tolerance dose for the OARs would suggest a better outcome or toxicity due to the dose underestimation. We have to be conscious of the level of accuracy achievable in the different dose levels, remembering that even the most accurate algorithm presents areas of high uncertainty that should be clinically considered.

10.8 Dose calculation with metallic objects

In general, cancer is a disease of patient age where implants of high-Z material, such as hip prostheses, dental filling or metallic fixation for the spine or breast implants are common. Managing metal prosthetics in radiation therapy treatments becomes an important issue. The common practice, due to the known uncertainty in properly evaluating the dose across those structures, as well as the increased electrons scattered by the metallic material, is to avoid irradiation through the implants, in particular in situations where they are located before the target volume. However, this is not always possible.

AAPM Task Group TG-63 [132] provided guidelines in managing prosthetic devices before the IMRT era. In this section, a summary of the results of the dosimetric consequences of irradiating metallic objects, using different dose calculation algorithms, is given. To exclude the problem of the artifacts generated by the metallic objects, in most of the studies, the CT numbers were corrected.

In 2003, Wieslander *et al* [133] evaluated different metal inserts in a phantom irradiated by a fixed beam of 6 or 18 MV, comparing pencil beam and collapsed cone algorithms against Monte Carlo simulations. At 6 cm beyond the steel insert, the calculated dose with the collapsed cone was within ~5% compared to the Monte Carlo, while it was ~12% and ~−41% for pencil beam calculations (6 and 18 MV, respectively). At the same point beyond titanium inserts, the difference for collapsed cone was within 1%, and within 4% for the pencil beam. The clear suggestion was the use of advanced algorithms for patients with prostheses.

Acuros and AAA calculations in the presence of metallic objects compared with Monte Carlo and measurements were published by Ojala *et al* [134] on VMAT plans for prostate treatments, and by Cheng *et al* [135] for spine SBRT with a metal fixation for spinal implants. In both publications, the accuracy was better achieved with Acuros than AAA, both inside and in the vicinity of the implants. Interesting is the case of the spinal implant as well as other situations; Cheng *et al* showed that the impact of the fixation device on the dose diminished with the increasing plan complexity or number of fields. This yielded to the result of an insignificant dose change near the spinal cord and tumor volume in the presence of the metallic device when 9-field IMRT was used, whereas the single open beam showed quite large dose.

The Monte Carlo based Monaco planning system was tested in the presence of metallic objects by Ade *et al* [136] and Byrnes *et al* [137]. In their work, Ade and colleagues compared film measurements also against the collapsed cone algorithm implemented in the XiO planning system. They concluded that, in the case of titanium prostheses, with an increase of the dose of 21%–30% at the entrance of the insert, and a fall-off of the dose at the exit of the same of 15%–21%, the accuracy for the collapsed cone was of ~1% in the entrance and ~23% in exit, while it was within 4% for Monaco Monte Carlo. Byrnes and colleagues, evaluated downstream a small metallic insert of aluminum and steel, an accuracy of −1% and −2%, respectively, for the Monte Carlo implemented in Monaco. Parenica and colleagues [138, 139] reported on a first study on VMAT prostate plans for patients with hip replacement using Monaco and collapsed cone (Pinnacle) with respect to ion chamber measurements, and on a second work on the effect of dental filling in head and neck treatments, with the same algorithms. For the prostate cases, they found an agreement in target coverage of ~0.2% with Monte Carlo, and of ~4.4% with collapsed cone, with the artifact corrected with known densities. For a dental implant, the agreement was of 3% for Monte Carlo, and 7% for collapsed cone. Interesting is the artifact correction analyzed in this last work and reported here in figure 10.21.

The dose difference between calculations with and without artifact overrides is shown (for collapsed cone and Monte Carlo) in figure 10.21. This underlines that other than the problem strictly related to the metallic insert, the artifact density corrections are of primarily dosimetric importance. It is not only the dose calculation algorithm generating an accurate dose distribution, but other factors

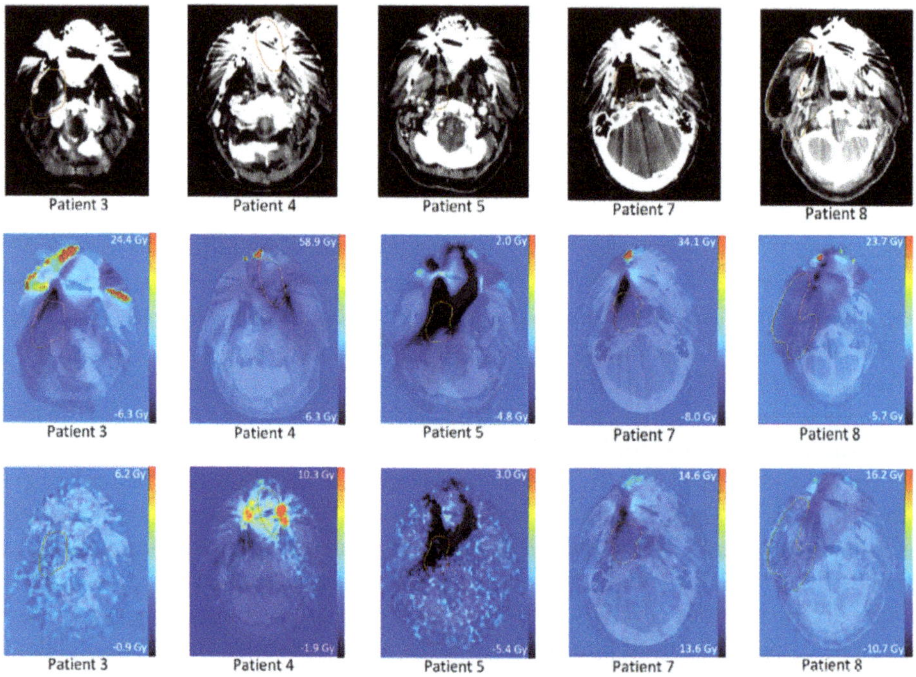

Figure 10.21. Top row: CT slices affected by severe image artifacts close to the PTV. Middle row: dose difference with collapsed cone calculation (Pinnacle) between plan computed with and without density overrides for the artifacts. Bottom row: dose difference with Monte Carlo calculation (Monaco) between plan computed with and without density overrides for artifacts. Adapted from Parenica *et al* [139], reproduced with permission from the American Association of Medical Dosimetrists.

(the CT accuracy in terms of density and material composition) must be taken into account to allow benefitting of the specific algorithm characteristics and keep the dosimetric uncertainty within the acceptable requirements. In this view, the metallic artifact reduction correction algorithms implemented in some CT scanners could have a substantial impact on the dose distribution estimation (as also described in chapter 8 on treatment planning of this book).

10.9 Other elements influencing the dose calculation accuracy

In the implementation of an algorithm for dose calculation, different factors could influence the dose estimation, the dose reporting, the dose evaluation. Here a few examples are briefly detailed, such as the dose calculation grid size, the slice spacing, the presence of contrast agents.

The possible consequences of a non-adequate *dose calculation grid size* have been analyzed, surprisingly rather recently, in different published works. As expected, the most significant influence was found for stereotactical treatments. The effect of the grid size can be easily pictured: the dose calculation with a finite number of calculation points (on a defined grid) inevitably lose the information of some peaks (resulting in an underestimation of the dose peaks); the opposite happens for the dose valleys (dose overestimation). In short, the coarse grid size would smooth the dose distribution. Bear in mind, the fluence is delivered to the patient without this artificial smoothing: it could be a case where a smoother (calculated) dose distribution is acceptable. In contrast, a very irregular dose distribution (delivered) could be not acceptable. On lung SBRT, Huang *et al* [140] evaluated the dose distribution for VMAT plans calculated by AAA and Acuros with two different grid sizes, 2.5 and 1 mm (using the same MUs), and reported the differences in the doses estimated in the PTV with soft tissue density, and in the portion of the PTV presenting lung density. The mean dose in the PTV in soft tissue was negligible using the two grid sizes, while a lower mean dose in the PTV in lung tissue by 1.5% with AAA and ~1% with Acuros was estimated for the finer grid. A possible clinical consequence is related to the plan normalization. For a dose prescribed to certain target coverage, being the PTV in lung region the external part of the target volume receiving a lower dose, a coarser grid size would possibly induce a shift toward higher delivered doses relative to a better, finer grid.

For spine stereotactic VMAT dose calculation with cord sparing, i.e., a situation opposite to the previous one concerning the tissue densities, Snyder *et al* [141] compared AAA calculations using grid sizes from 2.5 to 1 mm. The target coverage decreased by 0.7% as the PTV $D_{95\%}$, and, more important, the dose difference was 10% in the near-to-maximum dose to the cord, $D_{0.03cc}$, estimated as 11.5 and 10.5 Gy with 2.5 and 1 mm grid, respectively. Also, in this case, when the clinical decision is driven by the maximum dose to the spinal cord, a different treatment could be chosen if the same plan is computed with coarser or finer grid size.

Differences can also be found in non-stereotactic cases. Cases of prostate and head and neck have been studied by different groups, evaluating in some cases the biological more than the purely dosimetric consequence of using different dose calculation grid sizes. Concerning the prostate, Kim *et al* [142] analyzed VMAT treatments calculated with AAA and Acuros on the Eclipse planning system. Reducing the grid size from 3 to 1 mm, they reported a significant reduction of both TCP (−3%) and rectal NTCP (−24%) with Acuros calculations, while an increase of both TCP (+1%) and rectal NTCP (+9%) with AAA. Noteworthy is the TCP, and rectal NTCP spread for the same plans when a different algorithm and different gird size is used, ranging between 83.4 and 87.5% for TCP, and between 3.2% and 6.1% for NTCP, underlying the need for a high degree of accuracy to support the daily clinical decisions. Similarly, Chow *et al* [143] studied the prostate case with VMAT plans computed with AAA. They found, however, smaller discrepancies, resulting in a TCP variation of 0.06% per mm of grid size variation, and a rectal NTCP variation of 0.03% per mm of grid size variation.

Kawashima *et al* [144] reported tomotherapy prostate planning results with grid sizes defined as fine (2.73 mm), and standard (5.46 mm), finding a significant EUD (equivalent uniform dose) estimation and a near-to-maximum rectal dose increase when the grid size was changed from normal to the fine grid. The head and neck case was investigated by Srivastava *et al* [145] for step-and-shoot IMRT plans computed with AAA in the Eclipse planning system, showing, for a reduction of the grid size, a significant increase of the TCP and reduction of the NTCP. On Pinnacle (pencil beam), Chung *et al* [146] reported results on the phantom and clinical head and neck cases. A reduction of the grid size from 4 to 2 mm yielded a dose difference for the 95% region of interest of 4%–5% to be reduced to 0.5%–1% of the prescribed dose. These studies highlight that the dose calculation grid size clinically matters and a correct balance between accuracy (finer grid) and computation time (coarser grid) has to be found. The reported numbers showed that the only variation in the grid size could lead to non-compliance with the requirement related to the dose calculation accuracy.

A second point which could influence the dose calculation accuracy is the planning CT *slice thickness*. The most critical issue related to this element is the best determination of the volume of the delineated structures, especially the tiny ones. In consequence, a wrong estimation of the volume of an anatomical structure yields an incorrect estimate of the dosimetric parameters. The most simple example is the mean dose to a structure, that is the sum of the dose per pixel volume belonging to the structure, divided by the volume of the same structure. The accuracy of the mean dose determination depends on the structure volume delineation, which depends on the slice thickness and treatment planning system implementing the computation of volume [147].

Jacob and Kneschaurek [148] evaluated, on the iPlan planning system, the situation for two patients planned for stereotactical treatment in the brain, assessing planning CT with 2 mm thickness in the whole dataset, and with 2 mm at the target level and 4 mm elsewhere. In a non-coplanar setting of the fields, they reported maximum doses to the small volume critical structures, like the chiasm and the optic nerves, lower in the case of mixed 2 and 4 mm slice spacing relative to the 2 mm thicknesses. This was due to an underestimation of the contoured volumes. Again in the brain, Caivano *et al* [149], in the Eclipse planning system and pencil beam calculations, for a slice thickness varying from 1 to 10 mm, reported for small structures a volume reduction, a conformity index and a 95% isodose reduction when increasing the slice spacing. No differences were found for large structures (~90 cm^3).

Srivastava *et al* [147] reported IMRT plans on a phantom with controlled volume sizes. They evaluated different slice thicknesses, from 1 to 10 mm for different target sizes, ranging from 1 to 100 cm^3. The variability of the volumes with slice thickness was significant for the tiny structures. For a 1 cm^3 contour, the volume presented errors of 92% and 19% for the 10 mm and 1 mm slice thickness, respectively. Important differences were also found for volumes up to 20 cm^3. In consequence, the mean dose to the structure (as PTV) and the TCP decreased with increasing slice spacing, with maximum variations of ~5% and 2% in the mean dose and TCP, respectively, for slice thicknesses from 1 to 5 mm. For those cases, the homogeneity index increased by up to 163%, and the conformity index decreased by 4%. These results confirm the need to use an appropriate slice thickness to improve dose calculation accuracy, having proved that the smaller, the better. Also, in cases with not so small structure volumes, the slice thickness plays a role in the dose accuracy, although of lower magnitude, related to the reconstruction of the delineated contours. On the prostate, results have been reported by Tunio *et al* [150] and by

Olsson *et al* [151], showing differences in terms of TCP and NTCP. Similarly, Luo *et al* [152], on patients treated in the thorax region, reported volume errors, and significant heart dose reporting. Heart volume, for a slice thickness changing from 2 to 6 mm, was reduced by 3%, and the V_{30Gy} and V_{40Gy} increased by 18% and 47%, respectively. The authors also emphasized the effect that the volume reconstruction error, which also depends on the algorithm adopted, could have a significant impact on the GTV to CTV to PTV margin.

Regarding both elements of the grid size and the slice thickness, is noteworthy to consider that most of the planning systems use a dose calculation grid size as stated in the axial direction (on the slice plane). In contrast, on the longitudinal direction, a grid of the same size as the slice thickness is often used, or a multiple or sub-multiple of that value.

Another factor that could influence the dose calculation accuracy is the presence of *contrast* agent, or even the gastic air in bowel [153] in the CT planning images. The use of contrast-enhanced CT is often used to improve the delineation of the tumor volumes and the nodal regions, otherwise difficult to define in non-contrasted images accurately. This results in CT images with increased electron density in the vascular structures (for iodine-based intravenous injected contrast agent) and some of the nodes, or the bladder, stomach, intestine, colon, rectum for an oral contrast agent. The temporarily enhanced density, however (temporarily since it is not in the patient body during the treatment sessions), if it is on the same CT dataset used for delineation and dose calculation, in this second phase it could potentially affect the dose distribution and MU calculation, leading to a plan evaluation based on potentially inaccurate data. A number of publications reported the dose calculation differences in the case of intravenously injected contrast agent. The effect on patients treated for thoracic cancer (lung, esophagus) has been reported by different groups [154–160]. In general, the resulting differences in terms of MU calculation or mean, maximum, minimum doses were of a few percent. When the results showed non-significant or non-remarkable dosimetric differences, the clinical impact was judged negligible. However, although finding in most cases a minimal impact, attention has to be paid in some conditions, where for example the amount of contrast uptake is particularly high, or in some anatomical situations, like for oesophagal cancer, where Li *et al* [158] found differences larger than 2% in the estimation of the V_{40Gy} parameter for the heart. Also, Xiong *et al* [157] reported differences in the target coverage for oesophagal cancer approaching 2%, reaching 3% in minimum dose to the PTV. In summary, the uncertainty can be in most of cases considered acceptable, but with care. Lee *et al* [161] investigate the intravenous contrast on nasopharyngeal cancer patients, finding again a clinically insignificant effect.

In summary, the intravenous contrast agent affects the dosimetry significantly, but unremarkably. Different is the case of the oral contrast, which deserves more attention due to the large volumes interested by the density increase. Jing *et al* [162] investigated VMAT plans on pelvic treatments. In their work, they found a maximum difference in the prescription dose (PTV $D_{95\%}$) of 0.3%, and an average $V_{105\%}$ difference in the PTV of 1.5% (range −2%, +7%). More significant differences were found in the maximum dose to the intestine, in an average of 0.4 Gy (for a dose prescription of 50 Gy to the target), and a range of –0.1 Gy, +1.5 Gy. This potential uncertainty generated by the contrast agent could induce a risk of overdose to the PTV, but mainly to the bowels, suggesting a correction of the density in the contrast-enhanced areas. Similarly, another work on prostate treatment on patients with oral contrast showed differences in the bladder dose estimation [163].

Chandroth *et al* [74] evaluated IMRT and VMAT prostate plans with contrast agent in the bladder, with Monte Carlo calculations (in the Monaco planning system). They reported a $D_{98\%}$ variation for PTV and CTV as a function of the electron density of the contrast agent volume: in the case of dose-to-water reporting they found differences of ~1% in average with 1.8 relative electron density; conversely, in the case of dose-to-medium reporting, the mean differences increased from ~1% to ~8% with relative electron density increasing from 1.2 to 1.8. Similar behavior was reported for V_{40Gy} variations in the bladder. The authors suggested accounting for the contrast agents by contouring and forcing an appropriate electron density while planning. When high densities are included, as the contrast agent case, the correction of the contrast density is more crucial for dose-to-medium calculations due to the tissue that is associated with the density (HU values).

Let us consider an example of the contrast agent. In figure 10.22, the dose distribution for a pancreatic tumor is shown. The slices on the left have no contrast agent; those on the right were acquired after the contrast agent injection. The increased density is mostly shown in the kidneys and some regions of the target volume. Two points are shown: point A in the kidney, and point B in the target. The same VMAT plan is computed with the same MU with Acuros-XB with dose-to-medium reporting (as shown on the slices), and also as dose-to-water. The table on the bottom shows the characteristics of the two points A and B in terms of HU and density in the two conditions of absence or presence of the contrast. The supposed physical composition is also reported, automatically assigned by the system, by relating the HU and a pre-defined physical material table. The last columns report the calculated doses in all the conditions. When the dose is computed as dose-to-medium, the dose differences in points A (kidney) and B (PTV) are +0.2% and +1.5%, respectively. When the dose reporting is as dose-to-water, due to the supposed physical composition of cartilage and particularly bone, the dose differences in points A and B raise to +1.9% and +3.7%, respectively, differences possibly no more acceptable. With this simple example, we can have two conclusions. Firstly, the contrast agent, modifying the patient anatomy in terms of density, affects the calculated dose. The amount of the differences is significant, and maybe remarkable. Its clinical relevance is difficult to judge. However, it is an additional uncertainty that is added to the other uncertainties coming from different sources, and this specific error is systematic and in principle, quite correctable. Secondly, attention has to be paid if the dose-to-water reporting is chosen, since the contrast agent could easily present HU in the range of bone tissue, leading to the known overestimation of the dose.

In principle, since it is possible to correct for such uncertainty, it could be advised to correct those systematic errors in clinical practice.

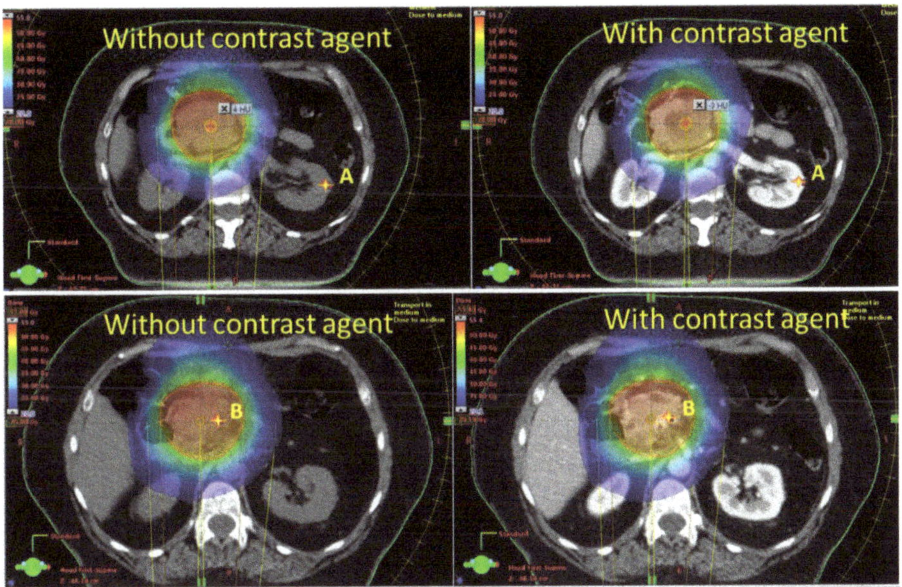

		HU	Relative electron density	Mass density g/cm³	Physical composition	Dose to Medium Gy	Dose to Water Gy
Kidney	A: no contrast	15	1.015	1.016	100% muscle	11.59	11.75
	A: contrast	204	1.150	1.144	91% cartilage 9% bone	11.61	11.97
PTV	B: no contrast	38	1.038	1.040	100% muscle	51.61	51.25
	B: contrast	257	1.175	1.175	85% cartilage 15% bone	52.36	53.15

Figure 10.22. Pancreatic VMAT plan with and without contrast agent.

References

[1] Brahme A 1984 Dosimetric precision requirements in radiation therapy *Acta Radiol. Oncol.* **23** 379–91

[2] ICRU 24 1976 Determination of absorbed dose in a patient irradiated by beams of X or Gamma rays in radiotherapy procedures (Washington, DC: International Commission on Radiation Units and Measurements)

[3] Brahme A (ed) 1988 Accuracy requirements and quality assurance of external beam therapy with photons and electrons *Acta Oncol.*

[4] Van Dyk J, Barnett R B, Cygler J E and Shragge P 1993 Commissioning and quality assurance of treatment planning computers *Int. J. Radiat. Oncol. Biol. Phys.* **26** 261–73

[5] ICRU Report 50 1993 *Prescribing, Recording, and Reporting Photon Beam Therapy* (Bethesda, MD: International Commission on Radiation Units and Measurements)

[6] ICRU Report 83 2010 *Prescribing, Recording, and Reporting Photon-beam Intensity-modulated Radiation Therapy (IMRT)* (Bethesda, MD: International Commission on Radiation Units and Measurements)

[7] Thwaites D 2013 Accuracy required and achievable in radiotherapy dosimetry: have modern technology and techniques changed our views? *J. Phys. Conf. Ser.* **444** 012006

[8] Mijnheer B J, Batterman J J and Wambersie A 1987 What degree of accuracy is required and can be achieved in photon and neutron therapy? *Radiother. Oncol.* **8** 237–52

[9] Boyer A L and Schultheiss T 1988 Effects of dosimetric and clinical uncertainty on complication-free local tumor control *Radiother. Oncol.* **11** 65–71

[10] Papanikolaou N and Stathakis S 2009 Dose-calculation algorithms in the context of inhomogeneity corrections for high energy photon beams *Med. Phys.* **36** 4765–75

[11] Fraass B A 1995 The development of conformal radiation therapy *Med. Phys.* **22** 1911–21

[12] Ahnesjö A and Aspradakis M M 1999 Dose calculations for external photon beams in radiotherapy *Phys. Med. Biol.* **44** R99–155

[13] Knöös T 2017 3D dose computation algorithms *J. Phys. Conf. Ser.* **847** 012037

[14] AAPM 85 2004 Tissue Inhomogeneity Corrections for MV Photon Beams Report of Task Group No. 65 of the Radiation Therapy Committee of the American Association of Physicists in Medicine. (Madison, WI: Medical Physics Publishing)

[15] International Atomic Energy Agency 2004 *Commissioning and Quality Assurance of Computerized Planning Systems for Radiation Treatment of cancer IAEA TRS-430* (Vienna: International Atomic Energy Agency)

[16] Knöös T, Wieslander E, Cozzi L, Brink C, Fogliata A and Albers D *et al* 2006 Comparison of dose calculation algorithms for treatment planning in external photon beam therapy for clinical situations *Phys. Med. Biol.* **51** 5785–807

[17] Johns H E and Cunningham J R 1969 *The Physics of Radiology* 3rd edn (Springfield, IL: Charles C. Thomas)

[18] Dutreix A, Bjärngard B E, Bridier A, Mijnheer B, Shaw J E and Svensson H 1997 Monitor Unit Calculation for High Energy Photon Beams. ESTRO Physics for Clinical Radiotherapy Booklet N. 3. ESTRO, Brussels

[19] Mijnheer B, Bridier A, Garibaldi C, Torzsok K and Venselaar J 2001 Monitor Unit Calculation for High Energy Photon Beams—Practical Examples. ESTRO Physics for Clinical Radiotherapy Booklet N. 6. ESTRO, Brussels

[20] Cunningham J R 1972 Scatter-air ratios *Phys. Med. Biol.* **17** 42–51

[21] Cunningham S R, Shrivastava P N and Wilkinson J M 1972 Program IRREG—calculation of dose from irregularly shaped radiation beams *Comp. Progr. Biomed.* **2** 192–99

[22] Clarkson J R 1941 A note on depth doses in fields of irregular shape *Br. J. Radiol.* **14** 265–8

[23] Sontag M R and Cunningham J R 1978 The equivalent tissue-air ratio method for making absorbed dose calculations in photon beam dose calculations in a heterogeneous medium *Radiology* **129** 787–94

[24] Sontag M R and Cunningham J R 1978 Clinical application of a CT based treatment planning system *Comput. Tomogr.* **2** 117–30

[25] O'Connor J E 1957 The variation of scattered X-Rays with density in an irradiated body *Phys. Med. Biol.* **1** 352–69

[26] Beaudoin L 1968 Analytical approach to the solution of the dosimetry in heterogeneous media *MSc Thesis* University of Toronto

[27] Wong J W and Henkelman R M 1983 A new approach to CT pixel-based photon dose calculations in heterogeneous media *Med. Phys.* **10** 199–208

[28] Batho H F 1964 Lung corrections in cobalt 60 beam therapy *J. Can. Assoc. Radiol.* **15** 79–83

[29] Young M E and Gaylord J D 1970 Experimental tests of corrections for tissue inhomogeneities in radiotherapy *Br. J. Radiol.* **43** 349–55

[30] Sontag M R and Cunningham J R 1977 Corrections to absorbed dose calculations for tissue inhomogeneities *Med. Phys.* **4** 431–6

[31] Boyer A L 1984 Shortening the calculation time of photon dose distributions in an inhomogeneous medium *Med. Phys.* **11** 552–4

[32] Boyer A and Mok E 1985 A photon dose distribution model employing convolution calculations *Med. Phys.* **12** 169–77

[33] Ulmer W and Harder D 1995 A triple Gaussian pencil beam model for photon beam treatment planning *Z. Med. Phys.* **5** 25–30

[34] Ulmer W and Harder D 1996 Applications of a triple Gaussian pencil beam model for photon beam treatment planning *Z. Med. Phys.* **6** 68–74

[35] Ulmer W and Kaissl W 2003 The inverse problem of a Gaussian convolution and its application to the finite size of the measurement chambers/detectors in photon and proton dosimetry *Phys. Med. Biol.* **48** 707–27

[36] Ulmer W, Pyyry J and Kaissl W 2005 A 3D photon superposition/convolution algorithm and its foundation on results of Monte Carlo calculations *Phys. Med. Biol.* **50** 1767–90

[37] Sievinen J, Ulmer W and Kaissl W AAA photon dose calculation model in Eclipse^{TM}. White paper Varian Medical Systems, RAD#7170A

[38] Ahnesjö A 1989 Collapsed cone convolution of radiant energy for photon dose calculation in heterogeneous media *Med. Phys.* **16** 577–92

[39] Ahnesjö A, Saxner M and Trepp A 1992 A pencil beam model for photon dose calculation *Med. Phys.* **19** 263–73

[40] Vassiliev O N, Wareing T A, McGhee J, Failla G, Salehpour M R and Mourtada F 2010 Validation of a new grid-based Boltzmann equation solver for dose calculation in radiotherapy with photon beams *Phys. Med. Biol.* **55** 581–98

[41] Petti P L, Goodman M S, Gabriel T A and Mohan R 1983 Investigation of buildup dose from electron contamination of clinical photon beams *Med. Phys.* **10** 18–24

[42] Mohan R, Chui C and Lidofsky L 1985 Energy and angular distributions of photons from medical linear accelerators *Med. Phys.* **12** 592–7

[43] Rogers D W O, Faddegon B, Ding G X, Ma C-M, We J and Mackie T R 1995 BEAM—a Monte Carlo code to simulate radiotherapy treatment units *Med. Phys.* **22** 503–24

[44] International Commission on Radiological Protection 1975 *Report of the Task Group on Reference Man. ICRP Publication 23* (Oxford: Pergamon)

[45] International Commission on Radiation Units and Measurements 1989 *Tissue Substitutes in Radiation Dosimetry and Measurement* (Report 44)

[46] International Commission on Radiation Units and Measurements 1992 *Photon, Electron, Proton and Neutron Interaction Data for Body Tissues* (Report 46)

[47] Andreo P 2018 Monte Carlo simulations in radiotherapy dosimetry *Radiat. Oncol.* **13** 121

[48] Reynaert N, van der Marck S C, Shaart D R, Van der Zee W, Van Vliet-Vroegindeweij C and Tomsej M *et al* 2007 Monte Carlo treatment planning for photon and electron beams *Radiat. Phys. Chem.* **76** 643–86

[49] Spezi E and Lewis G 2008 An overview of Monte Carlo treatment planning for radiotherapy *Radiat. Prot. Dosim.* **131** 123–9

[50] Fippel M 1999 Fast Monte Carlo dose calculation for photon beams based on the VMC electron algorithm *Med. Phys.* **26** 1466–75

[51] Kawrakow I 2001 VMC++, electron and photon Monte Carlo calculations optimized for radiation treatment planning: advanced Monte Carlo for radiation physics, particle transport simulation and applications *Proc. of the Monte Carlo 2000 Meeting, Lisbon* ed A Kling *et al* (Berlin: Springer) pp 229–36

[52] Sempau J, Wilderman S J and Bielajew A F 2000 DPM, a fast, accurate Monte Carlo code optimized for photon and electron radiotherapy treatment planning dose calculations *Phys. Med. Biol.* **45** 2263–91

[53] Rodriguez M, Sempau J and Brualla L 2013 PRIMO: a graphical environment for the Monte Carlo simulation of Varian and Elekta linacs *Strahlenther. Onkol.* **189** 881–6

[54] Wareing R A, McGhee J M, Morel J E and Pautz S D 2001 Discontinuous finite element S_N methods on three-dimensional unstructured grids *Nucl. Sci. Eng.* **138** 256–68

[55] Gifford K A, Horton J L, Wareing T A, Failla G and Mourtada F 2006 Comparison of a finite-element multigroup discrete-ordinates code with Monte Carlo for radiotherapy calculations *Phys. Med. Biol.* **51** 2253–65

[56] Vassiliev O N, Wareing T A, Davis I M, McGhee J, Barnett D and Horton J L *et al* 2008 Feasibility of a multigroup deterministic solution method for three-dimensional radiotherapy dose calculations *Int. J. Radiat. Oncol. Biol. Phys.* **72** 220–7

[57] Bedford J L 2019 Calculation of absorbed dose in radiotherapy by solution of the linear Boltzmann transport equations *Phys. Med. Biol.* **64** 02TR01

[58] Deng J, Jiang S B, Kapur A, Li J, Pawlicki T and Ma C M 2000 Photon beam characterization and modelling for Monte Carlo treatment planning *Phys. Med. Biol.* **45** 411–27

[59] Tillikainen L, Siljamäki S, Helminen H, Alakuijala J and Pyyry J 2007 Determination of parameters for multiple-source model of megavoltage photon beams using optimization methods *Phys. Med. Biol.* **52** 1441–67

[60] Ojala J J, Kapanen M K, Hyödynmaa S J, Wigren T K and Pitkänen M A 2014 Performance of dose calculation algorithms for three generations in lung SBRT: comparison with full Monte Carlo-based dose distribution *J. Appl. Clin. Med. Phys.* **15** 4–18

[61] Fogliata A and Cozzi L 2017 Dose calculation algorithm accuracy for small fields in non-homogeneous media: the lung SBRT case *Phys. Med.* **44** 157–62

[62] Jones A O and Das I J 2005 Comparison of inhomogeneity correction algorithms in small photon fields *Med. Phys.* **32** 766–76

[63] Timmermann R, Paulus R, Galvin J, Michalski J, Straube W and Bradley J *et al* 2010 Stereotactic body radiation therapy for inoperable early stage lung cancer *JAMA* **303** 1070–6

[64] Xiao Y, Papiez L, Paulus R, Timmerman R, Straube W L and Bosch W R *et al* 2009 Dosimetric evaluation of heterogeneity corrections for RTOG 0236: stereotactic body radiotherapy of inoperable stage I-II non-small-cell lung cancer *Int. J. Radiat. Oncol. Biol. Phys.* **73** 1235–42

[65] Akino Y, Das I J, Cardenes H R and Desrosiers C M 2014 Correlation between target volume and electron transport effects affecting heterogeneity corrections in stereotactic body radiotherapy for lung cancer *J. Radiat. Res.* **55** 754–76

[66] Siebers J V, Keall P J, Nahum A E and Mohan R 2000 Converting absorbed dose to medium to absorbed dose to water for Monte Carlo based photon beam dose calculations *Phys. Med. Biol.* **45** 983–95

[67] Kry S F, Feygelman V, Balter P, Knöös T, Ma C M C and Snyder M *et al* 2020 AAPM Task Group 329: reference dose specification for dose calculations: dose-to-water or dose-to-muscle? *Med. Phys.* **47** e52–64

[68] Reynaert N, Crop F, Sterpin E, Kawrakow I and Palmans H 2018 On the conversion of dose to bone to dose to water in radiotherapy treatment planning systems *Phys. Imag. Radiat. Oncol.* **5** 26–30

[69] Delbaere A, Younes T and Vieillevigne L 2019 On the conversion from dose-to-medium to dose-to-water in heterogeneous phantoms with Acuros XB and Monte Carlo calculations *Phys. Med. Biol.* **64** 195016

[70] Walters B R B, Kramer R and Kawrakow I 2010 Dose to medium versus dose to water as an estimator of dose to sensitive skeletal tissue *Phys. Med. Biol.* **55** 4535–46

[71] Dogan N, Siebers J V and Keall P J 2006 Clinical comparison of head and neck and prostate IMRT plans using absorbed dose to medium and absorbed dose to water *Phys. Med. Biol.* **51** 4967–80

[72] Radojčić Đ S, Kolacio M Š, Radojčić M, Rajlić D, Casar B, Faj D and Jurković S 2018 Comparison of calculated dose distributions reported as dose-to-water and dose-to-medium for intensity-modulated radiotherapy of nasopharyngeal cancer patients *Med. Dosim.* **43** 363–9

[73] Muñoz-Montplet C, Marruecos J, Buxó M, Jurado-Bruggeman D, Romera-Martínez I, Bueno M and Vilanova J C 2018 Dosimetric impact of Acuros XB dose-to-water and dose-to-medium reporting modes on VMAT planning for head and neck cancer *Phys. Med.* **55** 107–15

[74] Chandroth M M, Venning A, Chick B and Waller B 2016 Effects of contrast materials in IMRT and VMAT of prostate using a commercial Monte Carlo algorithm *Australas. Phys. Eng. Sci. Med.* **39** 547–56

[75] Zifodya J M, Challens C H C and Hsieh W L 2016 From AAA to Acuros XB-clinical implications of selecting either Acuros XB dose-to-water or dose-to-medium *Australas. Phys. Eng. Sci. Med.* **39** 431–9

[76] Hardcastle N, Montaseri A, Lydon J, Kron T, Osburne G and Casswell G *et al* 2019 Dose to medium in head and neck radiotherapy: clinical implications for target volume metrics *Phys. Imag. Radiat. Oncol.* **11** 92–7

[77] Fogliata A, De Rose F, Stravato A, Reggiori G, Tomatis S, Scorsetti M and Cozzi L 2018 Evaluation of target dose inhomogeneity in breast cancer treatment due to tissue elemental differences *Radiat. Oncol.* **13** 92

[78] Fogliata A, Nicolini G, Clivio A, Vanetti E and Cozzi L 2011 On the dosimetric impact of inhomogeneity management in the Acuros XB algorithm for breast treatment *Radiat. Oncol.* **6** 103

[79] Liu H H, Keall P and Hendee W R 2002 Point/Counterpoint: D_m rather than D_w should be used in Monte Carlo treatment planning *Med. Phys.* **29** 922–4

[80] Chetty I J, Curran B, Cygler J E, DeMarco J J, Ezzell G and Faddegon B A *et al* 2007 Report of the AAPM Task Group No. 105: issues associated with clinical implementation of Monte Carlo-based photon and electron external beam treatment planning *Med. Phys.* **34** 4818–53

[81] Andreo P 2015 Dose to 'water-like' media or dose to tissue in MV photons in radiotherapy treatment planning: still a matter of debate *Phys. Med. Biol.* **60** 309–37

[82] Ma C M and Li J 2011 Dose specification for radiation therapy: dose to water or dose to medium? *Phys. Med. Biol.* **56** 3073–89

[83] Fogliata A, Vanetti E, Albers D, Brink C, Clivio A and Knöös T *et al* 2007 On the dosimetric behaviour of photon dose calculation algorithms in the presence of simple geometric heterogeneities: comparison with Monte Carlo calculations *Phys. Med. Biol.* **52** 1363–85

[84] Shepard D M, Earl M A, Li X A, Naqvi S and Yu C 2002 Direct aperture optimization: a turnkey solution for step-and-shoot IMRT *Med. Phys.* **29** 1007–18

[85] Santvoort J P C V and Heijmen B J M 1996 Dynamic multileaf collimation without 'tongue-and-groove' underdosage effects *Phys. Med. Biol.* **41** 2091–105

[86] Webb S, Bortfeld T, Stein J and Convery D 1997 The effect of stair-step leaf transmission on the 'tongue-and-groove problem' in dynamic radiotherapy with a multileaf collimator *Phys. Med. Biol.* **42** 595–602

[87] Huq M S, Das I J, Steinberg T and Galvin J M 2002 A dosimetric comparison of various multileaf collimators *Phys. Med. Biol.* **47** N159–70

[88] Nakaguchi Y, Oono T, Araki F and Maruyama M 2013 Physical characterizations for an integrated 160-leaf multi-leaf collimator with a new concept design *Nihon Hoshasen Gijutsu Gakkai Zasshi* **69** 778–83

[89] Thompson C M, Weston S J, Covgrove V C and Thwaites D I 2014 A dosimetric characterization of a novel linear accelerator collimator *Med. Phys.* **41** 031713-1–11

[90] Szpala S, Cao F and Kohli K 2014 On using the dosimetric leaf gap to model the rounded leaf ends in VMAT/RapidArc plans *J. Appl. Clin. Med. Phys.* **15** 67–84

[91] Fogliata A, Lobefalo F, Reggiori G, Stravato A, Tomatis S, Scorsetti M and Cozzi L 2016 Evaluation of the dose calculation accuracy for small fields defined by jaw or MLC for AAA and Acuros XB algorithms *Med. Phys.* **43** 5685–94

[92] Younge K C, Roberts D, Janes L A, Anderson C, Moran J M and Matuszak M M 2016 Predicting deliverability of volumetric-modulated arc therapy (VMAT) plans using aperture complexity analysis *J. Appl. Clin. Med. Phys.* **17** 124–31

[93] Hernandez V, Vera-Sanchez J A, Vieillevigne L, Khamphan C and Saez J 2018 A new method for modelling the tongue-and-groove in treatment planning systems *Phys. Med. Biol.* **63** 245005

[94] Vieillevigne L, Khamphan C, Saez J and Hernandez V 2019 On the need for tuning the dosimetric leaf gap for stereotactic treatment plans in the Eclipse treatment planning system *J. Appl. Clin. Med. Phys.* **20** 68–77

[95] Han Z, Hacker F, Killoran J, Kukluk J and Aizer A *et al* 2020 Optimization of MLC parameters for TPS calculation and dosimetric verification: application to single isocenter radiosurgery of multiple brain lesions using VMAT *Biomed. Phys. Eng. Express* **6** 015004

[96] Koger B, Price R, Wang D, Toomeh D and Geneser S *et al* 2020 Impact of the MLC leaf-tip model in a commercial TPS: dose calculation limitations and IROC-H phantom failures *J. Appl. Clin. Med. Phys.* **21** 82–8

[97] Mei X, Nygren I and Villarreal-Barajas J E 2011 On the use of the MLC dosimetric leaf gap as a quality control tool for accurate dynamic IMRT delivery *Med. Phys.* **38** 2246–55

[98] Chen S, Yi B Y, Yang X, Xu H and Prado K L *et al* 2015 Optimizing the MLC model parameters for IMRT in the RayStation treatment planning system *J. Appl. Clin. Med. Phys.* **16** 322–32

[99] Yao W and Farr J B 2015 Determining the optimal dosimetric leaf gap setting for rounded leaf-end multileaf collimator systems by simple test fields *J. Appl. Clin. Med. Phys.* **16** 65–77
[100] Roche M, Crane R, Powers M and Crabtree T 2018 Agility MLC transmission optimization in the Monaco treatment planning system *J. Appl. Clin. Med. Phys.* **19** 473–82
[101] Snyder M, Halford R, Knill C, Adams J N, Bossenberger T and Nalichowski A *et al* 2016 Modeling the Agility MLC in the Monaco treatment planning system *J. Appl. Clin. Med. Phys.* **17** 190–202
[102] Gholampourkashi S, Cygler J E, Belec J, Vujicic M and Heath E 2019 Monte Carlo and analytic modelling of an Elekta Infinity linac with Agility MLC: investigating the significance of accurate model parameters for small radiation fields *J. Appl. Clin. Med. Phys.* **20** 55–67
[103] Bedford J L, Thomas M D R and Smyth G 2013 Beam modeling and VMAT performance with the Agility 160-leaf multileaf collimator *J. Appl. Clin. Med. Phys.* **14** 172–85
[104] Starkschall G, Steadham R E, Popple R A, Ahmad S and Rosen I I 2000 Beam-commissioning methodology for a three-dimensional convolution/superposition photon dose algorithm *J. Appl. Clin. Med. Phys.* **1** 8–27
[105] Feygelman V, Hunt D, Walker L, Mueller R, Demarco M L and Dilling T *et al* 2010 Validation of Pinnacle treatment planning system for use with Novalis delivery unit *J. Appl. Clin. Med. Phys.* **11** 135–53
[106] Young L A, Yang F, Cao N and Meyer J 2016 Rounded leaf end modeling in Pinnacle VMAT treatment planning for fixed jaw linacs *J. Appl. Clin. Med. Phys.* **17** 149–62
[107] Fogliata A, Nicolini G, Clivio A, Vanetti E and Cozzi L 2011 Accuray of Acuros XB and AAA dose calculation for small fields with reference to RapidArc stereotactic treatments *Med. Phys.* **38** 6228–37
[108] Kron T, Clivio A, Vanetti E, Nicolini G, Cramb J and Lonski P *et al* 2012 Small field segments surrounded by large areas only shielded by a multileaf collimator: comparison of experiments and dose calculation *Med. Phys.* **39** 7480–9
[109] Paganini L, Reggiori G, Stravato A, Palumbo V, Mancosu P and Lobefalo F *et al* 2019 MLC parameters from static fields to VMAT plans: an evaluation in a RT-dedicated MC environment (PRIMO) *Radiat. Oncol.* **14** 216
[110] Technical Reports Series No. 483 2017 *Dosimetry of Small Static Fields Used in External Beam Radiotherapy. An International Code of Practice for Reference and Relative Dose Determination* (Vienna: International Atomic Energy Agency)
[111] Das I J, Francescon P, Ahnesjö A, Moran J, Aspradakis M M and Cheng C W *et al* in review Small fields and non-equilibrium condition photon beam dosimetry: AAPM Task Group Report 155 *Med. Phys.*
[112] Kry S F, Salehpour M, Followill D S, Stovall M, Kuban D A, White R A and Rosen I I 2005 Out-of-field photon and neutron dose equivalents from step-and-shoot intensity-modulated radiation therapy *Int. J. Radiat. Oncol. Biol. Phys.* **62** 1204–16
[113] Kry S F, Titt U, Pönisch F, Followill D, Vassiliev O N and White R A *et al* 2006 A Monte Carlo model for calculating out-of-field dose from a Varian 6 MV beam *Med. Phys.* **33** 4405–13
[114] Kry S F, Titt U, Followill D, Pönisch F, Vassiliev O N and White R A *et al* 2007 A Monte Carlo model for out-of-field dose calculation from high-energy photon therapy *Med. Phys.* **34** 3489–99

[115] Bednarz B and Xu G 2009 Monte Carlo modeling of a 6 and 18 MV Varian Clinac medical accelerator for in-field and out-of-field dose calculation: development and validation *Phys. Med. Biol.* **54** N43–57
[116] Taylor M L and Kron T 2011 Consideration of the radiation dose delivered away from the treatment field to patients in radiotherapy *J. Med. Phys.* **36** 59–71
[117] Kry S F, Vassiliev O N and Mohan R 2010 Out-of-field photon dose following removal of the flattening filter from a medical accelerator *Phys. Med. Biol.* **55** 2155–66
[118] Lamberg S S, Frengen J and Lindmo T 2012 Monte Carlo study of in-field and out-of-field dose distributions from a linear accelerator operating with and without a flattening-filter *Med. Phys.* **39** 5194–203
[119] Wijesooriya K 2019 Part I: Out-of-field dose mapping for 6X and 6X-flattening filter-free beams on the TrueBeam for extended distances *Med. Phys.* **46** 868–76
[120] Wijesooriya K, Liyanage N K, Kaluarachchi M and Sawkey D 2019 Part II: Verification of the TrueBeam head shielding model in Varian VirtuaLinac via out-of-field doses *Med. Phys.* **46** 877–84
[121] Ruben J D, Lancaster C M, Jones P and Smith R L 2011 A comparison of out-of-field dose and its constituent components for intensity-modulated radiation therapy versus conformal radiation therapy: implications for carcinogenesis *Int. J. Radiat. Oncol. Biol. Phys.* **81** 1458–64
[122] Benadjaoud M A, Bezin J, Veres A, Lefkopoulos D, Chavaudra J and Bridier A *et al* 2012 A multi-plane source model for out-of-field head scatter dose calculations in external beam photon therapy *Phys. Med. Biol.* **57** 7725–39
[123] Howell R M, Scarboro S B, Kry S F and Yaldo D Z 2010 Accuracy of out-of-field dose calculations by a commercial treatment planning system *Phys. Med. Biol.* **55** 6999–7008
[124] Fogliata A, Clivio A, Vanetti E, Nicolini G, Belosi M F and Cozzi L 2013 Dosimetric evaluation of photon dose calculation under jaw and MLC shielding *Med. Phys.* **4** 101706-1–12
[125] Wang L and Ding G X 2014 The accuracy of the out-of-field dose calculations using a model based algorithm in a commercial treatment planning system *Phys. Med. Biol.* **59** N113–28
[126] Wang L and Ding G X 2018 Estimating the uncertainty of calculated out-of-field organ dose from a commercial treatment planning system *J. Appl. Clin. Med. Phys.* **19** 319–24
[127] Alghamdi S and Tajaldeen A 2019 Evaluation of dose calculation algorithms using different density materials for in-field and out-of-field conditions *Exp. Oncol.* **41** 46–52
[128] Shine N S, Paramu R, Gopinath M, Jaon Bos R C and Jayadevan P M 2019 Out-of-field dose calculation by a commercial treatment planning system and comparison by Monte Carlo simulation for Varian TrueBeam *J. Med. Phys.* **44** 156–75
[129] Huang J Y, Followill D S, Wang X A and Kry S F 2013 Accuracy and sources of error of out-of-field dose calculations by a commercial treatment planning system for intensity-modulated radiation therapy treatments *J. Appl. Clin. Med. Phys.* **14** 186–97
[130] Schneider U, Hälg R A, Hartmann M, Mack A, Storelli F and Joosten A *et al* 2014 Accuracy of out-of-field dose calculation of tomotherapy and cyberknife treatment planning systems: a dosimetric study *Z. Med. Phys.* **24** 211–5
[131] Colnot J, Barraux V, Loiseau C, Berejny P, Batalla A, Gschwind R and Huet C 2019 A new Monte Carlo model of a Cyberknife system for the precise determination of out-of-field doses *Phys. Med.Biol.* **64** 195008

[132] Reft C, Alecu R, Das I J, Gerbi B J, Keall P and Lief E *et al* 2003 Dosimetric considerations for patients with HIP prostheses undergoing pelvic irradiation. Report of the AAPM Radiation Therapy Committee Task Group 63 *Med. Phys.* **30** 1162–82

[133] Wieslander E and Knöös T 2003 Dose perturbation in the presence of metallic implants: treatment planning system versus Monte Carlo simulations *Phys. Med. Biol.* **48** 3295–305

[134] Ojala J, Kapanen M, Sipilä P, Hyödynmaa S and Pitkänen M 2014 The accuracy of Acuros XB algorithm for radiation beams traversing a metallic hip implant—comparison with measurements and Monte Carlo calculations *J. Appl. Clin. Med. Phys.* **15** 162–76

[135] Cheng Z J, Bromley R M, Oborn B, Carolan M and Booth J 2016 On the accuracy of dose prediction near metal fixation devices for spine SBRT *J. Appl. Clin. Med. Phys.* **17** 475–85

[136] Ade N and du Plessis F C P 2017 Dose comparison between Gafchromic film, XiO, and Monaco treatment planning systems in a novel pelvic phantom that contains a titanium hip prosthesis *J. Appl. Clin. Med. Phys.* **18** 162–73

[137] Byrnes K, Ford A and Bennie N 2019 Verification of the Elekta Monaco TPS Monte Carlo in modelling radiation transmission through metals in a water equivalent phantom *Australas. Phys. Eng. Sci. Med.* **42** 639–45

[138] Parenica H M, Mavroidis P, Jones W, Swanson G, Papanikolaou N and Stathakis S 2019 VMAT optimization and dose calculation in the presence of metallic hip prostheses *Technol. Cancer Res. Treat.* **18** 1–10

[139] Parenica H M, Ford J R, Mavroidis P, Li Y, Papanikolaou and Stathakis S 2019 Treatment planning dose accuracy improvement in the presence of dental implants *Med. Dos.* **44** 159–66

[140] Huang B, Wu L, Lin P and Chen C 2015 Dose calculation of Acuros XB and Anisotropic Analytical Algorithm in lung stereotactic body radiotherapy treatment with flattening filter free beams and the potential role of calculation grid size *Radiat. Oncol.* **10** 53

[141] Snyder K C, Liu M, Zhao B, Huang Y, Wen N, Chetty I J and Siddiqui M S 2017 Investigating the dosimetric effects of grid size on dose calculation accuracy using volumetric modulated arc therapy in spine stereotactic radiosurgery *J. Radiosurg. SBRT* **4** 303–13

[142] Kim K H, Chung J B, Suh T S, Kang S W, Kang S H and Eom K Y *et al* 2018 Dosimetric and radiobiological comparison in different dose calculation grid sizes between Acuros XB and anisotropic analytical algorithm for prostate VMAT *PLoS One* **13** e0207232

[143] Chow J C L and Jiang R 2018 Dose-volume and radiobiological dependence on the calculation grid size in prostate VMAT planning *Med. Dosim.* **43** 383–9

[144] Kawashima M, Kawamura H, Onishi M, Takakusagi Y, Okonogi N and Okazaki A *et al* 2017 The impact of the grid size on tomotherapy for prostate cancer *J. Med. Phys.* **42** 144–50

[145] Srivastava S P, Cheng C W and Das I J 2017 The dosimetric and radiobiological impact of calculation grid size on head and neck IMRT. Pract *Radiat. Oncol.* **7** 209–17

[146] Chung H, Jin H, Palta J, Suh T S and Kim S 2006 Dose variations with varying calculation grid size in head and neck IMRT *Phys. Med. Biol.* **51** 4841–56

[147] Srivastava S P, Cheng S W and Das I J 2016 The effect of slice thickness on target and organs at risk volumes, dosimetric coverage and radiobiological impact in IMRT planning *Clin. Transl. Oncol.* **18** 469–79

[148] Jacob V and Kneschaurek P 2009 Influence of the CT slice thickness on the dose calculation for stereotactic treatment planning ed O Dössel and W C Schlegel *Proceedings of the World*

Congress on Medical Physics and Biomedical Engineering, September 7–12 Munich IFMBE vol 25/1 (Berlin, Heidelberg: Springer)

[149] Caivano R, Fiorentino A, Pedicini P, Califano G and Fusco V 2014 The impact of computed tomography slice thickness on the assessment of stereotactic, 3D conformal and intensity-modulated radiotherapy for brain tumors *Clin. Transl. Oncol.* **16** 503–8

[150] Tunio M A, Rafi M, Ahmed Z, Ali S and Zameer A 2010 Influence of CT slice thickness on volume and dose uncertainty for different organs during treatment planning for early prostate cancer *Pakist. J. Radiol.* **20** 87–91

[151] Olsson C, Thor M, Liu M, Moiseenko V, Petersen S E and Høyer M *et al* 2014 Incluence of image slice thickness on rectal dose-response relationships following radiotherapy of prostate cancer *Phys. Med. Biol.* **59** 3749–59

[152] Luo H, He Y, Jin F, Yang D, Liu X, Ran X and Wang Y 2018 Inpact of CT slice thickness on volume and dose evaluation during thoracic cancer radiotherapy *Cancer Manag. Res.* **10** 3679–86

[153] Estabrook N C, Corn J B, Ewing M M, Cardenes H R and Das I J 2017 Dosimetric impact of gastrointestinal air column in radiation treatment of pancreatic cancer *Br. J. Radiol.* **91** 20170512

[154] Lees J, Holloway L, Fuller M and Forstner D 2005 Effect of intravenous contrast on treatment planning system dose calculations in the lung *Australas. Phys. Eng. Sci. Med.* **28** 190

[155] Burridge N A, Rowbottom C G and Burt P A 2006 Effect of contrast-enhanced CT scans on heterogeneity corrected dose computations in the lung *J. Appl. Clin. Med. Phys.* **7** 1–12

[156] Wo J Y, Mannarino E, Killoran J and Chen A B 2010 The impact of IV contrast on dose calculations in the treatment of lung cancer *Int. J. Radiat. Oncol. Biol. Phys.* **78** Suppl S750

[157] Ziong W, Huang D, Gewanter R and Burman C 2012 SU-E-T-545: dose comparison between intravenous contrast-enhanced CT and non contrast CT in treatment planning *Med. Phys.* **39** 3831

[158] Li H S, Chen J H, Zhang W, Shang D P, Li B S and Sun T *et al* 2013 Influence of intravenous contrast medium on dose calculation using CT in treatment planning for oesophageal cancer *Asian Pac. J. Cancer Prev.* **14** 1609–14

[159] Nasrollah J, Mikaeil M, Omid E, Mojtaba S S and Ahad Z 2014 Influence of intravenous contrast media on treatment planning dose calculations of lower esophageal and rectal cancers *J. Cancer Res. Ther.* **10** 147–52

[160] Li H, Bottani B, DeWees T, Low D A, Michalski J M and Mutic S *et al* 2014 Prospective study evaluating the use of IV contrast on IMRT treatment planning for lung cancer *Med. Phys.* **41** 031708-1–7

[161] Lee F K H, Chan C C L and Law C K 2009 Influence of CT contrast agent on dose calculation of intensity modulated radiation therapy plan for nasopharyngeal carcinoma *J. Med. Imag. Rad. Oncol.* **53** 114–8

[162] Jing H, Tian Y, Wang S L, Jin J and Li Y 2015 Oral contrast agent does have an impact on dose calculation of volumetric modulated arc therapy planning for pelvic irradiation: a reevaluation of intestine dose may be warranted *Int. J. Radiat. Oncol. Biol. Phys.* **93** Suppl E156–7

[163] Heydarheydari S, Farshchian N and Haghparast A 2016 Influence of the contrast agents on treatment planning dose calculations of prostate and rectal cancers *Rep. Pract. Oncol. Radiother.* **21** 441–6

Chapter 11

Plan variability

The variability in radiotherapy treatment plans is a complex issue. The same patient could be treated with the same technology (IMRT, for example) in different manners. Variability can occur during the contouring phase, which is subject to inter-observer skills, preferences and aims, as well as the imaging modalities used for delineating the various structures. Another significant source of variability is the treatment planning process. More specifically, the outcome of the inverse planning process depends on the different implementations of the optimization algorithms and their relative tools handling the dose-volume constraints. The planner's skill is another relevant source of variability complicated to model, impacting more the intensity-modulated techniques than the older 3DCRT. The foundation of the inverse optimization is based on the not straight translation of given clinical aims (e.g., complication or tumor control probabilities) into numerical input to the optimization (dose–volume) objectives. Additionally, the potential presence of conflicting aims/objectives generates the need for solving the trade-offs, which can require multiple (and time-consuming) planner's multiple iterations, whose results depend mainly on time and the operator's skills.

With the increasing use of the advanced techniques, IMRT in the early 2000s and VMAT ten years later, the need to homogenize the plan quality became, therefore, a concern. The possible approaches to reduce the variability observed in the plan quality were extensively investigated, aiming for the implementation of innovative and more automated methods for treatment planning. Similarly to the contouring process supported by auto-segmentation engines, the treatment planning could be supported by knowledge-based approaches with variable levels of automation with the final aim of harmonizing and improving the dosimetric quality of the plans as well as the efficiency.

An extensive plan variability, both at inter- and intra-center level, might affect the clinical outcome of the treatments. The final goal of a reduced plan variability

doi:10.1088/978-0-7503-1335-3ch11

should leverage the overall plan quality, also for centers with limited resources or expertize with a beneficial impact on the clinical outcome.

Hussein *et al* [1] in 2018, in their review paper, provide a glimpse of automation in intensity-modulated radiotherapy planning, showing the very sharp uplift in the number of publications starting when the first automated system was implemented in the commercial planning software, around 2008, after a first initial lag period of about five years.

Mainly three different approaches have been explored and applied over the years:

- knowledge-based planning
- template/protocol-based automation
- multi-criteria optimization

This chapter, starting from a picture of the plan variability arising from planners and technique implementations in the TPS, presents the available solutions to reduce this uncertainty and variability.

11.1 Dosimetric variation: the intra- and inter-planner and planning system sources

A large number of TPS are providing various forms of inverse planning used in IMRT with different fluence mapping and optimization routines, as well as different calculation engines and inhomogeneity handling. A collaborative study aiming to determine plan dosimetric variations was conducted in 2004 among eight different institutions using 11 TPS for IMRT planning. The plans were optimized on a pre-contoured CT dataset selected for prostate, lung, and head and neck cases, and used the same beam geometry (7, 5 and 9 equally spaced IMRT fields) [2]. The dosimetric variation is shown in figure 11.1, as the PTV DVHs for the head and neck case for the 11 analyzed TPS, showing a huge dosimetric variability.

The study continued on the same selected cases and beam arrangement, using one single TPS (Eclipse) and five planners [3] pursuing the same clinical goals and dose constraints. In figure 11.2 the DVHs for the three anatomical sites (PTV and OAR) are presented proving the inter-planner variation, standing as large as 20% in the PTV, and up to 60% in the OAR. Similar variations (up to 26%) were also noted for the intra-planner variability.

Such significant intra- and inter-planner variation indicates that the plan quality cannot be guaranteed to be of the same level. Hence the patient treatments are subject to random variations reflected with treatment planning processes which could vary significantly.

A similar work was done in the same years on IMRT planning for breast treatment including the internal mammary chain [4]. Datasets of five patients were distributed to different participants to plan ten different TPS or optimization modalities. The dosimetric variation is shown in figure 11.3 with DVH for the target and OAR.

These examples prove the wide variability in the plan quality despite the same clinical objectives having been used in all compared plans, enhancing the extreme

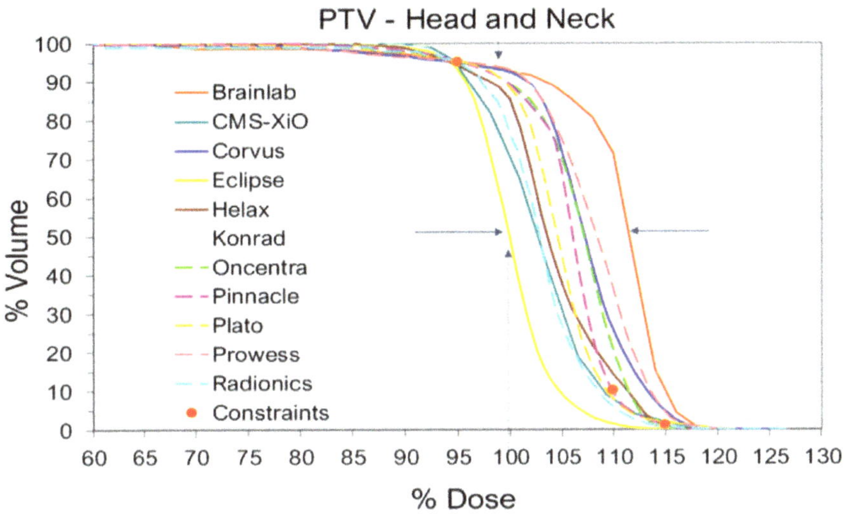

Figure 11.1. Plan variability for a single IMRT head and neck case planned on 11 different TPS. Courtesy of Indra Das.

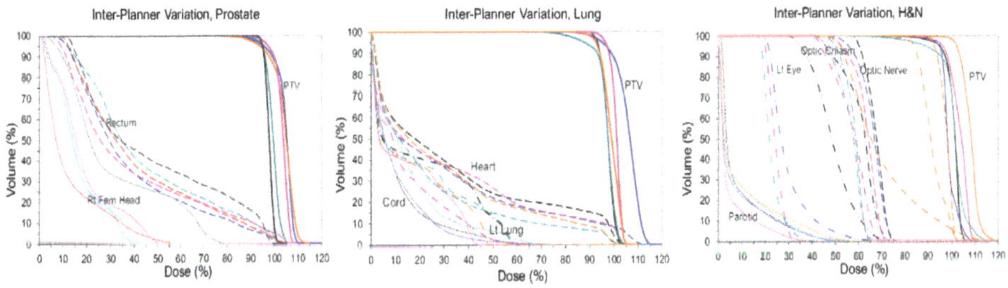

Figure 11.2. Plan variability of a prostate, a lung and a head and neck case planned with IMRT by five different planners on the same TPS (Eclipse). Courtesy of Indra Das.

need for an improved plan homogeneity when the same goals are defined. In the next section possible solutions to solve this issue are presented.

11.2 Knowledge-based planning

The *knowledge-based planning* approach aims at modeling historical data—which includes the best prior knowledge and experience on planning a specific anatomical site—into some predictive engine usable for new patients. The collection of knowledge needed for the models could be as simple as a database where planners can (manually or automatically) identify the representative case with the closest match (in terms of contouring and anatomical similarities) with any given new patient. This is the so-called *atlas-based* concept.

More properly *model-based* systems can better serve the planning needs. The foundation of this approach requires firstly the selection of (a large) number of clinically accepted plans and contours of high quality (the knowledge). Secondly, a

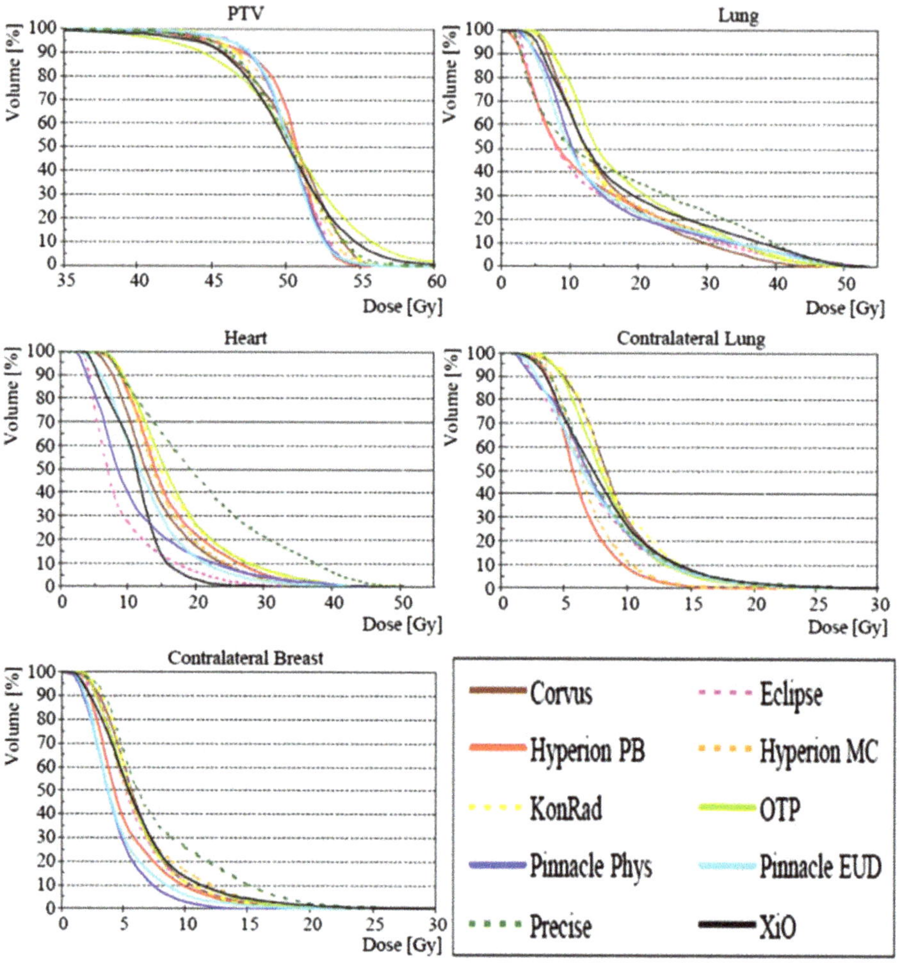

Figure 11.3. Plan variability for breast treatment with internal mammary chain, using different planning systems or different optimization or calculation methods. Adapted from Fogliata *et al* [4], reproduced with permission from Elsevier.

machine-learning training process identifies and parametrizes the relevant dosimetric, anatomical or geometrical characteristics which can be prospectively used to estimate the achievable dose distributions for new patients. The result is the generation of mathematical models capable of predicting the dose distributions, summarized by means of the DVHs, for the critical structures (if present in the predictive model) of any new patient. The plan quality should reflect those of the patients selected for training, while, at the same time, keeping the new patient specificity.

The first approaches were published by the group at Johns Hopkins University, who introduced a descriptor of PTV and OAR relationship: the overlap volume histogram (OVH) to measure the proximity of the OAR to the PTV [5]. In their concept, planners search through the database comparing the geometric relationships of the new patient with those of prior patients, guided by the OVH. This concept has been evaluated for head and neck [6], pancreas [7] and prostate cancer patients [8]. In the latter case, it was possible to predict the minimal achievable rectal dose ($D_{35\%}$).

Washington University investigated the correlation between the fraction of the OAR overlapping the PTV, and the OAR mean dose [9] and confirmed the evidence that one critical element contributing to the total plan quality was in the degree of overlap between PTV and OAR. This allowed a model to be developed to predict the OAR doses, applied on IMRT prostate and head and neck patients [10].

Both approaches paved the way to the possibility to semi-automatically predict the DVH of the OARs, facilitating the planner to drive the optimizer toward an 'ideal' or at least improved plan quality. The approach followed by the investigators at Duke University was, in the beginning, *atlas-based*. In their first works on knowledge-based planning [11, 12], they wanted to reduce the plan quality variation among different treatment centers, aiming to leverage the IMRT planning experience and to enable the automatic generation of high-quality plans. They explored the possibility to adapt plans from a high-quality dataset to other patients. Their approach was based on matching 2D beam's-eye-view projections of the structure contours to identify similar patients, by using a similarity metric for image matching. The treatment parameters of the selected expert case, as the beam geometry, the deformed fluence maps, the constraints were utilized to obtain the plan for the new patient. This approach was tested on 55 patients, achieving a superior or equivalent plan quality relative to the original plans in 95% of the cases, with increased plan quality homogeneity.

The same group at Duke University, developed, in a second phase, a *model-based* solution, starting from the concepts of the distance-to-target histogram (DTH, analogous to the OVH) and the 2D BEV matching. To select the most salient geometric and dosimetric features, they applied the principal component analysis (PCA) to the DTH (anatomical information) and the DVH (dosimetric information). This allowed collecting patient-specific information to input to the DVH estimation model [13]. This machine-learning approach was verified on prostate and head and neck patients [14].

Some investigations are, at present, exploring the possibility of building models with a voxel-based dose prediction instead of the DVH, in a sort of knowledge-guided dose prediction, and based on algorithms commonly used for auto-segmentation like the active shape model, or deep-learning artificial neural networks (described in chapter 7 of this book) [15–18].

The research conducted by the Duke and Washington University teams, led to the implementation of a knowledge-based planning engine in a commercial planning system, Eclipse, by Varian Medical Systems, known as the RapidPlan that uses DVH estimation algorithm, whose core is in the model-based approach of Duke University. Its implementation is based on the use of several plans (of a specific anatomical site) of high quality to build and train a model based on both geometric and dosimetric features of OARs to estimate their DVHs. For each OAR, the DVH

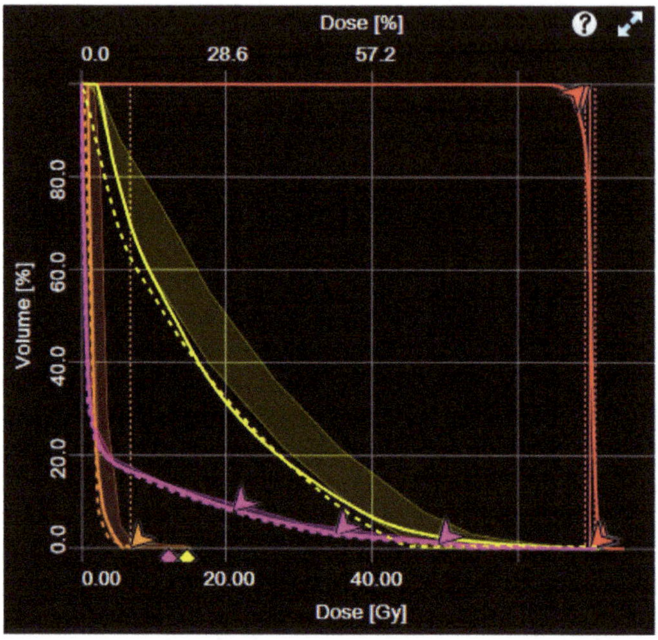

Figure 11.4. Example of a RapidPlan DVH range prediction (the colored bands), the optimization objectives (the dashed lines), and the DVH resulting from the optimization (the solid lines), for some OARs of a head and neck case.

is estimated to be within a range, and this result is used to feed the optimization engine with objectives driving the plan to achieve, or improve, those estimates. This is accomplished by applying an optimization objective as the lowest DVH in the calculated range, as shown in figure 11.4. RapidPlan has been evaluated before its clinical implementation by different groups, exploring a wide variety of anatomical sites: head and neck [19–21], esophagus [22], lung (advanced or SBRT) [23, 24], breast [25], liver [26, 27], pelvic treatment including prostate, rectum, gynecologic malignancies [23, 28–31].

Some publications refer to interesting applications of the RapidPlan engine. The knowledge-based planning models have been validated for mixed configuration, meaning that the plans used for training differed from what was adopted for the new patient plans. It was the case of patients in the prone position, planned with a model trained with patient anatomy in the supine position [32], or plans generated with IMRT technique using a model trained with VMAT plans [32], or, again, VMAT plans optimized with a model trained with TomoTherapy dose distribution plans [33]. Those results demonstrated the interesting usability of the models in a broad spectrum of patient and technique variety, not only restricted to the specific anatomies and techniques used for the patients and plans selected for the model training.

Another compelling utilization of the knowledge-based planning algorithms refers to the quality assurance of the clinical trials. Although the clinical trials' specifications are detailed in the protocols' guidelines, the dosimetric requests are generally given as tolerance dose levels for some OAR, one of the most critical points of the radiotherapy trials is the large variability in the plan quality. The need for reducing such plan variability could lead to the application of knowledge-based planning systems as a radiotherapy clinical trial plan quality control system. This has been positively explored, to give an example, by Li *et al* [34] on patients treated with IMRT according to the INTERTECC protocol for cervical cancer patients.

Some practical limitations are present for the model-based approaches. The main one is linked to the segmentation of the patient's anatomy. The predictive models can estimate the DVHs only for those structures included in the definition and training phase (and of course, contoured in the source data). Hence, the dose prediction of any other tissue/structure is not automated and included in the plan optimization. As a consequence, the overall dose distribution will still be manually controlled, including the appraisal of the conformality, the dose spillage, the dose gradients and any other relevant metrics. Lastly, since the dose information is based on the DVHs, the spatial information of the dose distribution in the various structures is not accounted for.

The quality of the dose distribution resulting in a new planned patient heavily depends on the quality of the plans selected for the training of the model [35]. The knowledge-based planning concept is based on DVH estimations. It drives the optimization of any new patient plan toward a plan with the same dose distribution strategy as the patients utilized to build the model, and no further attempt in improving the dose outside the target more than that determined by the DVH estimation is part of the process.

11.3 Protocol-based automation

The protocol-based approach relies on a different automation process, still aiming to obtain the highest plan quality. In general terms, the architecture of such a system requires as a first step the definition of a template inclusive of the dose prescription and the dose-volume objectives (clinical goals) with their priority needed to create the hierarchy to manage the trade-offs between target coverage and OAR sparing. The priorities can also be used to identify the structures requiring hard constraints (as could be the spinal cord example for head and neck case) or soft constraints in other structures. However, the information included in a template is static and if not well-tuned, could lead to suboptimal plans; further individualization and adjustments of the templates should, therefore, be applied, indicating that a simple template, however detailed, cannot be the solution for all patients with the same pathology. An automated approach of the protocol-based planning, starting from the initial clinically-determined and user-defined criteria, intends to improve the plan quality through iterative adjustments of the constraints attempting to lower the OAR doses to a maximum strength before compromising the criteria having higher priorities (figure 11.5). The main idea is to follow the typical planner working process. Often, during manual intensity-modulated planning, some non-anatomical structures are delineated: dummy structures, 'rings' or 'shells', ad-hoc contours

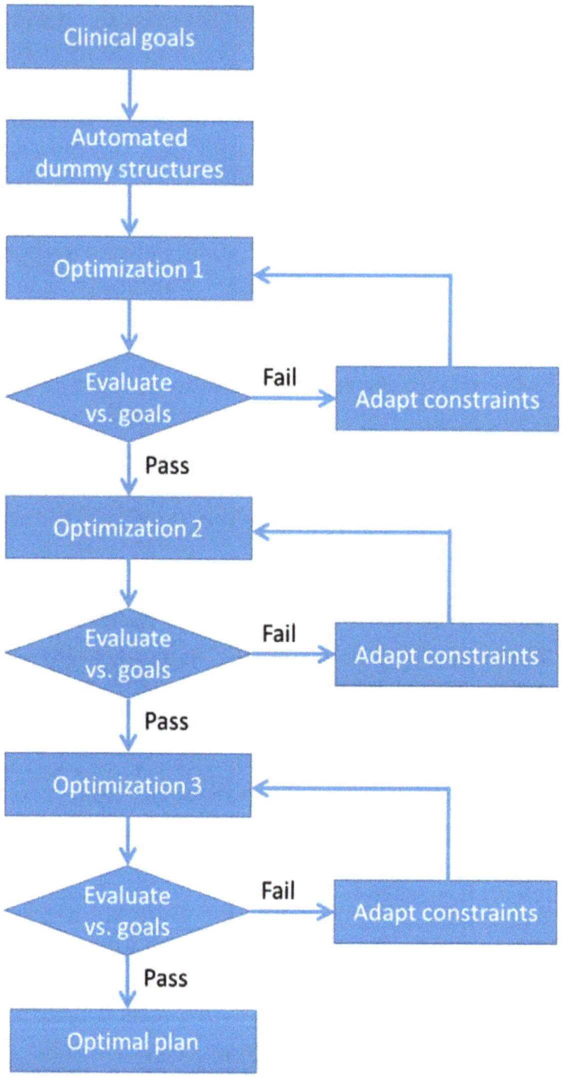

Figure 11.5. Schematic view of a possible flow of protocol-based planning automation.

obtained by Boolean operations from the anatomical delineations using or not margin between structures, etc. The automated process also intended to generate all those helping contours without the planner intervention and then apply the initial template with the desired priorities. Finally, the critical structure dose sparing is enforced.

Various efficient solutions have been proposed and applied, and some centers implemented their planned automation process, based on systems entirely developed in-house, or using the treatment planning scripting tools available in some commercial planning systems. This institutional approach of automation allows the entire process to be tailored according to the specific experience and clinical strategy.

In 2007, Wilkens *et al* [36] published their 'goal programming' approach presenting results on head and neck cases. The goals were addressed stepwise using a priority order. The achievement of a previous step was turned into hard constraints, allowing the lower priority goals optimization in the next level.

In 2011 Zhang *et al* [37] from the MD Anderson Cancer Center presented IMRT lung planning, their methodology implemented in an in-house system for inverse IMRT planning, following an automated sequence: (1) beam angle automation algorithm, (2) design the planning structures useful for the lung cancer cases, (3) automatically adjust the objectives of the cost function based on a parameter automation algorithm.

Many other methods and implementations for automated IMRT planning have been published [38, 39], each specifying the particular methodological flow. The automatic delineation of some dummy structures, mimicking the planner work conveniently, in some cases was also part of the implementations or proposals.

Most of the treatment planning systems allow implementing additional features to the system with the use of scripting directly connected to the system information, database, beam configurations. Those tools have been used by different authors to develop in-house planning automation directly using the clinical planning system. This has been for example the case of Boylan *et al* [40], using the Philips Pinnacle scripting tool, setting a three level procedure: first the PTV dose coverage and homogeneity, the second level focused on the OARs sparing, and thirdly the generation of dummy structure to lower the OAR dose, further than the clinical requirement. Several other investigators (Song *et al* [41] and Speer *et al* [42]) also used Pinnacle scripting and provided good results. Analogously, but on a different system, Winkel *et al* [43] developed automated planning based on the Elekta Monaco research automation toolkit which works as an application programming interface (API) enabling the development of applications communicating with the specific Monaco user interface.

A different and peculiar practical solution is the 'automatic interactive optimizer' proposed by Tol *et al* [44] on the Varian Eclipse system, aiming to automate the interactive guidance of the Progressive Resolution Optimizer. In their method, the authors realized a virtual robot controlling the mouse position and actions. The task of the robot was to 'observe' the evolution of the optimization process, i.e., the evolution of the DVH displayed in the optimization window and to automatically adjust (by unattended mouse actions) the position (i.e., the value) of the symbols corresponding to the dose-volume constraints in the user interface. This process is therefore in principle capable of continuously improving the OAR's DVH and can incorporate some logic to deal with trade-offs and to the convergence. The limitation of this work, making it unusable in a long term perspective, is its implementation based on the specific monitor display of specific optimization user interfaces.

The protocol-based concept of inverse plan automation led to a commercial clinical solution, the AutoPlanning, implemented in the Philips Pinnacle^3 planning system. Several publications compared the plan quality obtained by the

AutoPlanning engine with that from manual planning, showing a general improvement, especially in the OAR sparing. The most explored site, probably due to its intrinsic planning complexity, is the head and neck [42, 45–48]; other studies refer for example to esophageal cancer planning [49, 50], mediastinal Hodgkin lymphoma [51], and prostate [52].

Noteworthy is the application of AutoPlanning for the whole brain irradiation with hippocampus sparing for reducing the adverse neurocognitive effects, according to the RTOG 0933 trial [53], where the authors found significant improvement in fulfilling the protocol recommendations and homogenizing the brain dose, effectively leading to a standardized high plan quality. Speer *et al* [42] compared the conventional manual process, AutoPlanning, and a home automated planning script in the Pinnacle planning system. Both automated processes outperformed the manual work, particularly in the case of the home scripting, which probably better focused the institutional clinical criteria. However, the experienced planner gave the best results for particular cases, enhancing the fact that the plan automation is of help in common, although complex, cases, the planner's skills are still needed to allow proper treatments for very challenging anatomies, and ultimately to enable general improvement, development, and innovation.

The automated processes are well suited to the use of the artificial intelligence AI, with which the planners' knowledge and skills could be used for, e.g., artificial neural network training. Various studies developed systems mimicking the human planner actions during the plan optimization work, pioneered by Yan and colleagues [54–57]. Those are mainly based on the fuzzy logic, which is a common AI approach based on the observation of the people's actions (leading to setup procedures based on non-numerical and hence imprecise information).

The advantage of a protocol-based automation process in comparison with the knowledge-based approach previously described, atlas- or model-based, is that it is not necessaryily a prior database of successful and high-quality plans, but uses iterative processes for progressive optimization.

11.4 Multi-criteria optimization

Both the knowledge-based planning and the protocol-based automation cannot adequately address the compelling problem related to the trade-offs between the target coverage and the OAR sparing, or between OAR with conflicting potential for dose sparing. The multi-criteria optimization (MCO) strategy, based on the Pareto front concept, should allow the selection of an ideal solution from a set of Pareto-optimal plans. Tools enabling an easy (visual) navigation through the multi-dimensional surface constitute the end-user interface to this methodology [58–61].

In theory, the Pareto-optimal front can be defined after a vast number (in theory infinite) of plans has been optimized varying the constraints applied to each of the axes in the multi-dimensional space (one axis per OAR and objective). The plans which cannot improve the results on one axis (OAR/objective) without making the findings along any other axis deteriorate provides the set of Pareto-optimal solutions, as exemplified in figure 11.6, with a two-objectives problem with the mean doses of

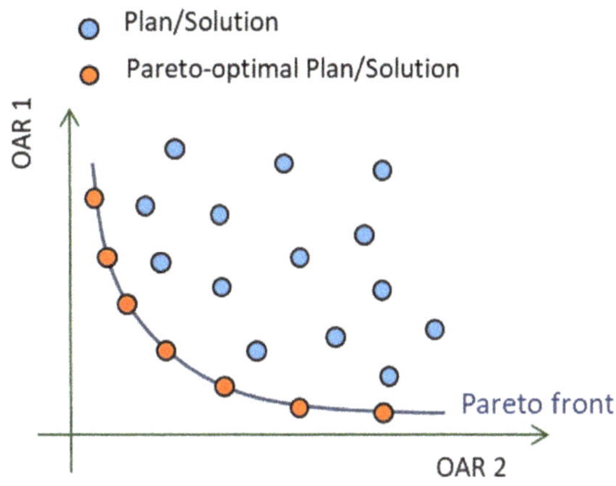

Figure 11.6. Example of the Pareto front.

OAR1 and OAR2 that has to be minimized. All feasible plans are located at the right of a line, called the Pareto front. The plans lying on the front (orange points) are the Pareto-optimal ones. All those at the right of the front (blue points) are suboptimal since both objectives could be simultaneously improved in the same plan.

The rationale for the implementation of this multi-criteria strategy is, therefore, the automated generation of solutions along the Pareto front and the implementation of some user interface for the selection of one of those better fitting the clinical preferences for the individual patient, according to predefined trade-offs, with the guarantee that no better global plan could be found. The key conceptual problem with this approach is the multiplicity of plans needed to identify the Pareto front.

11.5 MCO, *a posteriori*

The MCO can work on two different approaches. The first approach, called *a posteriori*, generates a high number of Pareto-optimal solutions and leaves the user the manual selection of the single plan meeting at best the requirements [58]. From the initial works of Thieke *et al* [60] and Monz *et al* [59], subsequent studies of the same group reported the research and development of this approach for the IMRT MCO planning [62, 63]. The drawback of the *a posteriori* approach is the vast amount of computations needed to generate the Pareto front. The minimum total number of plans sufficient to obtain the front was estimated to be $N + 1$, with N the number of objectives [64]. The higher the number of OAR and clinically desirable goals, the longer the computation time.

Clinical implementation of the *a posteriori* approach of MCO is currently RayNavigator in the RaySearch planning system, and more recently in MCO in the Varian Eclipse system. Almost the totality of the clinical studies implementing the *a posteriori* MCO refers to the RayStation system (since it appeared as the first commercial system released for clinical use). Similarly to the knowledge-based planning, different clinical sites were analyzed: prostate [65–69], head and neck [67, 70], brain [65, 71], lung [72], anal spine [73]. In general, the MCO produced comparable or better plans than with the manual planning procedure, in reduced planning time. Most of the studies compare MCO-based and manual plans through DVH metrics, while a few of them reported blinded review of the plans by clinicians.

The number of planning or clinical studies addressing the use of the MCO from the Eclipse system is, in contrast, and at the present time, still limited. Spalding *et al* [74] reported on fast dose calculation for MCO applied to VMAT plans on different anatomical sites. Miguel-Chumacero *et al* [75] published the results by combining the MCO to the knowledge-based planning RapidPlan for the selection of the optimization parameters to improve the trade-off between OAR sparing and target coverage for head and neck planning with VMAT.

A further limitation of the *a posteriori* MCO solution is that the Pareto-optimal plans might be not deliverable as they do not provide adequate constraints for the machine and MLC limitations. As a consequence, the plan chosen for delivery among the Pareto-optimal plans might need a 'finalization' which accounts for all the deliverability requirements. The resulting 'deliverable' plan—after final dose calculation—could more or less remarkably deviate from the selected Pareto-optimal one. In most cases, those differences may be negligible; however, in some cases, this new uncertainty might be more significant than what could be the result of a manual adjustment of the plan. It could compromise the clinical choice made during the navigation [69, 76]. This new kind of uncertainty should be taken into account with the latest planning approaches.

11.6 MCO, *a priori*

The second MCO approach is called *a priori*. This approach requires the computation of a single Pareto-optimal plan instead of the whole front. To allow this, the clinical trade-offs, according to the institutional protocol and strategy, are defined in a 'wish-list', where all the objectives are hierarchically listed together with their priorities and (hard) constraints [61, 77]. The wish-list alone is insufficient to guarantee that the resulting plan has the highest plan quality (i.e. is Pareto-optimal). To achieve this aim, it is necessary to perform an iterative process of minimization according to the priorities in the wish-list until the Pareto-optimal plan with the most favorable trade-offs is to be determined. The goal of the iterative process is to meet all the constraints, but in case of conflicts, the constraints with lower priorities are relaxed, so that those with higher priority are met. Then, starting from the constraints with the highest priorities, all the constraints are made more stringent to reach the Pareto front. This concept does not require any patient-specific adaptation of the wish-list. However, the same wish-list can be improved through an iterative procedure. A small group of patients is planned following an initial wish-list, and the resulting plans are evaluated with the objective of updating the wish-list. This is used for new plans, and again the result is evaluated to estimate any further improvement.

A clinical application of an *a priori* MCO approach has been developed and implemented at the Erasmus MC Cancer Institute in The Netherlands, called Erasmus-iCycle. Currently, it is implemented in the Elekta Monaco planning system. The validation of the Erasmus-iCycle MCO on different anatomical sites:

head and neck [78], lung [79], spinal metastases [80], prostate [81], cervix [82], gastric cancer [83] have been successfully implemented.

Improved plan quality was also associated with a considerable reduction of the treatment time (to the limit toward zero when no human interaction is required). On the Monaco implementation of the *a priori* MCO, there are for example the works of Buschmann *et al* [84] on prostate planning, and Clements *et al* [85] describing the Monaco planning system tools for optimization purposes.

11.7 Plan variability conclusion

All the three modalities discussed in this chapter aimed at reducing the plan variability and can be used as a basis for the automation of the plan optimization procedures. This is an essential step toward the adaptive radiotherapy in providing converging or a unique plan. The planning processes need to be automated, and only the high quality of the resulting plans will give successful adaptive radiotherapy.

Attention has to be also paid to the specific configuration of the planning tools. For example, in the case of the knowledge-based planning, a bad choice of the plan quality, or an adverse selection of the specific objectives to use during the optimization could lead to a poor model due to a suboptimal configuration. The same knowledge-based planning process, using good plans and objectives would result in a good model able to obtain good plans.

Similarly, in the case of the *a posteriori* MCO, the final plan could not reflect the navigation on the Pareto front due to machine limitations not included in the process. Or, again, navigating on the Pareto front, the institutional strategy could be disregarded. With the clinical use of these rather new planning approaches, we have to start considering the uncertainties linked to the new concepts. It is in this frame essential to keep in mind the imperative goal of maximizing the accuracy and the knowledge of the dose delivered to the patients: it is only through this that we can correctly correlate the patient outcomes and improve the radiotherapy treatments.

References

[1] Hussein M, Heijmen B J M, Verellen D and Nisbet A 2018 Automation in intensity modulated radiotherapy planning—a review of recent innovations *Br. J. Radiol.* **91** 20180270

[2] Das I, Bieda M, Cheng C W, Chopra K, Hasson B and Olch A *et al* 2004 Dosimetric comparison of inverse treatment planning system for IMRT: a collaborative study *Med. Phys.* **31** 1750

[3] Das I, Cashon K, Chopra K, Khadivi K, Malhotra H and Mayo C 2005 Intra- and inter-treatment planner dosimetric variation in inverse planning of IMRT *Med. Phys.* **32** 2147

[4] Fogliata A, Nicolini G, Alber M, Asell M, Dobler B and El-Haddad *et al* 2005 IMRT for breast. A planning study *Radiother. Oncol.* **76** 300–10

[5] Wu B, Ricchetti F, Sanguineti G, Kazhdan M, Simari P and Chuang M *et al* 2009 Patient geometry-driven information retrieval for IMRT treatment plan quality control *Med. Phys.* **36** 5497–505

[6] Wu B, Ricchetti F, Sanguineti G, Kazhdan M, Simari P and Jacques R *et al* 2011 Data-driven approach to generating achievable dose-volume histogram objectives in intensity-modulated radiotherapy planning *Int. J. Radiat. Oncol. Biol. Phys.* **79** 1241–7

[7] Petit S F, Wu B, Kazhdan M, Dekker A, Simari P and Kumar R *et al* 2012 Increased organ sparing using shape-based treatment plan optimization for intensity modulated radiation therapy of pancreatic adenocarcinoma *Radiother. Oncol.* **102** 38–44

[8] Wang Y, Zolnay A, Incrocci L, Joosten H, McNutt T, Heijmen B and Petit S 2013 A quality control model that uses PTV-rectal distances to predict the lowest achievable rectum dose, improves IMRT planning for patients with prostate cancer *Radiother. Oncol.* **107** 352–7

[9] Moore K L, Brame R S, Low D A and Mutic S 2011 Experience-based quality control of clinical intensity-modulated radiotherapy planning *Int. J. Radiat. Oncol. Biol. Phys.* **81** 545–51

[10] Appenzoller L M, Michalski J M, Thorstad W L and Mutic S 2012 Predicting dose-volume histograms for organs-at-risk in IMRT planning *Med. Phys.* **39** 7446–61

[11] Chanyavanich V, Das S K, Lee W R and Lo J Y 2011 Knowledge-based IMRT treatment planning for prostate cancer *Med. Phys.* **38** 2515–22

[12] Good D, Lo J, Lee W R, Wu Q J, Yin F F and Das S K 2013 A knowledge-based approach to improving and homogenizing intensity modulated radiation therapy planning quality among treatment centers: an example application to prostate cancer planning *Int. J. Radiat. Oncol. Biol. Phys.* **87** 176–81

[13] Zhu Z, Ge Y, Li T, Thongphiew D, Yin F F and Wu Q J 2011 A planning quality evaluation tool for prostate adaptive IMRT based on machine learning *Med. Phys.* **38** 719–26

[14] Yuan L, Ge Y, Lee W R, Yin F F, Kirkpatrick J P and Wu Q J 2012 Quantitative analysis of the factors which affect the interpatient organ-at-risk dose sparing variation in IMRT plans *Med. Phys.* **39** 6868–78

[15] Shiraishi S and Moore K L 2016 Knowledge based prediction of three-dimensional dose distributions for external beam radiotherapy *Med. Phys.* **43** 378–87

[16] Liu J, Wu Q J, Kirkpatrick J P, Yin F-F, Yuan L and Ge Y 2015 From active shape model to active optical flow model: a shape-based approach to predicting voxel-level dose distributions in spine SBRT *Phys. Med. Biol.* **60** N83–92

[17] McIntosh C and Purdie T G 2017 Voxel-based dose prediction with multi-patient atlas selection for automated radiotherapy treatment planning *Phys. Med. Biol.* **62** 415–31

[18] McIntosh C, Welch M, McNiven A, Jaffray D A and Purdie T G 2017 Fully automated treatment planning for head and neck radiotherapy using a voxel-based dose prediction and dose mimicking method *Phys. Med. Biol.* **62** 5926–44

[19] Tol J P, Delaney A R, Dahele M, Slotman B J and Verbakel W F A R 2015 Evaluation of a knowledge-based planning solution for head and neck cancer *Int. J. Radiat. Oncol. Biol. Phys.* **91** 612–20

[20] Chang A R Y, Hung A W M, Cheung F W K, Lee M C H, Chan O S H and Philips H *et al* 2016 Comparison of planning quality and efficiency between conventional and knowledge-based algorithms in nasopharyngeal cancer patients using intensity modulated radiation therapy *Int. J. Radiat. Oncol. Biol. Phys.* **95** 981–90

[21] Fogliata A, Reggiori G, Stravato A, Lobefalo F, Franzese C and Franceschini D *et al* 2017 RapidPlan head and neck model: the objectives and possible clinical benefit *Radiat. Oncol.* **12** 73

[22] Fogliata A, Nicolini G, Clivio A, Vanetti E, Laksar S and Tozzi A *et al* 2015 A broad scope knowledge based model for optimization of VMAT in esophageal cancer: validation and assessment of plan quality among different centers *Radiat. Oncol.* **10** 220

[23] Fogliata A, Belosi F, Clivio A, Navarria P, Nicolini G and Scorsetti M *et al* 2014 On the pre-clinical validation of a commercial model-based optimisation engine: application to volumetric modulated arc therapy for patients with lung or prostate cancer *Radiother. Oncol.* **113** 385–91

[24] Snyder K C, Kim J, Reding A, Fraser C, Gordon J and Ajlouni M *et al* 2016 Development and evaluation of a clinical model for lung cancer patients using stereotactic body radiotherapy (SBRT) within a knowledge-based algorithm for treatment planning *J. Appl. Clin. Med. Phys.* **17** 263–75
[25] Fogliata A, Nicolini G, Bourgier C, Clivio A, De Rose F and Fenoglietto P *et al* 2015 Performance of a knowledge-based model for optimization of volumetric modulated arc therapy plans for single and bilateral breast irradiation *PLoS One* **10** e0145137
[26] Fogliata A, Wang P M, Belosi F, Clivio A, Nicolini G, Vanetti E and Cozzi L 2014 Assessment of a model based optimization engine for volumetric modulated arc therapy for patients with advanced hepatocellular cancer *Radiat. Oncol.* **9** 236
[27] Yu G, Li Y, Feng Z, Tao C, Yu Z, Li B and Li D 2018 Knowledge-based IMRT planning for individual liver cancer patients using a novel specific model *Radiat. Oncol.* **13** 52
[28] Hussein M, South C P, Barry M A, Adams E J, Jordan T J, Stewart A J and Nisbet A 2016 Clinical validation and benchmarking of knowledge-based IMRT and VMAT treatment planning in pelvic anatomy *Radiother. Oncol.* **120** 473–9
[29] Wu H, Jiang F, Yue H, Li S and Zhang Y 2016 A dosimetric evaluation of knowledge-based VMAT planning with simultaneous integrated boosting for rectal cancer patients *J. Appl. Clin. Med. Phys.* **17** 78–85
[30] Panettieri V, Ball D, Chapman A, Cristofaro N, Gawthrop J and Griffin P *et al* 2019 Development of a multicentre automated model to reduce planning variability in radiotherapy of prostate cancer *Phys. Imag. Rad. Onc.* **11** 34–40
[31] Castriconi R, Fiorino C, Broggi S, Cozzarini C, Di Muzio N, Calandrino R and Cattaneo G M 2019 Comprehensive intra-institution stepping validation of knowledge-based models for automatic plan optimization *Phys. Med.* **57** 231–7
[32] Wu H, Jiang F, Yue H, Zhang H, Wang K and Zhang Y 2016 Applying a RapidPlan model trained on a technique and orientation to another: a feasibility and dosimetric evaluation *Radiat. Oncol.* **11** 108
[33] Cagni E, Botti A, Micera R, Galeandro M, Sghedoni R and Orlandi M *et al* 2017 Knowledge-based treatment planning: an inter-technique and inter-system feasibility study for prostate cancer *Phys. Med.* **36** 38–45
[34] Li N, Carmona R, Sirak I, Kasaova, Followill D and Michalski J *et al* 2017 Highly efficient training, refinement, and validation of a knowledge-based planning quality-control system for radiation therapy clinical trials *Int. J. Radiat. Oncol. Biol. Phys.* **97** 164–72
[35] Fogliata A, Cozzi L, Reggiori G, Stravato A, Lobefalo F and Franzese C *et al* 2019 RapidPlan knowledge based planning: iterative learning process and model ability to steer planning strategies *Radiat. Oncol.* **14** 187
[36] Wilkens J J, Alaly J R, Zakarian K, Thorstad W L and Deasy J O 2007 IMRT treatment planning based on prioritizing prescription goals *Phys. Med. Biol.* **52** 1675–92
[37] Zhang X, Li X, Quan E M, Pan X and Li Y 2011 A methodology for automatic intensity modulated radiation treatment planning for lung cancer *Phys. Med. Biol.* **56** 3873–93
[38] Purdie T G, Dinniwell R E, Fyles A and Sharpe M B 2014 Automation and intensity modulated radiation therapy for individualized high-quality tangent breast treatment plans *Int. J. Radiat. Oncol. Biol. Phys.* **90** 688–95
[39] Xhaferllari I, Wong E, Bzdusek K, Lock M and Chen J 2013 Automated IMRT planning with regional optimization using planning scripts *J. Appl. Clin. Med. Phys.* **14** 176–91

[40] Boylan C and Rowbottom C 2014 A bias-free, automated planning tool for technique comparison in radiotherapy—application to nasopharyngeal carcinoma treatments *J. Appl. Clin. Med. Phys.* **15** 213–25

[41] Song Y, Wang Q, Jiang X, Liu S, Zhang Y and Bai S 2016 Fully automatic volumetric modulated arc therapy plan generation for rectal cancer *Radiother. Oncol.* **119** 531–6

[42] Speer S, Klein A, Kober L, Weiss A, Yohannes I and Bert C 2017 Automation of radiation treatment planning: evaluation of head and neck cancer patient plans created by the Pinnacle^3 scripting and Auto-Planning functions *Strahlenther. Onkol.* **193** 656–65

[43] Winkel D, Bol G H, van Asselen B, Hes J, Scholten V and Kerkmeijer L G W *et al* 2016 Development and clinical introduction of automated radiotherapy treatment planning for prostate cancer *Phys. Med. Biol.* **61** 8587–95

[44] Tol J P, Dahele M, Peltola J, Nord J, Slotman B J and Verbakel W F A R 2015 Automatic interactive optimization for volumetric modulated arc therapy planning *Radiat. Oncol.* **10** 75

[45] Hazell I, Bzdusek K, Kumar P, Hansen C R, Bertelsen A and Eriksen J G *et al* 2016 Automatic planning of head and neck treatment plans *J. Appl. Clin. Med. Phys.* **17** 272–82

[46] Hansen C R, Bertelsen A, Hazell I, Zukauskaite R, Gyldenkerne N and Johansen J *et al* 2016 Automatic treatment planning improves the clinical quality of head and neck cancer treatment plans *Clin. Transl. Radiat. Oncol.* **1** 2–8

[47] Gintz D, Latifi K, Caudell J, Nelms B, Zhang G and Moros E *et al* 2016 Initial evaluation of automated treatment planning software *J. Appl. Clin. Med. Phys.* **17** 331–46

[48] Kusters J M A M, Bzdusek K, Kumar P, van Kollenburg P G M, Kunze-Busch M C and Wendling M *et al* 2017 Automated IMRT planning in Pinnacle *Strahlenther. Onkol.* **193** 1031–8

[49] Li X, Wang L, Wang J, Han X, Xia B and Wu S *et al* 2017 Dosimetric benefits of automation in the treatment of lower thoracic esophageal cancer: is manual planning still an alternative option? *Med. Dosim.* **42** 289–95

[50] Hansen C R, Nielsen M, Bertelsen A S, Hazell I, Holtved E and Zukauskaite R *et al* 2017 Automatic treatment planning facilitates fast generation of high-quality treatment plans for esophageal cancer *Acta Oncol.* **56** 1495–500

[51] Clemente S, Oliviero C, Palma G, D'Avino V, Liuzzi R and Conson M *et al* 2018 Auto-versus human-driven plan in mediastinal Hodgkin lymphoma radiation treatment *Radiat. Oncol.* **13** 202

[52] Nawa K, Haga A, Nomoto A, Sarmiento R A, Shiraishi K and Yamashita H *et al* 2017 Evaluation of a commercial automatic treatment planning system for prostate cancers *Med. Dosim.* **42** 203–9

[53] Krayenbuehl J, Di Martino M, Guckenberger M and Andratschke N 2017 Improved plan quality with automated radiotherapy planning for whole brain with hippocampus sparing: a comparison to the RTOG 0933 trial *Radiat. Oncol.* **12** 1–7

[54] Yan H, Yin F-F, Guan H and Kim J H 2003 Fuzzy logic guided inverse treatment planning *Med. Phys.* **30** 2675–85

[55] Yan H, Yin F-F, Guan H-q and Kim J H 2003 AI-guided parameter optimization in inverse treatment planning *Phys. Med. Biol.* **48** 3565–80

[56] Yan H, Yin F-F and Willett C 2007 Evaluation of an artificial intelligence guided inverse planning system: clinical case study *Radiother. Oncol.* **83** 76–85

[57] Stieler F, Yan H, Lohr F, Wenz F and Yin F-F 2009 Development of a neuro-fuzzy technique for automated parameter optimization of inverse treatment planning *Radiat. Oncol.* **4** 39

[58] Lahanas M, Schreibmann E and Baltas D 2003 Multiobjective inverse planning for intensity modulated radiotherapy with constraint-free gradient-based optimization algorithms *Phys. Med. Biol.* **48** 2843–71
[59] Monz M, Küfer K H, Bortfeld T R and Thieke C 2008 Pareto navigation—algorithmic foundation of interactive multi-criteria IMRT planning *Phys. Med. Biol.* **53** 985–98
[60] Thieke C, Küfer K-H, Monz M, Scherrer A, Alonso F and Oelfke U *et al* 2007 A new concept for interactive radiotherapy planning with multicriteria optimization: first clinical evaluation *Radiother. Oncol.* **85** 292–8
[61] Breedveld S, Storchi P R M, Keijzer M, Heemink A W and Heijmen B J M 2007 A novel approach to multi-criteria inverse planning for IMRT *Phys. Med. Biol.* **52** 6339–53
[62] Serna J I, Monz M, Küfer K H and Thieke C 2009 Trade-off bounds for the Pareto surface approximation in multi-criteria IMRT planning *Phys. Med. Biol.* **54** 6299–311
[63] Teichert K, Süss P, Serna J I, Monz M, Küfer K H and Thieke C 2011 Comparative analysis of Pareto surfaces in multi-criteria IMRT planning *Phys. Med. Biol.* **56** 3669–84
[64] Craft D and Bortfeld T 2008 How many plans are needed in an IMRT multi-objective plan database? *Phys. Med. Biol.* **53** 2785–96
[65] Müller B S, Shih H A, Efstathiou J A, Bortfeld T and Craft D 2017 Multicriteria plan optimization in the hands of physicians: a pilot study in prostate cancer and brain tumors *Radiat. Oncol.* **12** 168
[66] Wala J, Craft D, Paly J, Zietman A and Efstathiou J 2013 Maximizing dosimetric benefits of IMRT in the treatment of localized prostate cancer through multicriteria optimization planning *Med. Dosim.* **38** 298–303
[67] Chen H, Craft D L and Gierga D P 2014 Multicriteria optimization informed VMAT planning *Med. Dosim.* **39** 64–73
[68] Ghandour S, Matzinger O and Pachoud M 2015 Volumetric-modulated arc therapy planning using multicriteria optimization for localized prostate cancer *J. Appl. Clin. Med. Phys.* **16** 258–69
[69] McGarry C K, Bokrantz R, O'Sullivan J M and Hounsell A R 2014 Advantages and limitations of navigation-based multicriteria optimization (MCO) for localized prostate cancer IMRT planning *Med. Dosim.* **39** 205–11
[70] Kierkels R G J, Visser R, Bijl H P, Langendijk J A, van 't Veld A A and Steenbakkers R J H M *et al* 2015 Multicriteria optimization enables less experienced planners to efficiently produce high quality treatment plans in head and neck cancer radiotherapy *Radiat. Oncol.* **10** 87
[71] Zieminzki S, Khandekar M and Wang Y 2018 Assessment of multi-criteria optimization (MCO) for volumetric modulated arc therapy (VMAT) in hippocampal avoidance whole brain radiation therapy (HA-WBRT) *J. Appl. Clin. Med. Phys.* **19** 184–90
[72] Kamran S C, Mueller B S, Paetzold P, Dunlap J, Niemierko A and Bortfeld T *et al* 2016 Multicriteria optimization achieves superior normal tissue sparing in a planning study of intensity-modulated radiation therapy for RTOG 1308-eligible non-small cell lung cancer patients *Radiother. Oncol.* **118** 515–20
[73] Rønde H S, Wee L, Pløen J and Appelt A L 2017 Feasibility of preference-driven radiotherapy dose treatment planning to support shared decision making in anal cancer *Acta Oncol.* **56** 1277–85
[74] Spalding M, Walsh A, Clarke H and Aland T 2020 Evaluation of a new hybrid VMAT-IMRT multi-criteria optimization plan generation algorithm *Med. Dosim.* **45** 41–5

[75] Miguel-Chumacero E, Currie G, Johnston A and Currie S 2018 Effectiveness of multi-criteria optimization-based trade-off exploration in combination with RapidPlan for head & neck radiotherapy planning *Radiat. Oncol.* **13** 229

[76] Kyroudi A, Petersson K, Ghandour S, Pachoud M, Matzinger O and Ozsahin M *et al* 2016 Discrepancies between selected Pareto optimal plans and final deliverable plans in radiotherapy multi-criteria optimization *Radiother. Oncol.* **120** 346–8

[77] Breedveld S, Storchi P R M, Voet P W J and Heijmen B J M 2012 iCycle: integrated, multicriterial beam angle, and profile optimization for generation of coplanar and non-coplanar IMRT plans *Med. Phys.* **39** 951–63

[78] Voet P W J, Dirkx M L P, Breedveld S, Fransen D, Levendag P C and Heijmen B J M 2013 Toward fully automated multicriterial plan generation: a prospective clinical study *Int. J. Radiat. Oncol. Biol. Phys.* **85** 866872

[79] Della Gala G, Dirkx M L P, Hoekstra N, Fransen D, Lanconelli N and van de Pol M *et al* 2017 Fully automated VMAT treatment planning for advanced-stage NSCLC patients *Strahlenther. Onkol.* **193** 402409

[80] Buergy D, Sharfo A W M, Heijmen B J M, Voet P W J, Breedveld S and Wenz F *et al* 2017 Fully automated treatment planning of spinal metastases—A comparison to manual planning of Volumetric Modulated Arc Therapy for conventionally fractionated irradiation *Radiat. Oncol.* **12** 33

[81] Voet P W J, Dirkx M L P, Breedveld S, Al-Mamgani A, Incrocci L and Heijmen B J M 2014 Fully automated volumetric modulated arc therapy plan generation for prostate cancer patients *Int. J. Radiat. Oncol. Biol. Phys.* **88** 1175–9

[82] Sharfo A W M, Breedveld S, Voet P W J, Heijkoop S T, Mens J-W M and Hoogeman M S *et al* 2016 Validation of fully automated VMAT plan generation for library-based plan-of-the-day cervical cancer radiotherapy *PLoS One* **11** e0169202

[83] Sharfo A W M, Stieler F, Kupfer O, Heijmen B J M, Dirkx M L P and Breedveld S *et al* 2018 Automated VMAT planning for postoperative adjuvant treatment of advanced gastric cancer *Radiat. Oncol.* **13** 74

[84] Buschmann M, Sharfo A W M, Penninkhof J, Seppenwoolde Y, Goldner G and Georg D *et al* 2018 Automated volumetric modulated arc therapy planning for whole pelvic prostate radiotherapy *Strahlenther. Onkol.* **194** 333–42

[85] Clements M, Schupp N, Tattersall M, Brown A and Larson R 2018 Monaco treatment planning system tools and optimization processes *Med. Dosim.* **43** 106–17

Chapter 12

Quality assurance and verification

There are two main types of treatment errors: human and machine. Human errors are due to negligence, ignorance, lack of training, and fatigue that could be minimized. Machines in general cannot make errors unless there is a problem with their software or if their execution of a plan happens in the wrong sequence. Such was the case of the Therac-25 incidence in Tyler, Texas which killed eight patients [1]. There are many other radiation incidences in every country that impact patient safety [2, 3]. As such, ASTRO decided to tackle this issue in a special publication [4]. IMRT/VMAT is very complex process and any error or mistake has huge consequences for a patient. Modern treatments are all computer-controlled with minimal input from the user. However, certain signs and warnings on the control panel cannot be ignored. Such a case was associated with an incident in New York where several patients lost their lives; this was described in detail by Bogdanich [5, 6]. In this incident, the MLC leaves did not go to their programmed position; rather, the machine opened the jaw to the widest position. As mentioned before, IMRT delivers nearly 3–5 times Monitor Unit (MU), so the patient received 5 times the radiation to a wide area exposed by the open jaws. In IMRT, a very small fraction of MU is normally delivered in the subfields. This incident created the international caution that each IMRT field must be visually verified before treatment. Such a process is counterproductive with reduced throughput. The compromise of inspecting each treatment field/subfield was challenging, so vendors stepped in to provide an extra safety net in the software so that an incident like the one in New York would not happen again.

After the radiation incident that happened in New York and was widely reported by the New York Times, most radiation societies, including ACR, ASTRO and AAPM, recommended that all modulated treatment plans must be independently verified [7, 8]. The importance of the measurement process for IMRT QA has been debated by physicists, as some of them do not feel that is it necessary for each plan to be checked. However, currently verifying the treatment plan with measurements is

doi:10.1088/978-0-7503-1335-3ch12

still continuing in some form. Other issues that are often debated include whether the measurement process is superior to other methods [9–11]. It is not the intent of this chapter to debate one method versus another but instead to provide guidelines as to how one can implement measurement or any other methods to verify their IMRT plans before patient treatment.

The need for verification and the regulatory issues associated with the incidents created extra work for medical physicists; thus, IMRT pretreatment quality assurance was introduced. By an insurance or regulatory mandate, each treatment should be verified by the patient-specific quality assurance (PSQA) that has become the standard of care. An AAPM task group, TG-218 [12], was formed to evaluate the PSQA issues and more importantly to provide guidance on the limit of accuracy that should be followed in IMRT.

The IMRT QA process in some form is universally adopted. The QA is not performed on patients to verify the dose, unlike TLD, Diode, IVD devices in 3D; rather, a pseudo-approach is adapted. Once the patient plan is evaluated and approved by a physician, the 3D dose matrix is transferred to a phantom. Without optimization, the dose calculation is performed (forward dose) at a fine resolution with the same gantry, beamlets, and MU. The phantom data is then sent with the beam parameters to a record and verify system in the same way that the patient's data is sent for the treatment. Often, a detector (a small volume) at the isocenter is placed along with a 2D detector (a film) at a given plane (1–2.5 cm away from detector). Later, the film and ion chamber measurements are replaced with electronic devices; this will be discussed in further detail later in this chapter. The treatment is then performed for the phantom with a given MU and the rest of the IMRT parameters that have been imported. The film or detector results of the phantom measurements are reflective of patient dosimetry (indirectly), which is compared with the calculated data in the same plane with that of the detector.

In general, IMRT QA does not provide an assurance of the plan quality or safety of the treatment [13–15], but there are no other alternatives but to check the minimum requirements. The question then is how to verify IMRT plans that vary from institution to institution? In general, one can divide this process into four broad categories as below:

1. In Silico (second calculation);
2. Measurement-based;
3. Machine log-file;
4. Artificial intelligence.

12.1 Theory of comparison

12.1.1 Statistical analysis

The simplest approach for comparing two sets of independent data is by statistical analysis, which calculates the mean or average of the data points to give a central value. The spread is computed in terms of the standard deviation (SD), which is the distance from the mean. Another quantity, standard error (SE) of the mean provides additional information on two samples for similarity. The average values should be the same and the SD should be minimal, i.e., the spread is narrow or minimum. One can further evaluate this in terms of the interquartile range for a meaningful comparison. Other tools such as the range (maximum–minimum) also provide the spread of the data. Additionally, one can use a *t*-test based on the average and SD; this will provide a unique number that differentiates the two data sets and a *p*-value that gives the statistical significance if the data is similar or not. These analyses are mainly used for 2D data and have limited application in our dosimetric comparison.

12.1.2 Dice Similarity Coefficient (DSC)

Dice similarity coefficient (DSC) is a modern approach to compare large sets of data, especially comparing imaging features or in artificial intelligence training data to compare the resultant data. DSC is mainly computed using high-level software like Python or Matlab. Image comparisons are now performed using DSC with the help of ITK software too. The theory behind DSC was originally developed by Dice [16] and later modified by Sørensen [17] to evaluate the similarity in two population systems. If X and Y are two discrete data sets and $|X|$ and $|Y|$ are their respective cardinalities data, then DSC is defined as:

$$\mathrm{DSC} = 2\frac{\lfloor X \rfloor \cap \lfloor Y \rfloor}{\lfloor X \rfloor + \lfloor Y \rfloor} \tag{12.1}$$

This equation can be written for a Boolean data type using the definition of true positive (TP), false positive (FP), and false negative (FN) as is done in a receiver operating characteristic (ROC) curve:

$$\mathrm{DSC} = \frac{2\mathrm{TP}}{(2\mathrm{TP} + \mathrm{FP} + \mathrm{FN})} \tag{12.2}$$

Along with the Dice–Sorenson coefficient, there are additional tools such as the Jaccard Coefficient (JC) and the Cosine Coefficient (CC), which are defined as below, and are used in many imaging and AI applications.

$$\mathrm{JC} = \frac{\lfloor X \rfloor \cap \lfloor Y \rfloor}{\lfloor X \rfloor \cup \lfloor Y \rfloor} = \frac{\lfloor X \rfloor \cap \lfloor Y \rfloor}{\lfloor X \rfloor + \lfloor Y \rfloor - \lfloor X \rfloor \cap \lfloor Y \rfloor} \tag{12.3}$$

$$\mathrm{CC} = \frac{X \cdot Y}{\lfloor X \rfloor \cdot \lfloor Y \rfloor} \tag{12.4}$$

In IMRT/VMAT, the two sets of data are the 3D TPS calculated data and the derived or measured data. There is no effort to use the above applications in the IMRT QA. To make a comparison, not only the magnitude of the data but also its position needs to be verified, which is discussed in the following section.

12.1.3 Gamma index

The most common practice in comparing two sets of data is to look at their pattern in 2D or 3D. The concept of distance to agreement (DTA) was originated by

Van Dyk *et al* [18] in the context of TPS quality assurance. The DTA provided a distance (x) where the reference or measured dose (D_m) and calculated dose (D_c) data points have same value. Mathematically, it can be written as:

$$X \rightarrow \text{DTA} \quad \text{when } D_m - D_c = \Delta D \approx 0 \tag{12.5}$$

The dose difference ΔD has a practical value for an acceptance, usually 3% or 5%, which is treated as close to zero. Generally, the criteria of ΔD as 3% and DTA as 2 mm are acceptable. The DTA concept was later expanded upon by Low *et al* [19] who provided the concept of a gamma index option for the difficult task of comparing calculated and measured dose matrices in 3D (figure 12.1). Additionally, this concept was applied to clinical cases and shown to be satisfactory when the criterion of 5% 3 mm DTA was applied due to noise in the gamma index [20].

12.2 Silico method

Silico is a phrase used to denote 'performed on computer or via computer simulation.' In this process, the IMRT treatment plan is sent to a different computer system or different methodology for a comparison of the results. This ensures that the algorithm used in treatment planning produces an accurate dose calculation. The two plans are then compared in terms of MU, dose, and distribution. In this methodology, the QA is performed on a different machine than the one that is treating the patient. Some purists will negate this approach as it does not verify that the plan is deliverable on the actual treatment machine, which is one of the checks that should be performed especially to verify if the MLC travel is smooth in the planned IMRT gantry angles.

The Silico approach has been used in many institutions that feel comfortable with PSQA. Various research has been reported with a multi-center approach and indicated in many diseases for a successful outcome. These approaches include an

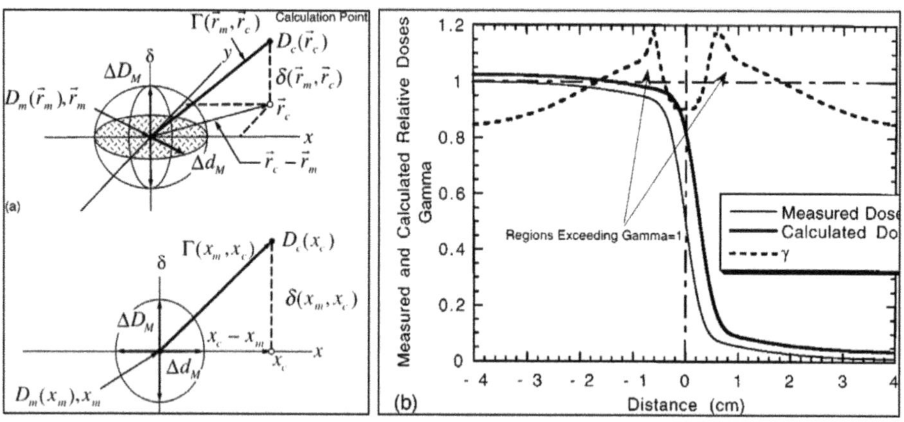

Figure 12.1. Concept of gamma index and distance to agreement (DTA); (a) top panel 2D and lower 1D representation of dose difference and DTA and (b) evaluation of profiles of measured and calculated dose and respective gamma index. Adapted with permission from Low *et al* [19] John Wiley & Sons. Copyright 1998 American Association of Physicists in Medicine.

in-house treatment planning system, the Monte Carlo simulation, a machine log-file, and radiomics features [21–27]. This methodology certainly requires a different high-order skill that most clinical physicists will not feel comfortable to adopt or will not have the tools to verify the QA themselves. Kry *et al* [28] showed that an independent recalculation method is superior in detecting errors in the IMRT process compared to measurements using the EPID, MapCheck, and Mobius log files. In any case, clinical physicists would find that the simplest approach is to measure the PSQA using various devices; this is discussed below.

12.3 Measurements

Miften *et al* [12] provided a comprehensive comparison of devices and their roles in the IMRT QA process. Every radiation detector vendor has stepped on this process for verification by providing measurement-related QA devices, which will be discussed in a later section. In this section, a broad category of measuring devices is presented but this is not an exhaustive list. Among all of these QA methods, Esposito *et al* [29] showed that only a few are sensitive enough for SBRT QA.

There are many approaches to IMRT QA, and a wide range of literature has been published on every aspect of IMRT validation. In the beginning of IMRT QA, most institutions relied on single-point measurements using an ion chamber as the gold standard. The data from Dong *et al* [30] showed the initial approach and what we can expect in various disease sites. Agreement within 3.5% was obtained in 97% of 751 cases, representing nine different treatment sites. Figure 12.2 summarizes the MD Anderson Cancer Center, Houston, data for each disease site, indicating a relatively good agreement with the measurements despite the rather large standard deviation (±3%). For the pediatric cases, the dose deviation is 3% with +4% standard deviation, which is even larger compared to other diseases.

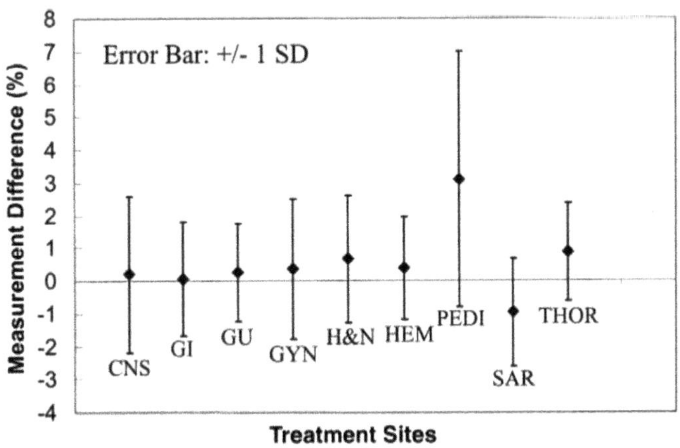

Figure 12.2. Comparison of point dose measurement and calculation in nine different treatment sites for a total of 751 cases using a special water tank fitted with an ion chamber. Results are summarized for each disease site. Adopted from Dong *et al* [30] with permission from Elsevier.

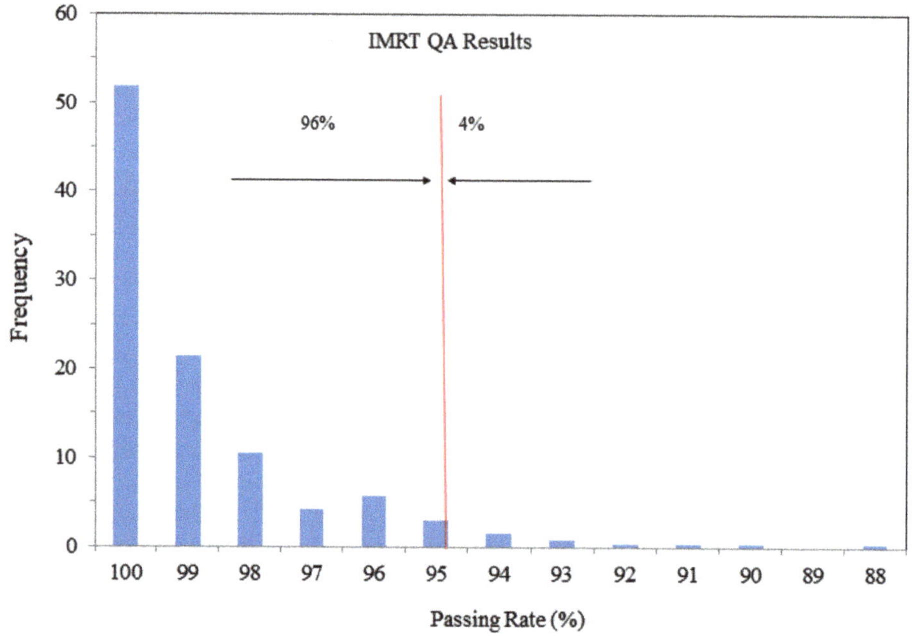

Figure 12.3. Frequency distribution of a typical PSQA passing rate in a typical clinic. This data is from 800 cases analyzed from the author's institution.

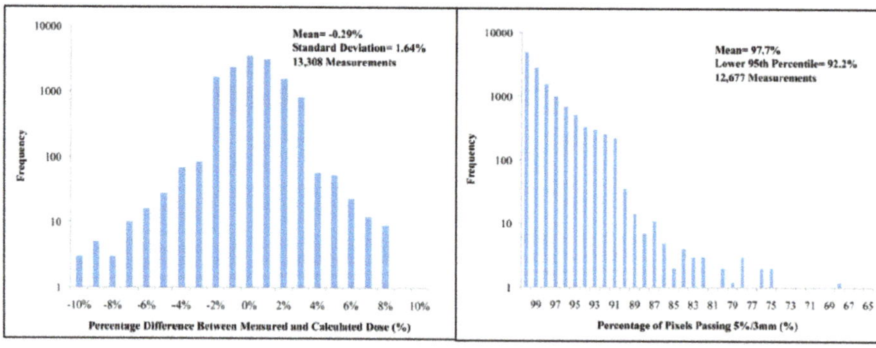

Figure 12.4. Analysis of IMRT measured QA data of over 13 000 patients. Adapted from Pulliam *et al* [31] copyright 2014 the authors. Open access CC BY 3.0.

Figure 12.3 provides a typical passing rate of IMRT QA for 95% of the cases. This can be increased if the passing criterion can be increased to 90% for 3% and 3 mm DTA. In very complex and highly modulated beams such as those used in head and neck cancer, the criterion for 5% and 5 mm DTA has also been used. The arbitrary change in the passing criterion from 5% to 10% and in the gamma index and DTA from 3% to 5% and 3 mm to 5 mm, respectively, is not uncommon [20].

An analysis of over 13 000 patients over a six year period from MD Anderson Cancer Center, Houston, was presented by Pulliam *et al* [31], as shown in figure 12.4. It provided the complexity of IMRT QA and its passing rate. A typical failure rate, as shown in figure 12.3, is observed by Pulliam *et al* too. The data spread is up to ±10%, which is typically adapted in a clinical practice. The other panel in figure 12.4 shows the frequency distribution indicating the 5%/3 mm criterion with a mean of 97.7% and a 95th percentile of 92.2%. There were a few cases where the differences were extremely large. It was pointed out that with iterative processes (repeated measurements or planning), the passing rate can be improved. Basran and Woo [32] provided the Canadian experience in terms of IMRT acceptability. It was shown that for non-head and neck cancer 3% and 3 mm can easily be achieved in 90% of the cases; however, for head and neck, this criteria will be only possible for 88% of the cases. The TG-218 [12] has provided guidelines for the gamma passing rate; the universal acceptance limit is the 95% passing criterion 3%/2 mm with a 10% threshold and an action plan when it is ⩾ 90% 3%/2 mm with a 10% threshold.

Eventually, it was realized that point dose was not adequate and volumetric analysis was needed. In this context, the IMRT community immediately adapted film measurement even though using it has many difficulties including energy dependence, film processing, linearity, and the dose range of films [33, 34]. In the beginning, dose measurements were performed with mainly Kodak XV radiographic films in combination with various phantoms. Ion chambers were used in combination with films for simultaneously measuring absolute dose and dose distribution. Due to the larger MU needed, there was evolution in film development. An extended dose range (EDR) film was introduced [35–38] that provided a good dose range and immediately became a successful device for IMRT QA. As mentioned before, there were many problems with film and latent imaging; as such, timing was critical when instantaneous results were needed. Additionally, single-point measurements were not suitable, as they needed to provide confidence that MLC leaves were working properly with the correct dose distribution.

Industry came to our help and developed many types of planar dose measurement devices. The first such device was made by Sun Nuclear (FL) who made MapCheck using the uniquely patented diodes that they specialized in. This device became an instantaneous success as it could provide direct results in terms of composite fields or for a field-by-field dose approach.

Imaging and Radiation Oncology Core (IROC), Houston, provided an outreach phantom study based on the individual measurements of a single head and neck phantom [15]. It was found that with even the relatively large criteria (7% and 4 mm DTA), only 77% intuitions were able to pass. Surprisingly, the dosimetric variability was very large. Measurement-based QA is not able to detect various types of error as noted by Nelm *et al* [13]. It was found that the gamma passing rate did not indicate the passing criterion of an IMRT clinical setting. On a similar note, Kry *et al* [14] also concluded that IMRT QA does not predict unacceptable plan delivery. Comparative studies have been conducted for nearly all electronic PSQA devices, including PTW, SunNuclear, IBA, and Delta4 [39–41].

There are various other devices in different countries such as IQM that have been compared with traditional devices [42–44]. It is the user's preference to select a device that meets the ease of operation and comfort in data collection in their respective place of work. The following sections are in no way any endorsement, rather an example of the measurement process in IMRT QA.

12.3.1 Film dosimetry

As mentioned above, historically film was a suitable medium for the comprehensive evaluation of an IMRT plan. It included radiographic and radiochromic films [45]. Radiochromic films became popular as they did not need film processing, which had been quickly disappearing from hospitals, and they had a higher dose range. The details of the evolution of radiochromic films can be found in the reference [45]. Films were placed in a phantom and exposed with the IMRT plans of either individual beams or combined beams in a single gantry angle. The latter option was more convenient as it saved time in the PSQA process. Various types of software were developed for image analysis in terms of 2D dose distributions. Figure 12.5 provides images and analysis of the dose distributions.

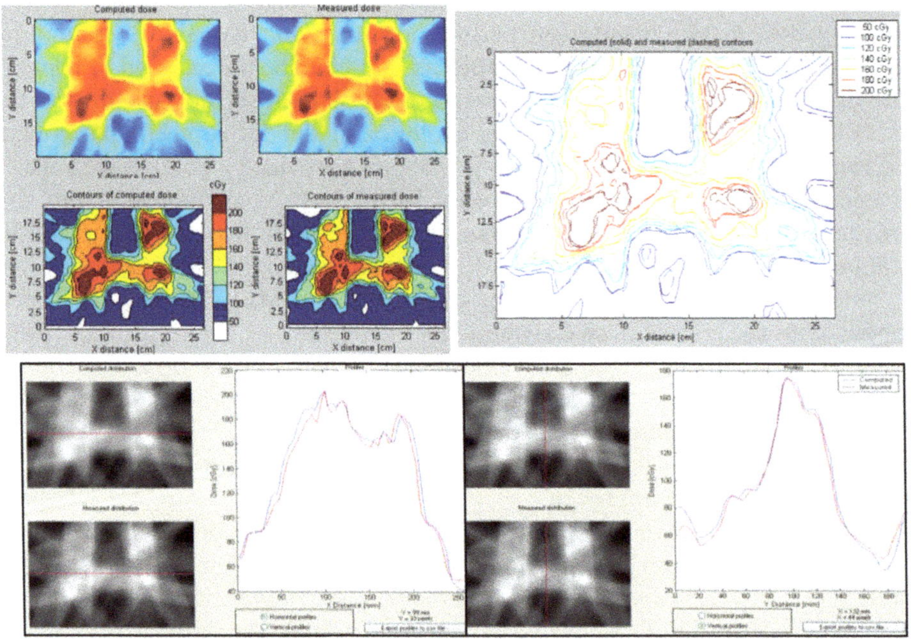

Figure 12.5. Film analysis of a prostate cancer IMRT QA showing various representations of color-wash data of computed and measured dose distributions on a selected plane (usually the isocenter). Visual display of dose difference and line graphs are also shown in x and y directions.

12.3.2 Sun nuclear map check

Electronic devices were needed so that instantaneous dose display and analysis could be performed unlike with film. Vendors stepped in to provide electronic IMRT QA devices with various unique features.

The MapCheck device was introduced by the Sun Nuclear Corporation and has evolved from MapCheck 1 to 3, but essentially, the fundamental features remain the same. It is a 2D detector array intended to measure a radiation dose distribution. The array has 1527 diode detectors embedded in a polymethyl methacrylate (PMMA) phantom with a detector spacing of 7.07 mm in an array size of 32 cm × 26 cm. Additionally, the software provides the interpolated data in mm resolution. Figure 12.6 provides an image of MapCheck 2. This device is extremely simple, easy to set, and collects data quickly via an RS232 cable, which is used for most daily QA devices in radiation oncology. The diode detectors are a unique proprietary feature of Sun Nuclear and are used in many of their other devices. These are also radio-resistance and have minimal directional dependence.

The data analysis is performed using the MapCheck software. The calculated dose distribution in DICOM format is transferred to software that compares it with the collected (measured) dose distribution. It provides a quick analysis of the collected data based on the gamma index and DTA, which is shown in figure 12.6 and in various references [32, 46–49]. There are many options for the displays of the analysis, either in the form of histograms or other graphical representations, based on the user's selection. Finally, it provides the % dose difference and DTA in mm for quick review and sign off. In case of QA failures, individual fields can be analyzed. Based on this technology, Sun Nuclear also introduced another successful device ArcCheck, which is used for VMAT verification [42, 50, 51]. Instead of having diodes on a planer device, the detectors are arranged on a cylindrical phantom.

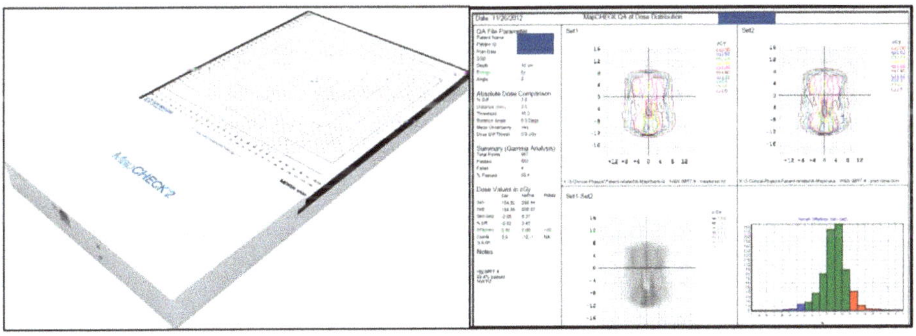

Figure 12.6. Picture of MapCheck 2 device for IMRT QA (https://www.sunnuclear.com/) Image provided courtesy of Sun Nuclear Corporation. Also shown is a typical display of IMRT QA indicating the dose distributions of Set 1 and Set 2 representing calculated and measured dose distribution. The bottom panel shows the dose difference, dose-histogram analysis at various dose bins. The left side of the display shows the actual analysis indicating gamma index, DTA and % passing rate for quick review and sign off.

12.3.3 IBA MatriXX

For the purists who would like to have an ion chamber-based device for PSQA, the IBA MatriXX is such a device for them. It has an array of ion chambers placed in a solid phantom. It consists of 1020 vented parallel plate ion chambers arranged in

32 × 32 cm grid except for the four in the corner positions. The active measurement area is 24.4 × 24 cm^2. The ion chamber specifications are 4.5 mm in diameter and 5 mm in height with the chamber volume of 18 mm^3. The distance between detectors is 7.62 mm from center-to center. It operates at 500 ± 30 V with a sensitivity of 2.4 nC/Gy. It provides dose linearity within 1% in the range of 0.02–12 Gy. The ion chambers are embedded at a depth of 3 mm in solid Tecaran with a density of 1.06 g cm^{-3}. Hence, this provides a 3.1 mm thickness on the top of the detector that needs to be accounted for in depth. The MatriXX device is used in various applications including proton beam therapy [52, 53] and in IMRT QA [41] in the dose range of 0.02–12 Gy min^{-1}. For the FFF beams, this device has been slightly modified to provide data up to 48 Gy min^{-1}.

The device comes with associated software (OmniPro ImRT) for PSQA data analysis in terms of gamma index and DTA based on a planner measurement. Since it is an ion chamber-based device, it requires temperature and pressure correction at each measurement. With proper calibration, the device can provide absolute dose and dose distribution. Figure 12.7 shows the device and its associated display as well as its analysis of gamma and DTA. A detailed comparison of this device with other devices is presented by Chandraraj *et al* [41]. IBA is no longer developing software associated with OmniPro rather all development related to patient QA is performed in myQA Patients software. A display is shown in figure 12.7 right panel.

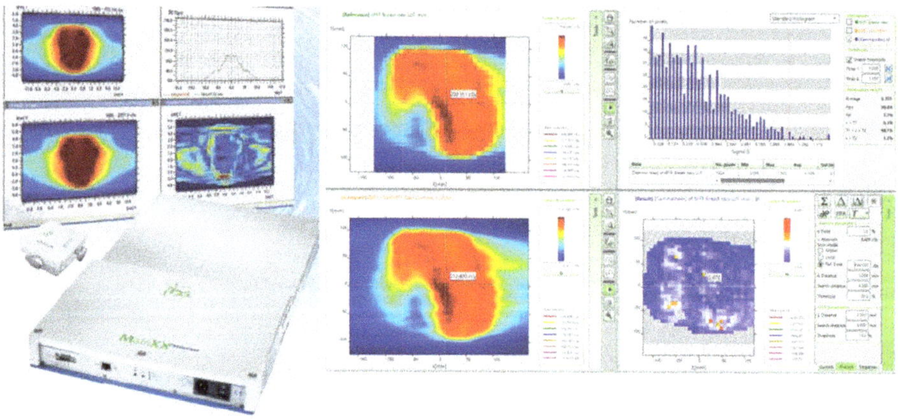

Figure 12.7. The MatriXX device and associated display for IMRT QA. On the right panel, display associated with the new platform myQA Patients (https://www.iba-dosimetry.com/product/matrixx-universal-detector-array/).

12.3.4 PTW Octavius

The PTW Octavius detector system is an ion chamber-based device for IMRT QA and quality control in photon and proton beams. Some traditionalist physicists would prefer such a device since it is ionization chamber based and can provide the absolute dose with proper calibration and correction of temperature and pressure. The ion chambers are made of parallel plates 4.4 × 4.4 × 3 mm^3 in size with a center-to-center spacing of 7.1 mm. It has 1405 ion chambers in a chessboard matrix providing a maximum field size of 27 × 27 cm^2. The device can read the entire dose in a hundred milliseconds. This device can provide a real time analysis of any beam profile. There is no radiation damage as it is an ion chamber-based device. The device comes with a software program called Verisoft or MultiCheck that provides QA processes for IMRT and proton beams. Figure 12.8 shows the device, its operational method, and beam analysis. Details of IMRT QA by the PTW Octavius have been reported in the literature [39, 54].

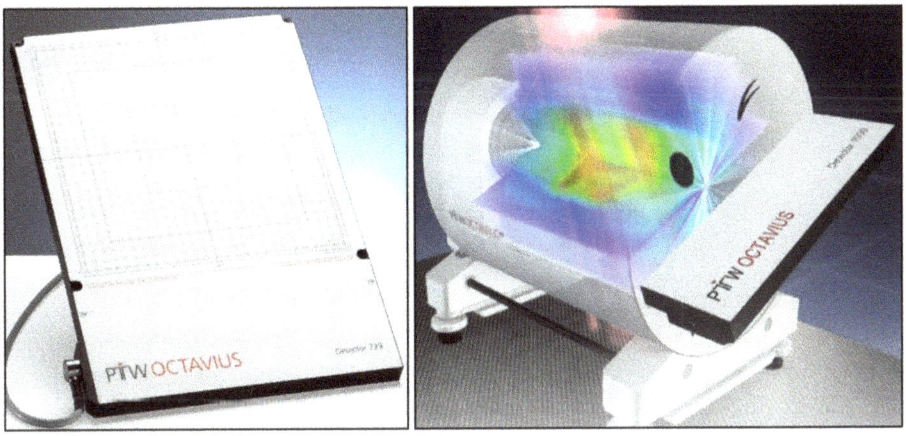

Figure 12.8. PTW Octavius device for QA in photon and proton beam. https://www.ptwdosimetry.com/en/products/octavius-4d/.

12.3.5 Scandidos Delta4

The Delta4 device by Scandidos is a solid phantom base that contains 1069 *p*-type diodes arranged in a matrix along two orthogonal planes [40]. It is a family of products for machine QA, IMRT QA, and DVH analysis. The device and plan analysis is shown in figure 12.9. A detailed comparison of this device is also reported in many references [40, 44, 50].

12.3.6 Electronic Portal Imaging Dosimetry (EPID)

Radiographic film has been the backbone of radiation since its invention, but since film is a passive device, it requires processing time and the images cannot be manipulated. This gave birth to electronic devices for portal imaging. Original panels were ionization chambers first developed in the Netherlands [55–57]. It was refined with flat panels as described in the historical view by Antonuk *et al* [58, 59]. With the development of EPID imaging using amorphous silicon (aSi), high-quality detector panels were introduced for KV and MV imaging that are used now in modern linear accelerators.

Soon after the EPID developments, Kirby *et al* [60, 61] realized that these imaging panels could be used for exit dosimetry. The Mijnheer group in the

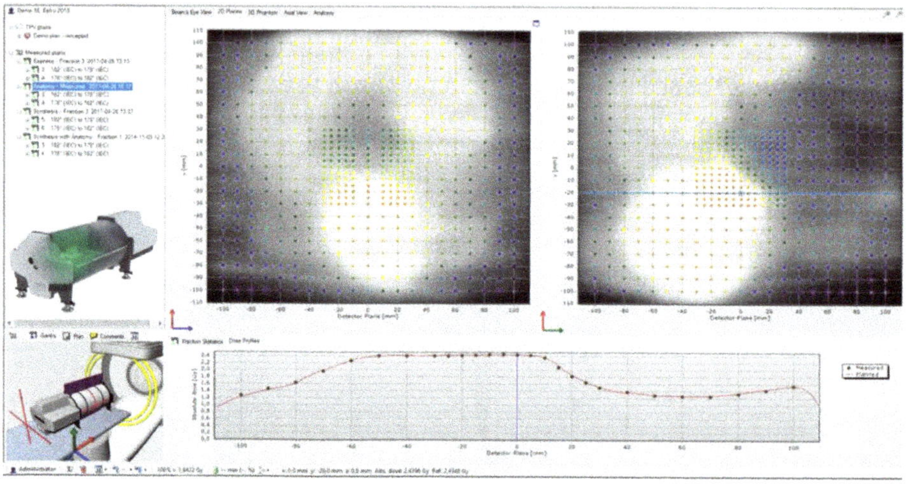

Figure 12.9. Delta[4] Phantom+ measurement phantom and a sample result. Images approved for use by ScandiDos AB.

Netherlands provided a vast amount of literature based on their experience with EPID in dosimetry [62–64]. In the early days, image quality was very poor and hence dosimetry was not very successful. However, with aSi, imaging contrast and resolution can be of a very high-quality and consequently, many vendors saw the opportunity for its use in MLC QA that led to its development in IMRT/VMAT QA. With proper EPID QA software, as discussed in the literature [65, 66], image quality can be maintained over a period of time. Every machine vendor with aSi-based panel has provided software on their accelerator for dosimetry (figure 12.10). A large number of publications have dealt with various aspects of IMRT QA using EPID [67–76].

For a successful implementation of the EPID in IMRT QA, many factors have to be considered including Kernel selection, scatter contribution with and without the phantom, scaling due to distance, backscatter, and pixel sensitivity. Most of these factors have been studied and resolved with proper calibration used in the software. However, proper and periodic calibration of the EPID is needed for satisfactory use in IMRT QA. It is also realized that even though the resolution of aSi is very high, the error detection in EPID-based QA is relatively poor. It is a well-known fact that in EPID-based IMRT QA, the passing rate is relatively very high.

There are a large number of advantages in EPID-based QA, as it saves a significant amount of time for the physics staff. It provides direct QA for the MLC leaves for the dynamic positions used in VMAT and it ensures that patient treatment will not be at fault by MLC errors. The QA run can be performed by any therapist with the knowledge of the machine's operation at any time of the day. Additionally, depending on the software, the analysis does not take a significant amount of time; thus, for a busy department with a heavy load of IMRT/VMAT, EPID-based QA could be cost-effective and the preferred choice.

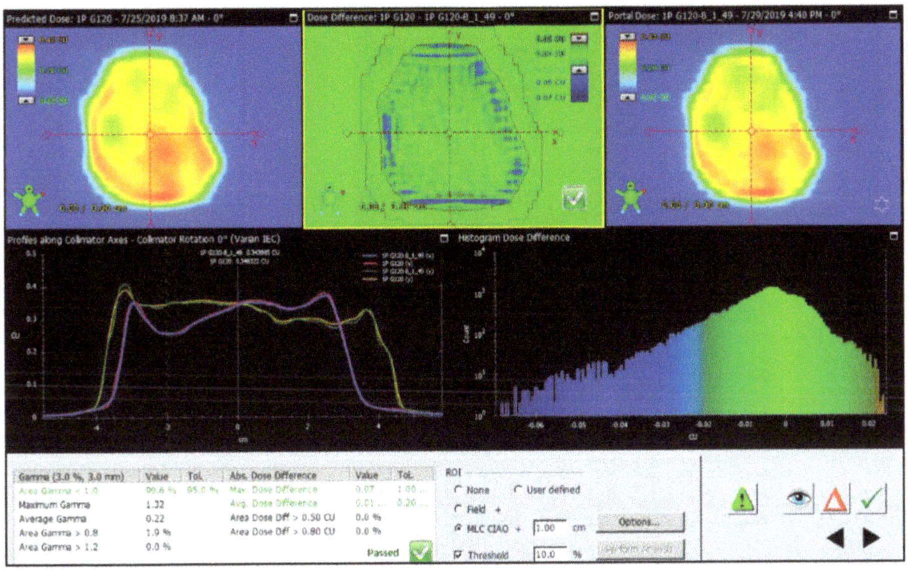

Figure 12.10. Illustration of the Varian Portal Dosimetry derived IMRT QA of a prostate patient. Various panels indicate calculated, portal dose, and difference plot. The analysis with gamma and DTA as well as line profile and histograms are shown.

12.4 Log-file approach

In general, modern digital linear accelerators contain information about the machine's performance such as dose rate, MLC position, gantry angle, collimator angle, etc in their log files; this data is stored in intervals of milliseconds. The log files are generated in a binary format and proprietary to the vendors, as such they may require conversion prior to processing and analyzing. Stell *et al* [11] showed that MLC leaf errors in IMRT can easily be detected from machine log files. A growing interest in using machine log files and independent treatment planning system (TPS) dose recalculation for IMRT QA has been proposed by various investigators [10, 77, 78]. It has been reported that log-file-based QA is able to provide insight into machine parameters that may not be possible with phantom-based QA and to improve the efficiency of patient-specific QA.

Traditionally, the pretreatment IMRT QA has been carried out by irradiating a phantom and detector combination to measure the consistency between the delivered and calculated dose distributions as shown in previous sections. However, studies have pointed out that phantom measurement-based QA may not be able to detect some types of failures in the IMRT process, such as dose calculation errors, plan transfer errors, etc [28, 79]. Additionally, the use of water-equivalent phantoms for dose recalculation and delivery oversimplifies the QA processes, because water-equivalent phantoms do not represent the real geometry and tissue heterogeneities. As discussed earlier, the biggest shortcoming of measurement-based QA is that it is a labor-intensive and time-consuming process for most

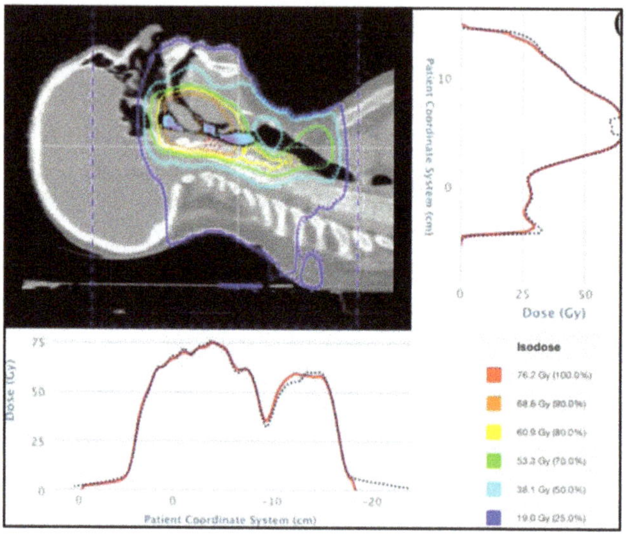

Figure 12.11. Display of isodose for a head and neck cancer case. The solid line is calculated by the TPS and the dashed line is calculated from the log-file. The line profiles are nearly identical indicating that Mobius can be used for IMRT QA. Adopted from Fontenot *et al* [24] copyright 2014 the authors. Open access CC BY 3.0.

busy departments where access to machines could be limited, especially in the USA where required certifications make it very restrictive to acquire new machines.

Additionally, log-file-based QA could assess the actual delivered dose by reconstructing the dose on patients' original CT images. However, the accuracy of log-file-based QA has also been questioned and it has been reported that in some cases the recorded MLC position in the log files did not agree with the observed positions. Currently, there is still no consensus on whether the log files and independent TPS dose checks are effective enough to be an alternative to phantom measurement-based QA. Kry *et al* [28] analyzed data for IROC head and neck phantom and compared it with institutional data. It was shown that a simple recalculation based on Mobius log files outperformed the measurement-based IMRT QA for detecting unacceptable plans. These findings highlight the value of an independent recalculation, and raise further questions about the current standard of measurement-based IMRT QA.

There is however a great deal of acceptance of log-file-based QA, since the offshoot company Mobius3D (Mobius Medical System LP, Houston, TX, USA), which was used for plan verification, was acquired by the Varian Medical system. The efficacy of this program is successfully used and reported in various publications [24, 25, 28, 77, 78, 80–83]. Figure 12.11 shows the data for a head and neck patient where the isodose is displayed from TPS and calculated from Mobius3D (dashed line). The line profiles in the x and y planes are also shown. The software also provides the percentage passing rate, gamma index, and DTA, which is comparable with other systems.

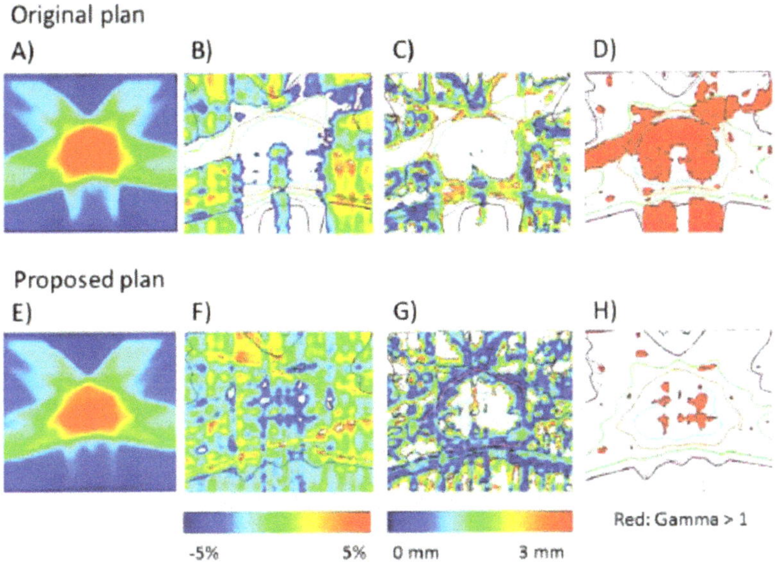

Figure 12.12. Measure and proposed model dose distribution with various passing rate. Adopted from Sumida *et al* [96] copyright 2014 the authors. Open access CC BY 3.0.

12.5 Artificial intelligence

As mentioned earlier, the time requirement for IMRT/VMAT PSQA is extremely large and could be prohibitive in a busy department. Also the workload is steadily increasing for the modulated treatments to nearly 60% of the case load in the majority of centers today. Given the financial strain, additional staffing for QA and machine time may not be readily available. In this context, the log-file approach and the use of AI in radiation oncology is growing rapidly. There are many groups working on machine and deep learning algorithms that have proposed their use for IMRT QA [84–86]. Machine learning algorithms are based on probabilities, and in radiation oncology, most tasks can be performed based on probability as well. In this context, AI is being proposed for contouring [87–91], knowledge-based treatment planning [92–94], chart checks [84], and IMRT QA [85, 86, 95]. Li *et al* [95] showed that a convolution neural network (CNN) could be used to validate the random forest approach and derive the gamma passing rate in VMAT. The model was compared with the measured data that was used as training data. In a similar approach, Sumida *et al* [96] showed that using a 2D measured data set, 3D data could be predicted, as shown in figure 12.12, where utilizing an AI approach indicated significant improvement in the dose distribution.

12.6 Outlook

The process described in this chapter is dynamic and may change with technology and newer techniques that are being developed. In a recent paper, Mehrens *et al* [97] analyzed the practice of IMRT QA conducted by IROC. They analyzed IMRT QA process from 2861 institutions from 2011–2018 via questionnaire. The 2D diode array, EPID and 2D ion chamber based devices for QA were 52.8%, 27.4% and 23.9%, respectively. The passing rate criterion for gamma index varied from 5%/5 mm to 1%/2 mm for ⩾ 90% of the data points. Obviously, this analysis was earlier than the publication of TG-218 [12]. It will be worth noting the trend post TG-218 report. Also, when QA fails, the strategy applied varied among institutions either repeating the QA or re-planning the IMRT. Additional recommendation or use of AI could be the way for IMRT QA but time will tell which way we are moving in this labor-intensive IMRT QA process.

References

[1] Leveson N G and Turner C S 1993 An investigation of the Therac-25 accidents *IEEE Comput.* **26** 18–41

[2] Bourguignon M, Simon J M and Peiffert D *et al* 2009 Radiothérapie: les leçons à tirer des accidents d'Épinal et de Toulouse *Radioprotecion* **44** 417–29

[3] Derreumaux S, Etard C and Huet C *et al* 2008 Lessons from recent accidents in radiation therapy in France *Radiat. Prot. Dosimetry.* **131** 130–5

[4] Zietman A L, Palta J R and Steinberg M L (ed) 2012 *Saftey Is No Accident: A Framework for Quality Radiation Oncology and Care* (Fairfax, VA: American Society for Radiation Oncology)

[5] Bogdanich W 2010 Radiation offers new cures, and ways to do harm *The New York Times* http://www.nytimes.com/2010/01/24/health/24radiation.html

[6] Bogdanich W and Rebelo K 2010 A pinpoint beam strays invisibly, harming instead of healing *The New York Times.* http://www.nytimes.com/2010/12/29/health/29radiation.html?_r=0

[7] Ezzell G A, Galvin J M and Low D *et al* 2003 Guidance document on delivery, treatment planning, and clinical implementation of IMRT: report of the IMRT Subcommittee of the AAPM Radiation Therapy Committee *Med. Phys.* **30** 2089–115

[8] Hartford A C, Galvin J M and Beyer D C *et al* 2012 American College of Radiology (ACR) and American Society for Radiation Oncology (ASTRO) Practice Guideline for Intensity-modulated Radiation Therapy (IMRT) *Am. J. Clin. Oncol.* **35** 612–7

[9] Agnew A, Agnew C E and Grattan M W *et al* 2014 Monitoring daily MLC positional errors using trajectory log files and EPID measurements for IMRT and VMAT deliveries *Phys. Med. Biol.* **59** N49–63

[10] Rangaraj D, Zhu M and Yang D *et al* 2013 Catching errors with patient-specific pretreatment machine log file analysis *Pract. Radiat. Oncol.* **3** 80–90

[11] Stell A M, Li J G and Zeidan O A *et al* 2004 An extensive log-file analysis of step-and-shoot intensity modulated radiation therapy segment delivery errors *Med. Phys.* **31** 1593–602

[12] Miften M, Olch A and Mihailidis D *et al* 2018 Tolerance limits and methodologies for IMRT measurement-based verification QA: recommendations of AAPM Task Group No. 218 *Med. Phys.* **45** e53–83

[13] Nelms B E, Zhen H and Tomé W A 2011 Per-beam, planar IMRT QA passing rates do not predict clinically relevant patient dose errors *Med. Phys.* **38** 1037–44

[14] Kry S F, Molineu A and Kerns J R *et al* 2014 Institutional patient-specific IMRT QA does not predict unacceptable plan delivery *Int. J. Radiat. Oncol. Biol. Phys.* **90** 1195–201

[15] Carson M E, Molineu A and Taylor P A *et al* 2016 Examining credentialing criteria and poor performance indicators for IROC Houston's anthropomorphic head and neck phantom *Med. Phys.* **43** 6491–6
[16] Dice L R 1945 Measures of the amount of ecologic association between species *Ecology* **26** 297–302
[17] Sørensen T 1948 A method of establishing groups of equal amplitude in plant sociology based on similarity of species and its application to analyses of the vegetation on Danish commons *K.dansk. Vid. Selsk. Skr.* **5** 1–34
[18] Van Dyk J, Barnett R B and Cygler J E *et al* 1993 Commissioning and quality assurance of treatment planning computers *Int. J. Radiat. Oncol. Biol. Phys.* **26** 261–73
[19] Low D A, Harms W B and Mutic S *et al* 1998 A technique for the quantitative evaluation of dose distributions *Med. Phys.* **25** 656–61
[20] Low D A and Dempsey J F 2003 Evaluation of the gamma dose distribution comparison method *Med. Phys.* **30** 2455–64
[21] Francescon P, Cora S and Chiovati P 2003 Dose verification of an IMRT treatment planning system with the BEAM EGS4-based Monte Carlo code *Med. Phys.* **30** 144–57
[22] Paganini L, Reggiori G and Stravato A *et al* 2019 MLC parameters from static fields to VMAT plans: an evaluation in a RT-dedicated MC environment (PRIMO) *Radiat. Oncol.* **14** 216
[23] Fan J, Li J and Chen L *et al* 2006 A practical Monte Carlo MU verification tool for IMRT quality assurance *Phys. Med. Biol.* **51** 2503–15
[24] Fontenot J D 2014 Evaluation of a novel secondary check tool for intensity-modulated radiotherapy treatment planning *J. Appl. Clin. Med. Phys.* **15** 207–15
[25] Teichmann T, Salz H and Schwedas M *et al* 2020 A multi-institutional initiative on patient-related quality assurance: independent computational dose verification of fluence-modulated treatment techniques *Z. Med. Phys.* **30** 155–65
[26] Kamima T, Baba H and Takahashi R *et al* 2018 Multi-institutional comparison of computer-based independent dose calculation for intensity modulated radiation therapy and volumetric modulated arc therapy *Phys. Med.* **45** 72–81
[27] Nyflot M J, Thammasorn P and Wootton L S *et al* 2019 Deep learning for patient-specific quality assurance: identifying errors in radiotherapy delivery by radiomic analysis of gamma images with convolutional neural networks *Med. Phys.* **46** 456–64
[28] Kry S F, Glenn M C and Peterson C B *et al* 2019 Independent recalculation outperforms traditional measurement-based IMRT QA methods in detecting unacceptable plans *Med. Phys.* **46** 3700–8
[29] Esposito M, Villaggi E and Bresciani S *et al* 2020 Estimating dose delivery accuracy in stereotactic body radiation therapy: a review of in-vivo measurement methods *Radiother. Oncol.* **149** 158–67
[30] Dong L, Antolak J and Salehpour *et al* 2003 Patient-specific point dose measurement for IMRT monitor unit verification *Int. J. Radiat. Oncol. Biol. Phys.* **56** 867–77
[31] Pulliam K B, Followill D and Court L *et al* 2014 A six-year review of more than 13,000 patient-specific IMRT QA results from 13 different treatment sites *J. Appl. Clin. Med. Phys.* **15** 196–206
[32] Basran P S and Woo M K 2008 An analysis of tolerance levels in IMRT quality assurance procedures *Med. Phys.* **35** 2300–7

[33] Pai S, Das I J and Dempsey J F *et al* 2007 TG-69: radiographic film for megavoltage beam dosimetry *Med. Phys.* **34** 2228–58

[34] Das I J 2009 Radiographic film ed D W O Rogers and J E Cyglar *Clinical Dosimetry Measurements in Radiotherapy* (Madison, WI: Medical Physics Publishing) pp 865–90

[35] Chetty I and Charland P 2002 Investigation of Kodak extended dose range (EDR) film for megavoltage photon beam dosimetry *Phys. Med. Biol.* **47** 3629–41

[36] Childress N L, Dong L and Rosen I I 2002 Rapid radiographic film calibration for IMRT verification using automated MLC fields *Med. Phys.* **29** 2384–90

[37] Dogan N, Leybovich L B and Sethi A 2002 Comparative evaluation of Kodak EDR2 and XV2 films for verification of intensity modulated radiation therapy *Phys. Med. Biol.* **47** 4121–30

[38] Childress N L, Salehpour M and Dong L *et al* 2005 Dosimetric accuracy of Kodak EDR2 film for IMRT verifications *Med. Phys.* **32** 539–48

[39] Hussein M, Adams E J and Jordan T J *et al* 2013 A critical evaluation of the PTW 2D-ARRAY seven29 and OCTAVIUS II phantom for IMRT and VMAT verification *J. Appl. Clin. Med. Phys.* **14** 274–92

[40] Sadagopan R, Bencomo J A and Martin R L *et al* 2009 Characterization and clinical evaluation of a novel IMRT quality assurance system *J. Appl. Clin. Med. Phys.* **10** 104–19

[41] Chandraraj V, Stathakis S and Manickam R *et al* 2011 Comparison of four commercial devices for RapidArc and sliding window IMRT QA *J. Appl. Clin. Med. Phys.* **12** 338–49

[42] Saito M, Kadoya N and Sato K *et al* 2017 Comparison of DVH-based plan verification methods for VMAT: ArcCHECK-3DVH system and dynalog-based dose reconstruction *J. Appl. Clin. Med. Phys.* **18** 206–14

[43] Kadoya N, Saito M and Ogasawara M *et al* 2015 Evaluation of patient DVH-based QA metrics for prostate VMAT: correlation between accuracy of estimated 3D patient dose and magnitude of MLC misalignment *J. Appl. Clin. Med. Phys.* **16** 179–89

[44] Saito M, Sano N and Shibata Y *et al* 2018 Comparison of MLC error sensitivity of various commercial devices for VMAT pre-treatment quality assurance *J. Appl. Clin. Med. Phys.* **19** 87–93

[45] Das I J 2017 *Advances in Radiochromic Film for Radiation Dosimetry: Role and Clinical Applications* (Boca Raton, FL: CRC Press| Taylor & Francis Group)

[46] Xu Z, Wang I Z and Kumaraswamy L K *et al* 2016 Evaluation of dosimetric effect caused by slowing with multi-leaf collimator (MLC) leaves for volumetric modulated arc therapy (VMAT) *Radiol. Oncol.* **50** 121–8

[47] McKenzie E M, Balter P A and Stingo F C *et al* 2014 Toward optimizing patient-specific IMRT QA techniques in the accurate detection of dosimetrically acceptable and unacceptable patient plans *Med. Phys.* **41** 121702

[48] Andenna C, Benassi M and Caccia B *et al* 2006 Comparison of dose distributions in IMRT planning using the gamma function *J. Exp. Clin. Cancer Res.* **25** 229–34

[49] Jursinic P A and Nelms B E 2003 A 2-D diode array and analysis software for verification of intensity modulated radiation therapy delivery *Med. Phys.* **30** 870–9

[50] Hussein M, Rowshanfarzad P and Ebert M A *et al* 2013 A comparison of the gamma index analysis in various commercial IMRT/VMAT QA systems *Radiother. Oncol.* **109** 370–6

[51] Coleman L and Skourou C 2013 Sensitivity of volumetric modulated arc therapy patient specific QA results to multileaf collimator errors and correlation to dose volume histogram based metrics *Med. Phys.* **40** 111715

[52] Lin Y, Bentefour H and Flanz J *et al* 2018 Design of a QA method to characterize submillimeter-sized PBS beam properties using a 2D ionization chamber array *Phys. Med. Biol.* **63** 105007

[53] Arjomandy B, Sahoo N and Ding X *et al* 2008 Use of a two-dimensional ionization chamber array for proton therapy beam quality assurance *Med. Phys.* **35** 3889–94

[54] Stathakis S, Myers P and Esquivel C *et al* 2013 Characterization of a novel 2D array dosimeter for patient-specific quality assurance with volumetric arc therapy *Med. Phys.* **40** 071731

[55] van Herk M and Meertens H 1988 A matrix ionisation chamber imaging device for on-line patient setup verification during radiotherapy *Radiother. Oncol.* **11** 369–78

[56] Meertens J, Bijhold J and Strackee J 1990 A method for the measurement of field placement variations in digital portal images *Phys. Med. Biol.* **35** 299–323

[57] Meertens H, van Herk M and Bijhold J *et al* 1990 First clinical experience with a newly developed electronic portal imaging device *Int. J. Radiat. Oncol. Biol. Phys.* **18** 1173–81

[58] Antonuk L E 2002 Electronic portal imaging devices: a review and historical perspective of contemporary technologies and research *Phys. Med. Biol.* **47** R31–65

[59] Antonuk L, Yorkston J and Huang W *et al* 1996 Megavoltage imaging with a large-area, flat-panel, amorphous silicon imager *Int. J. Radiat. Oncol. Biol. Phys.* **36** 661–72

[60] Kirby M C and Williams P C 1993 Measurement possibilities using an electronic portal imaging device *Radiother. Oncol.* **29** 237–43

[61] Kirby M C and Williams P C 1995 The use of an electronic portal imaging device for exit dosimetry and quality control measurements *Int. J. Radiat. Onol. Biol. Phys.* **31** 593–603

[62] van Elmpt W, McDermott L and Nijsten S *et al* 2008 A literature review of electronic portal imaging for radiotherapy dosimetry *Radiother. Oncol.* **88** 289–309

[63] Mijnheer B, Beddar S and Izewska J *et al* 2013 *In vivo* dosimetry in external beam radiotherapy *Med. Phys.* **40** 070903

[64] Olaciregui-Ruiz I, Vivas-Maiques B and Kaas J *et al* 2019 Transit and non-transit 3D EPID dosimetry versus detector arrays for patient specific QA *J. Appl. Clin. Med. Phys.* **20** 79–90

[65] Pesznyák C, Fekete G and Mózes A *et al* 2009 Quality control of portal imaging with PTW EPID QC PHANTOM *Strahlenther. Onkol.* **185** 56–60

[66] Das I J, Cao M and Cheng C W *et al* 2011 A quality assurance phantom for electronic portal imaging devices *J. Appl. Clin. Med. Phys.* **12** 391–402

[67] Warkentin B, Steciw S and Rathee S *et al* 2003 Dosimetric IMRT verification with a flat-panel EPID *Med. Phys.* **30** 3143–55

[68] Chang J, Obcemea C H and Sillanpaa J *et al* 2004 Use of EPID for leaf position accuracy QA of dynamic multi-leaf collimator (DMLC) treatment *Med. Phys.* **31** 2091–06

[69] Van Esch A, Depuydt T and Huyskens D P 2004 The use of an aSi-based EPID for routine absolute dosimetric pre-treatment verification of dynamic IMRT fields *Radiother. Oncol.* **71** 223–34

[70] McDermott L N, Wendling M and van Asselen B *et al* 2006 Clinical experience with EPID dosimetry for prostate IMRT pre-treatment dose verification *Med. Phys.* **33** 3921–30

[71] Talamonti C, Casati M and Bucciolini M 2006 Pretreatment verification of IMRT absolute dose distributions using a commercial a-Si EPID *Med. Phys.* **33** 4367–78

[72] Nelms B E, Rasmussen K H and Tome W A 2010 Evaluation of a fast method of EPID-based dosimetry for intensity-modulated radiation therapy *J. Appl. Clin. Med. Phys.* **11** 140–57

[73] Bojechko C, Phillps M and Kalet A *et al* 2015 A quantification of the effectiveness of EPID dosimetry and software-based plan verification systems in detecting incidents in radiotherapy *Med. Phys.* **42** 5363–9
[74] Miri N, Keller P and Zwan B J *et al* 2016 EPID-based dosimetry to verify IMRT planar dose distribution for the aS1200 EPID and FFF beams *J. Appl. Clin. Med. Phys.* **17** 292–304
[75] Alhazmi A, Gianoli C and Neppl S *et al* 2018 A novel approach to EPID-based 3D volumetric dosimetry for IMRT and VMAT QA *Phys. Med. Biol.* **63** 115002
[76] Nailon W H, Welsh D and McDonald K *et al* 2019 EPID-based *in vivo* dosimetry using Dosimetry Check™: overview and clinical experience in a 5-yr study including breast, lung, prostate, and head and neck cancer patients *J. Appl. Clin. Med. Phys.* **20** 6–16
[77] Defoor D L, Stathakis S and Roring J E *et al* 2017 Investigation of error detection capabilities of phantom, EPID and MLC log file based IMRT QA methods *J. Appl. Clin. Med. Phys.* **18** 172–9
[78] Calvo-Ortega J F, Teke T and Moragues S *et al* 2014 A Varian DynaLog file-based procedure for patient dose-volume histogram-based IMRT QA *J. Appl. Clin. Med. Phys.* **15** 100–9
[79] Nelms B E, Chan M F and Jarry G *et al* 2013 Evaluating IMRT and VMAT dose accuracy: practical examples of failure to detect systematic errors when applying a commonly used metric and action levels *Med. Phys.* **40** 111722
[80] Zhang Y, Le A H and Tian Z *et al* 2019 Modeling Elekta VersaHD using the Varian Eclipse treatment planning system for photon beams: a single-institution experience *J. Appl. Clin. Med. Phys.* **20** 33–42
[81] Kabat C N, Defoor D L and Myers P *et al* 2019 Evaluation of the Elekta Agility MLC performance using high-resolution log files *Med. Phys.* **46** 1397–407
[82] Childress N, Chen Q and Rong Y 2015 Parallel/Opposed: IMRT QA using treatment log files is superior to conventional measurement-based method *J. Appl. Clin. Med. Phys.* **16** 5385
[83] Song J Y, Jeong J U and Yoon M S *et al* 2017 Dosimetric evaluation of MobiusFX in the RapidArc delivery quality assurance comparing with 3DVH *PLoS One* **12** e0183165
[84] Kalet A M, Luk S M H and Phillips M H 2020 Radiation therapy quality assurance tasks and tools: the many roles of machine learning *Med. Phys.* **47** e168–77
[85] Mahdavi S R, Tavakol A and Sanei M *et al* 2019 Use of artificial neural network for pretreatment verification of intensity modulation radiation therapy fields *Br. J. Radiol.* **92** 20190355
[86] Mahdavi S R, Bakhshandeh M and Rostami A *et al* 2018 2D dose reconstruction by artificial neural network for pretreatment verification of IMRT fields *J. Med. Imag. Radiat. Sci.* **49** 286–92
[87] Thong W, Kadoury S and Piche N *et al* 2018 Convolutional networks for kidney segmentation in contrast-enchanced CT-scans *Comp. Meth. Biomech. Biomed. Eng. Imag. Visul.* **6** 277–82
[88] Lustberg T, van Soest J and Gooding M *et al* 2018 Clinical evaluation of atlas and deep learning based automatic contouring for lung cancer *Radiother. Oncol.* **126** 312–7
[89] Gooding M J, Smith A J and Tariq M *et al* 2018 Comparative evaluation of autocontouring in clinical practice: a practical method using the Turing test *Med. Phys.* **45** 5105–15

[90] Shen C, Nguyen D and Chen L *et al* 2020 Operating a treatment planning system using a deep-reinforcement learning-based virtual treatment planner for prostate cancer intensity-modulated radiation therapy treatment planning *Med. Phys.* **47** 2329–36

[91] Fan J, Wang J and Chen Z *et al* 2019 Automatic treatment planning based on three-dimensional dose distribution predicted from deep learning technique *Med. Phys.* **46** 370–81

[92] Archambault Y, Boylan C and Bullock D *et al* 2020 Making on-line adaptive radiotherapy possible using artificial intelligence and machine learning for efficient daily re-planning *Med. Phys. Int.* **8** 77–86

[93] Hussein M, Heijmen B J M and Verellen D *et al* 2018 Automation in intensity modulated radiotherapy treatment planning-a review of recent innovations *Br. J. Radiol.* **91** 20180270

[94] Hussein M, South C P and Barry M A *et al* 2016 Clinical validation and benchmarking of knowledge-based IMRT and VMAT treatment planning in pelvic anatomy *Radiother. Oncol.* **120** 473–9

[95] Li J, Wang L and Zhang X *et al* 2019 Machine learning for patient-specific quality assurance of VMAT: prediction and classification accuracy *Int. J. Radiat. Oncol. Biol. Phys.* **105** 893–902

[96] Sumida I, Yamaguchi H and Kizaki H *et al* 2014 Three-dimensional dose prediction based on two-dimensional verification measurements for IMRT *J. Appl. Clin. Med. Phys.* **15** 133–46

[97] Mehrens H, Taylor P and Followill D S *et al* 2020 Survey results of 3D-CRT and IMRT quality assurance practice *J. Appl. Clin. Med. Phys.* **21** 70–6

Chapter 13

IMRT dose prescription and recording

Imagine a perfect scenario where every cell in a tumor volume gets the prescribed dose and the dose-volume histogram looks like a step function. Unfortunately, such a scenario is ideal but probably cannot be realized. This is because the dose delivery is not a perfect process. Even though the treatment plan can provide such an option, the delivered dose often deviates from perfect due to the nature of photon interactions and electron transport, which make the dose spill over from the target volume. Now look at figure 13.1(a), where several possible scenarios are described with four dose-volume histogram (DVH) graphs by four different planners. Which graph should a clinician choose and which dose point would represent a good treatment? This was the rather difficult task in the beginning of the IMRT implementation, when the community had little experience with IMRT and what little we knew was from 3DCRT. On the other hand, let us look at figure 13.1(b), and compare one DVH with four points for dose prescriptions: D_{100}, D_{98}, D_{95}, and D_{50} indicating the dose where 100%, 98%, 95% and 50% volumes are covered, respectively. In fact, one can use as many points as one chooses on this graph. In these scenarios, one could argue their respective point of view for choosing a point for prescription without being able to provide a clear rationale for such a selection. This indifferent point selection precipitates to a large variation in the delivered dose in each mode of prescription. Although intuitively one would prefer curve 'B' in figure 13.1(b) where 100% PTV volume is covered by the prescription dose, later it will be shown that such a selection is not prudent and not advisable. In this figure, one can also see that there is ΔD that differentiates the two curves and may have a significant impact in a clinical trial.

So what does it matter if one chooses curve A or B? The answer is clear: the outcome of the patients treated with options A and B from two institutions cannot be compared, as the dose prescriptions are very different. This has huge implications for scientific and clinical knowledge, as the reporting process of outcomes cannot be certain. Additionally, the knowledge of the dose that provides a cure for a certain

doi:10.1088/978-0-7503-1335-3ch13

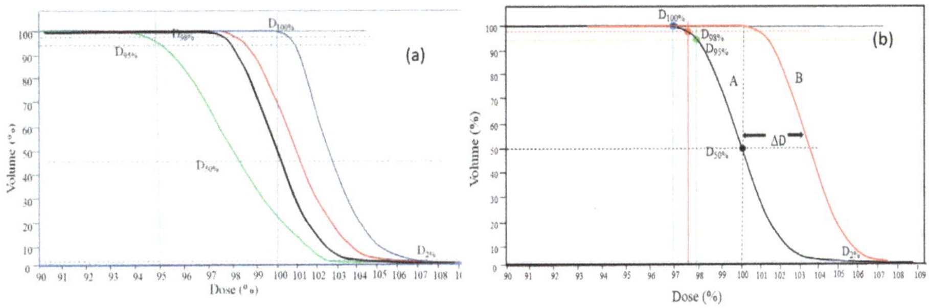

Figure 13.1. (a) Four DVH curves by four planners indicating variability. (b) DVH (A) shows various points D_{100}, D_{98}, D_{95}, and D_{50} for dose prescription. ICRU-83 recommends using D_{50} for the prescription. In such a case, a portion of tumor volume will get less dose and other parts will get higher dose. However, some people prefer curve (B) where 100% volume is covered. It is clear that there is a difference of dose (ΔD) between curve A and B, and this could be detrimental for the outcome.

disease is lost. For any international or national protocols where the clinical outcome has to be reproduced from one institution to another, the delivered dose has to be accurate.

We all agree to some extent that a unified approach for prescribing the dose should be adopted, so that outcome data from one institution to the other can be compared. In this chapter, we will discuss the rationales as how one should prescribe dose in IMRT. In this context, similar to the ICRU-50 [1] and ICRU-62 [2] for the case of 3DCRT conformal therapy, ICRU-83 [3] provided guidelines for IMRT prescriptions. Unfortunately, these international recommendations have not been universally followed over a long period of time. Das *et al* [4] provided an early overview of the state of IMRT prescriptions and delivery among several academic institutions and reported a large variation among them. The same work was later extended with over 5000 patients and 10 institutions for the adoption of the ICRU-83 guidelines [5].

13.1 Planning variability

Variability in IMRT planning and the consequential results were felt early on in the implementation process throughout the community, as results are dependent on the optimization routine and its robustness in solving the global minimum of the cost function. This was inherent in the inverse planning process, as an exact and unique solution cannot be found. As early as 2008, Das *et al* [4] compared data from 805 IMRT patients treated across five institutions using five treatment planning systems. This study was conducted to see if the IMRT plans from multiple institutions could be compared and if they were identical. The dose in terms of maximum, minimum, median, and isocenter to PTV was compared. The largest variation was noted in the isocenter dose (precursor to the ICRU-50) as a reference point. This shows that in IMRT, using the isocenter as a reference point cannot be meaningful because it can be placed out of PTV with negligible dose. So unlike 3DCRT, the isocenter dose should be avoided from IMRT. It was also noted that a large variation in the maximum and minimum dose was seen amongst various institutions.

Figure 13.2 shows such patterns in the two most common malignancies for IMRT treatment: prostate and head and neck. It shows the prescribed data (symbol) and delivered dose representing maximum and minimum dose in PTV by the error bars. However, the median dose in the PTV was consistently and uniformly unique in most treatment planning systems. Based on this observation [4], ICRU-83 [3] made it a seminal point to recommend that in IMRT, the dose should be prescribed to the median point. This aspect will be discussed further in section 13.3.

We have come a long way in terms of accuracy of radiation dose. The dose is defined by international guidelines, and it is now universally accepted that ±2% dose accuracy can be maintained for any radiation machine, which can be done during the machine calibration based on one of the guidelines [6, 7]. However, such guidelines cannot be maintained for the dose delivery, especially in IMRT. The dosimetric variations were quite large during days of 3DCRT when ICRU-50 and ICRU-62 played an important role in defining tumor volumes and dose prescription [1, 2]. The dosimetric uniformity in IMRT is equally hard to achieve unless strict guidelines are adopted. In this context, AAPM Task Group 119 [8] stated that in IMRT, the dose is never perfect but the question is 'how close to perfect can we achieve?' Using multicenter data from a phantom study, they compared the IMRT point dose and provided guidance that institutions should compare their data with TG-119. The task group, however, did not address the dose prescription points. Additionally, ASTRO IMRT [9] guideline is silent on the dose prescription as well. This is a seminal question with a huge societal cost, as trust amongst institutions providing IMRT could be lost if the IMRT prescription dose is not unique and the same for a given probability of cure/outcome.

13.2 ICRU-83 guidelines

Seventeen years after the publication of ICRU-50 [1] for a comprehensive dose prescription, in 2010 ICRU-83 [3] was published to provide guidance and recommendations for IMRT. It emphasized defining target volumes using imaging technologies such as CT, MRI, and PET, which are developed enough to be utilized in target volume delineation. Additionally, functional imaging should be incorporated for defining the volume. The concept of sub-volumes was introduced to define a meaningful volume for IMRT optimization in dose painting. These volumes can be used as the intersections of volumes to be used for optimization. It was realized that CTV must be associated with GTV for malignant tumors. ICRU-83 also emphasized the need for delineating the organs at risk (OAR) and extended the concept of extension for OAR, which is called planning organs at risk volume (PRV). Additional terminology such as remaining value at risk (RVR) was also introduced. The RVR is defined as volumes not included in OAR and CTV that can be contoured for optimization purposes.

There was a huge paradigm shift from 3DCRT dose prescription to IMRT. ICRU-50 recommended that the dose to be delivered to a point (the reference point

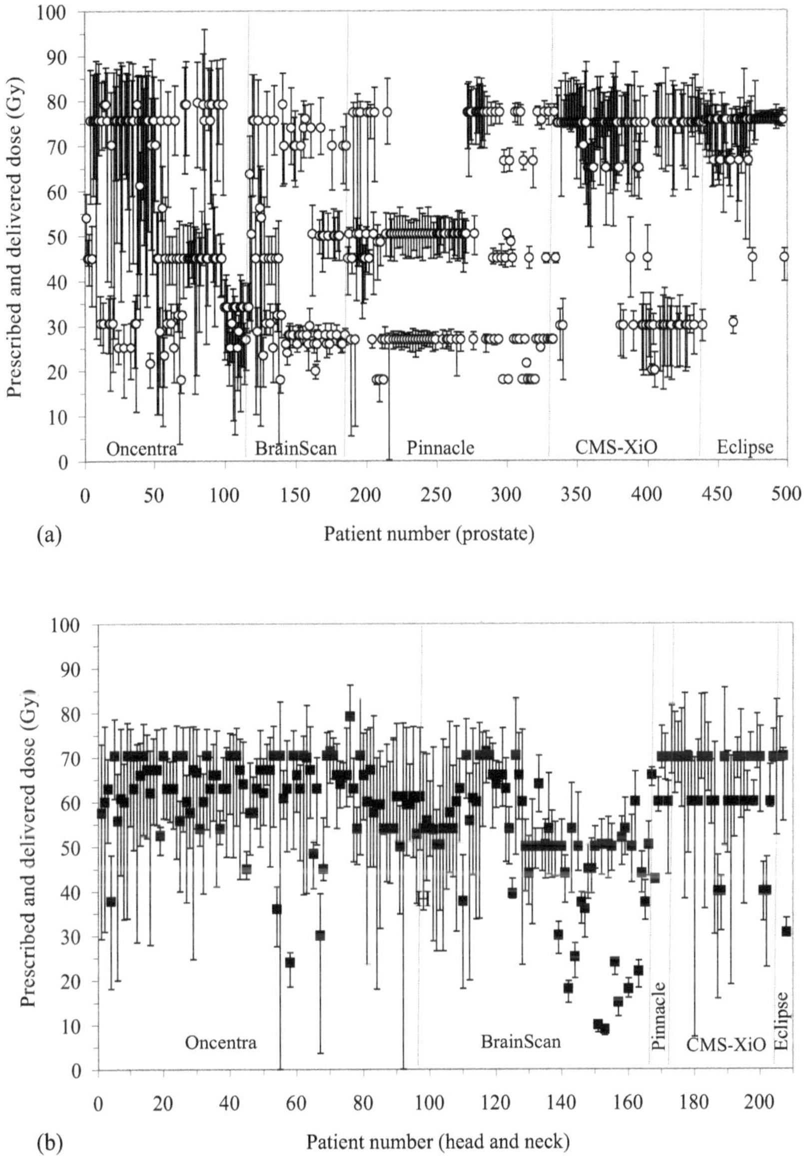

Figure 13.2. (a) Variation of prescription dose (symbol) with error bars representing the minimum and maximum delivered dose to the prostate target volume among different treatment planning systems. These data include dose to original (45–50 Gy) and sequential cone down (30 Gy) treatment volumes. The larger the error bars, the higher the dose variation is in delivery. (b) Variation of prescription dose (symbol) with error bars representing minimum and maximum delivered dose to the PTV in head and neck patients among different treatment planning systems for 70 Gy treatments. These data include dose to original and sequential cone down treatment volumes. The larger the error bars, the greater the variation.

typically was the isocenter), whereas ICRU-83 recommended that the dose should be given to a volume and evaluated based on the DVH. ICRU-83 introduced several new dosimetric terms for reporting purposes to represent the minimum, maximum and medium dose in the volume: D_{98}, D_2 and D_{50}, respectively (see figure 13.1). It also recommended that D_{50} should be treated as the reference point and the IMRT dose should be specified at D_{50}. ICRU-83 defined the low gradient (⩽20%/cm) and high-gradient (⩾20%/cm) regions and gave enough emphasis on quality assurance in IMRT in terms of the gamma index and DTA, which has been already discussed previously in chapter 12 of this book. ICRU-83 also specified that biological indices should be evaluated in terms for TCP and NTCP for the evaluation of the plan. Various terms discussed above are defined below and several new terms such as homogeneity index (HI) and conformity index (CI) are defined and emphasized. A summary of recommendations is as follows:

- IMRT plans should not be performed without DVH constraints;
- Uncertainty and confidence intervals should be evaluated;
- Dose should be reported to OAR and PRV along with PTV;
- Maximum dose is defined as $D_{2\%}$ which is different from ICRU-50;
- Median dose, $D_{50\%}$ is close to the prescription dose and should be treated as the reference dose;
- ICRU-83 stated that the median absorbed dose is close to the mean absorbed dose for a target volume;
- $D_{98\%,}$ is considered the minimum dose in PTV;
- Defined homogeneity index (HI) as below:

$$\mathrm{HI} = \frac{[D_2 - D_{98}]}{D_{50}} \tag{13.1}$$

It is clear that for an ideal plan HI should be near zero when the maximum and minimum dose in a PTV volume is same and the DVH curve is close to a step function.

Very similar to ICRU-50, importance is given to Conformity Index (CI) as:

$$\mathrm{CI}_{\mathrm{iso}} = \frac{\text{TV Covered by \% isodose}}{\text{Planning target volume}} \tag{13.2}$$

It is clear that CI should be close to 100% when the entire PTV is covered by the chosen isodose line. So with the help of HI and CI, a planner can opt for the following,

$$\begin{cases} \mathrm{HI} \rightarrow 0.0 \\ \mathrm{CI} \rightarrow 1.0 \end{cases} \tag{13.3}$$

ICRU-83 also emphasized and provided rationales for using clinical and biological evaluations with well-known parameters as TCP: Tumor control probability; NTCP: Normal tissue complication probability; and EUD: Equivalent uniform dose as defined in literature [10, 11]. In terms of surviving fraction (SF) of the cells to a radiation dose, D, and using linear quadratic parameters α and β, d is fractional dose and γ_{50} is slope at 50% cell survival SF is given by

$$\mathrm{SF} = e^{-n(\alpha d+\beta d^2)} \tag{13.4}$$

$$\mathrm{TCP} = e^{(-N\cdot \mathrm{SF})} \tag{13.5}$$

$$\mathrm{TCP} = e^{(-N\cdot \mathrm{SF})} \tag{13.6}$$

$$\mathrm{TCP} = \left[1 + \left(\frac{d_{50}}{D}\right)^{4\gamma_{50}}\right]^{-1} \tag{13.7}$$

$$\mathrm{TCP} = \prod_i \left(e^{n_i \mathrm{SF}(D\cdot d_i)}\right) \tag{13.8}$$

With all these efforts, ICRU-83 tried to unify many topics, including target volume delineation, DVH constraints, DVH evaluations, dose prescription, and recordings. This was all done so that a meaningful comparison could be made when a patient is treated with a modulated beam or inversely planned.

13.3 State of compliance

The state of dose delivery and prescription in IMRT has been discussed by many groups indicating poor compliance [4, 12, 13]. With such a rate, clinical trials or comparing IMRT outcome data is very uncertain. To evaluate this further, Das *et al* [5] undertook a large study comparing dosimetry and IMRT performance among several academic institutions. They found that the majority of institutions still followed their old guidelines, similar to the days of 3DCRT, and prescribed 95% dose delivery to the 95% volume of the target. In IMRT, such a practice is unacceptable and unjustifiable because in IMRT, the dose distribution can be achieved by forcing the optimization routine to deliver dose as required to the target volume. Figure 13.3 was supposed to reveal the compliance of IMRT prescriptions with ICRU-83; however, it is not observed.

Further analysis showed that a majority of the institutions still follow D_{95} as a common practice, as indicated in figure 13.4. If there were compliance with ICRU-83, the D_{50} graph in figure 13.4 would be the highest and most narrowly peaked, but what we observed was that unexpectedly D_{95} had highest peak. This indicates that old habits die hard. We carry over our thought processes from 3DCRT where the dose was typically prescribed as 95% isodose to 95% volume. Another observation notes that the 100% dose as expected (curve 'B' from figure 13.1(b)) should have been pointier and sharper but instead it was rather low frequency and spread out, indicating that very few clinicians prescribe in that way. This is in contrast to the thought process of 'cold spot' where Tomé *et al* [14] showed that even a small amount of cold spot can reduce the TCP significantly. This point is well-known and it was also shown by Goitein *et al* in 1996 that a small amount of under dosage lowers the TCP precipitously [15]. In spite of this, ICRU-83 stated that the prescription is a scaling process similar to normalization in 3DCRT. Hence, one has to draw a line somewhere and ICRU decided that prescription point should be at D_{50}.

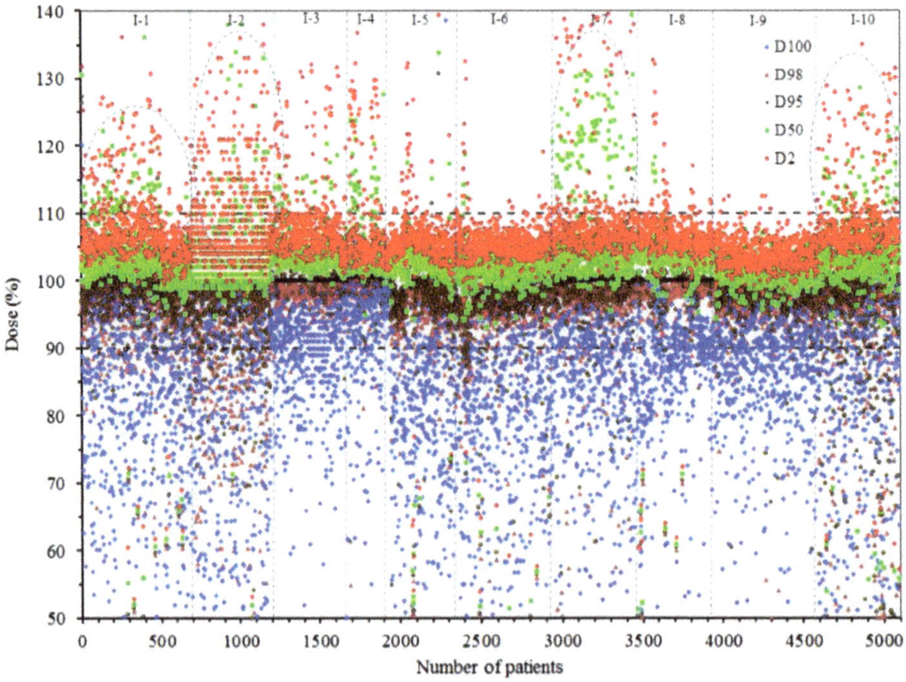

Figure 13.3. Prescription and recording dose from ten academic institutions for 5100 patients. Various dose parameters D_{100}, D_{98}, D_{95}, D_{50} and D_2 are plotted. Two lines with ±10% dose are also shown along with the 100% line where dose is presumed to be delivered. Adapted from Das *et al* [5] with permission from the American Society of Radiation Oncology.

As IMRT can be delivered in many ways (IMRT, VMAT, tomotherapy, and SBRT), it is good to know if one device is better than others in terms of dose prescriptions. This question was undertaken during a study conducted in a multi-institutional trial of IMRT compliance [5]. Figure 13.5 shows the findings with respect to IMRT parameters. IMRT and VMAT are nearly identical in terms of dose delivery to any one of these points. More uniformity is visible in tomotherapy and it seems better with respect to the shape of DVH, indicating a steeper curve reflective of a relatively small difference in dose parameters. On the other hand, greater variation is observed in SBRT; this is likely because of the small volumes and large gradients. It shows a wide variation and significant differences in dosimetric parameters. Such variability has also been alluded to by several investigators [16–18] who have emphasized the need for consensus in dose prescription.

13.4 Essentiality in IMRT

In general, the multicenter clinical trials provided mixed results due to the variability in many parameters but mostly due to non-compliance of the protocols. It is often noted that radiation therapy deviations are one of the most important factors in primary end-point evaluations amounting to 2/3 of the studies [19]. In these studies,

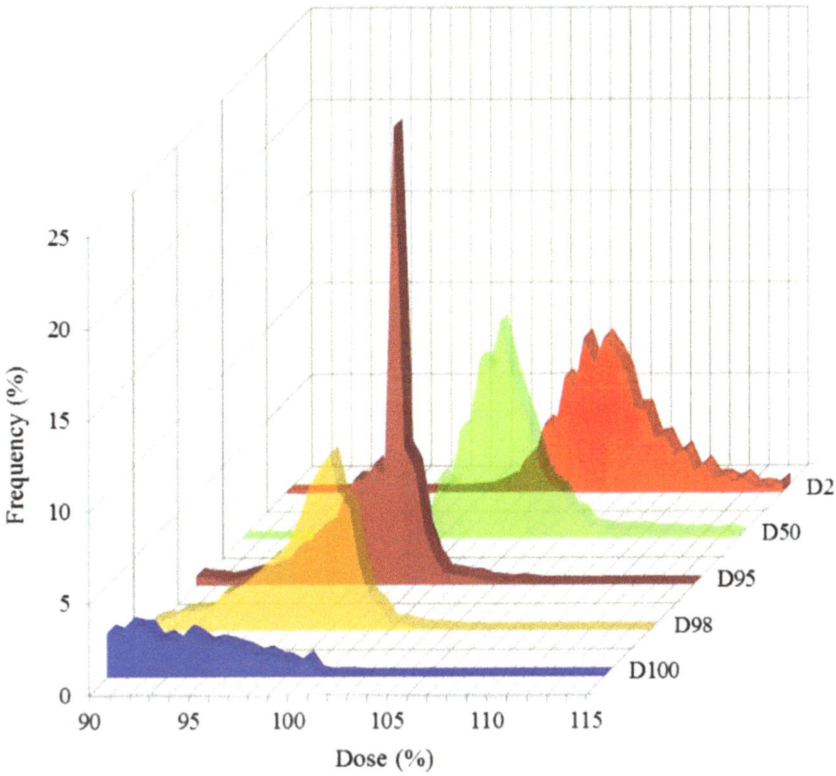

Figure 13.4. Frequency distribution of dosimetric parameters D_{100}, D_{98}, D_{95}, D_{50}, and D_2 in over 5000 patients. D_{100} a logically suitable choice is widely distributed whereas D_{95} seems to have a peak distribution centered at 100% with 97.1% ± 8.3% dose. The ICRU-83 recommended D_{50} peaks at around 103% (102.9% ± 9.4%) and much wider. Adapted from Das *et al* [5] with permission from the American Society for Radiation Oncology.

dose prescription is not one of the factors, but it is likely that deviation in dose (related to prescription) is one of the parameters. Compliance in a trial is a minimum requirement and even that cannot be met between 11.8% and 48% of the trials [20]. Moore *et al* [21] showed that better plans can be created in the majority of the cases even though they have met the criterion for clinical trials. Unlike 3DCRT where dose is fixed to a reference point that is typically the isocenter, in IMRT the dose is uncertain and not exact. It is an iterative process due to inverse planning and it takes a significant amount of time to achieve a plan of acceptable quality [22].

In IMRT, it is imperative that target volume and OAR should be drawn before the beginning of the planning process. Leaving aside the variability in delineation in target volumes, which has been discussed in chapter 7 of this book and by various groups [23–29], in each disease site a planner should try to create a plan with a step gradient such that the boundaries between various dose parameters (D_{100}, D_{95}, D_{50}, etc) start to become blurry. For a steep DVH, the differences in dosimetric

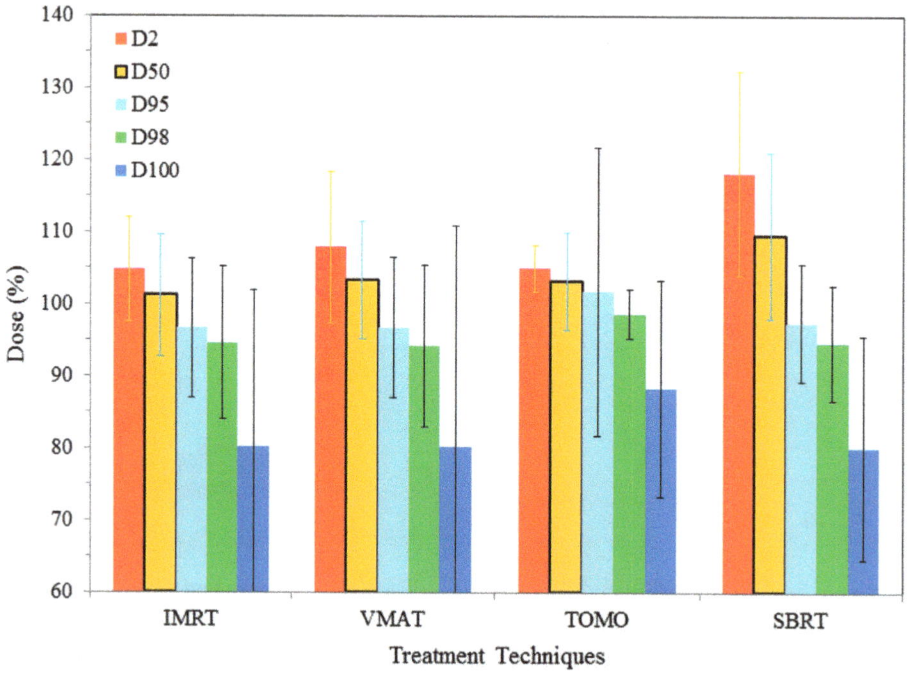

Figure 13.5. Variability in dose prescription parameters in different treatment modalities. Adapted from Das *et al* [5] with permission from the American Society for Radiation Oncology.

parameters are relatively small and one may not worry about the choice of prescriptions. In any case, the prescription must be uniform and should be uniquely qualified, so that the clinical outcomes can be compared between two institutions. The outcome without an identical dose prescription is a meaningless concept. If the planned DVH is steep, it can provide the best option for clinicians to deliver a higher dose to the target volume and reduce the dose to the OARs; this is the central theme of radiation treatment. Some other salient features are highlighted here:

- The target volume nomenclature should be clearly adapted, as has been proposed by various groups [5, 30, 31]. This will help compare clinical data from one institution to another without any interpretation.
- Reduce variability in the target volume delineation, which is a common theme from various papers [23, 24]. This is more of a chronic problem in radiation oncology that has been discussed in chapter 7 of this book.
- Acceptable criterion for DVH constraints can be found from Quantec [32] and documentation can be adapted from ASTRO guidelines [9].
- The dose prescription in PTV should be based on D_{50} as discussed in ICRU-83 [3].
- Clinical trials should emphasize the need for compliance because the criterion for most clinical trials are minimum goals and superior results can be achieved, as shown by Moore *et al* [21]. Also the protocol-compliance studies

provide superior overall survival, and likely contributes to the ability of collected data to answer the central trial question [19].

- There is no need for dose normalization, unlike in 3DCRT plans. Let inverse planning takes care as it should be incorporated in DVH constraints.

References

[1] ICRU Report 50 1993 *Prescribing, Recording, and Reporting Photon Beam Therapy* (Bethesda, MD: International Commission on Radiation Units and Measurements)

[2] ICRU 62 1999 *Prescribing, Recording and Reporting Photon Beam Therapy (Supplement to ICRU Report 50)* (Bethesda, MD: International Commission on Radiation Units and Measurements)

[3] ICRU Report 83 2010 *Prescribing, Recording, and Reporting Intensity-Modulated Photon-Beam Therapy (IMRT)(ICRU Report 83)* (Bethesda, MD: International Commission on Radiation Units and Measurements)

[4] Das I J, Cheng C W and Chopra K L *et al* 2008 Intensity-modulated radiation therapy dose prescription, recording and delivery: Patterns of variability among institutions and planning systems *J. Natl Cancer Inst.* **100** 300–7

[5] Das I J, Andersen A and Chen Z J *et al* 2017 State of dose prescription and compliance to international standard (ICRU-83) in intensity modulated radiation therapy among academic institutions *Pract. Radiat. Oncol.* **7** e145–55

[6] Almond P R, Biggs P J and Coursey B M *et al* 1999 AAPM's TG-51 protocol for clinical reference dosimetry of high-energy photon and electron beams *Med. Phys.* **26** 1847–70

[7] IAEA TRS 398 2000 Absorbed Dose Determination in External Beam Radiotherapy: An International Code of Practice for Dosimetry Based on Standards of Absorbed Dose to Water *Technical Reports Series No. 398* (Vienna, Austria: International Atomic Energy Agency)

[8] Ezzell G A, Burmeister J W and Dogan N *et al* 2009 IMRT commissioning: multiple institution planning and dosimetry comparisons, a report from AAPM Task Group 119 *Med. Phys.* **36** 5359–73

[9] IMRT Documentation Working Group, Holmes T and Das R *et al* 2009 American Society of Radiation Oncology recommendations for documenting intensity-modulated radiation therapy treatments *Int. J. Radiat. Oncol. Biol. Phys.* **74** 1311–8

[10] Drzymala R E, Mohan R and Brewster L *et al* 1991 Dose-volume histograms *Int. J. Radiat. Oncol. Biol. Phys.* **21** 71–8

[11] Niemierko A and Goitein M 1993 Implementation of a model for estimating tumor control probability for an inhomogeneously irradiated tumor *Radiother. Oncol.* **29** 140–7

[12] Yaparpalvi R, Hong L and Mah D *et al* 2008 ICRU reference dose in an era of intensity-modulated radiation therapy clinical trials: correlation with planning target volume mean dose and suitability for intensity-modulated radiation therapy dose prescription *Radiother. Oncol.* **89** 347–52

[13] Shepherd A, James S S and Rengan R 2018 The practicality of ICRU and considerations for future ICRU definitions *Semin. Radiat. Oncol.* **28** 201–6

[14] Tomé W A and Fowler J F 2002 On cold spots in tumor subvolumes *Med. Phys.* **29** 1590–8

[15] Goitein M and Niemierko A 1996 Intensity modulated therapy and inhomogeneous dose to the tumor: a note of caution *Int. J. Radiat. Oncol. Biol. Phys.* **36** 519–22

[16] Eaton D J, Naismith O F and Henry A M 2015 Need for consensus when prescribing stereotactic body radiation therapy for prostate cancer *Int. J. Radiat. Oncol. Biol. Phys.* **91** 239–41

[17] Esposito M, Maggi G and Marino C *et al* 2016 Multicentre treatment planning inter-comparison in a national context: the liver stereotactic ablative radiotherapy case *Phys. Med.* **32** 277–83

[18] Giglioli F R, Garibaldi C and Blanck O *et al* 2020 Dosimetric multicenter planning comparison studies for stereotactic body radiation therapy: methodology and future perspectives *Int. J. Radiat. Oncol. Biol. Phys.* **106** 403–12

[19] Fairchild A, Straube W and Laurie F *et al* 2013 Does quality of radiation therapy predict outcomes of multicenter cooperative group trials? A literature review *Int. J. Radiat. Oncol. Biol. Phys.* **87** 246–60

[20] Weber D C, Tomsej M and Melidis C *et al* 2012 QA makes a clinical trial stronger: evidence-based medicine in radiation therapy *Radiother. Oncol.* **105** 4–8

[21] Moore K L, Schmidt R and Moiseenko V *et al* 2015 Quantifying unnecessary normal tissue complication risks due to suuboptimal planning: a secondary study of RTOG 0126 *Int. J. Radiat. Oncol. Biol. Phys.* **92** 228–35

[22] Das I J, Moskvin V and Johnstone P A 2009 Analysis of treatment planning time among systems and planners for intensity-modulated radiation therapy *J. Am. Coll. Radiol.* **6** 514–7

[23] Hong T S, Bosch W R and Krishnan S *et al* 2014 Interobserver variability in target definition for hepatocellular carcinoma with and without portal vein thrombus: radiation therapy oncology group consensus guidelines *Int. J. Radiat. Oncol. Biol. Phys.* **89** 804–13

[24] Lim K, Erickson B and Jurgenliemk-Schulz I M *et al* 2015 Variability in clinical target volume delineation for intensity modulated radiation therapy in 3 challenging cervix cancer scenarios *Pract. Radiat. Oncol.* **5** e557–65

[25] Leunens G, Menten J and Weltens C *et al* 1993 Quality assessment of medical decision making in radiation oncology: variability in target volume delineation for brain tumors *Radiother. Oncol.* **28** 169–75

[26] Louie A V, Rodrigues G and Olsthoorn J *et al* 2010 Inter-observer and intra-observer reliability for lung cancer target volume delineation in the 4D-CT era *Radiother. Oncol.* **95** 166–71

[27] Caldwell C B, Mah K and Ung Y C *et al* 2001 Observer variation in contouring gross tumor volume in patients with poorly defined non-small-cell lung tumors on CT: the impact of 18FDG-hybrid PET fusion *Int. J. Radiat. Oncol. Biol. Phys.* **51** 923–31

[28] Weltens C, Menten J and Feron M *et al* 2001 Interobserver variations in gross tumor volume delineation of brain tumors on computed tomography and impact of magnetic resonance imaging *Radiother. Oncol.* **60** 49–59

[29] Fiorino C, Vavassori V and Sanguineti G *et al* 2002 Rectum contouring variability in patients treated for prostate cancer: impact on rectum dose-volume histograms and normal tissue complication probability *Radiother. Oncol.* **63** 249–55

[30] Bosch W R 2009 Uniform tissue names for use in RTOG advanced technology clinical trials http://atc.wustl.edu/resources/RTOG-ATIC/ATIC-ATC_Uniform_Tissue_Names.pdf

[31] Mayo C S, Moran J M and Bosch W *et al* 2018 American Association of Physicists in Medicine Task Group 263: standardizing nomenclatures in radiation oncology *Int. J. Radiat. Oncol. Biol. Phys.* **100** 1057–66

[32] Marks L B and Ten Haken R K 2010 K. MM Quantitative analyses of normal tissue effects in the clinic (QUANTEC) *Int. J. Radiat. Oncol. Biol. Phys.* **76** S1–60

IOP Publishing

Intensity Modulated Radiation Therapy
A clinical overview
Indra J Das, Nicholas J Sanfilippo, Antonella Fogliata and Luca Cozzi

Chapter 14

Tumors of the central nervous system

The primary audience of this textbook is the medical physicist. However, we believe it is imperative to provide clinical context of how IMRT is used and describe clinical data on it's efficacy. Accordingly, we have included the following chapters on the primary disease sites where IMRT is utilized. These chapters provide a general description of the epidemiology and clinical presentation of the disease and how each tumor is evaluated for treatment with radiation therapy. Anatomic considerations are then described since the basis of IMRT is maximizing tumor dose while sparing normal organs. Different tumors have different patterns of spread and, accordingly, can result in different toxicities, which are described in some detail. Finally, clinical trials, both retrospective and prospective, are reviewed so that the physicist may understand the degree of available evidence to justify the use of IMRT and quantify the benefit that it may confer.

14.1 Epidemiology

According to the Surveillance, Epidemiology and End Results Program (SEER) of the National Institutes of Health, there will be 23 770 new cases of primary central nervous system tumors in the United States [1]. Brain and other nervous system cancer is the tenth leading cause of cancer death and the number of deaths was 4.3 per 100 000 men and women per year based on 2009–2013 deaths. An evaluation of risk factors was conducted by the Brain Tumor Epidemiology Consortium [2]. Established risk factors include exposure to high-dose radiation and certain hereditary syndromes such as neurofibromatosis and von Hippel–Lindau disease. Increasing age and male versus female gender are risk factors for glioma while female gender is a risk factor for meningioma. Family history of a particular histologic tumor type is considered a probable risk factor. Environmental exposures such as filtered cigarette smoking, alcohol consumption, and diagnostic radiation, are probably not risk factors. The use of cellular telephones has been questioned as a contributing factor to brain tumor development. The World Health Organization

(WHO) previously classified radiofrequency electromagnetic fields, such as those emanated by cell phones, as a possibly carcinogenic to humans based on limited clinical evidence [3]. However, subsequently three large epidemiologic studies have examined the possible association between cell phone use and cancer. Interphone was a case-control study conducted by a team of researchers from 13 countries where questionnaires were filled out by study participants [4]. The Danish Study, a cohort study, linked billing information from more than 358 000 cell phone subscribers with brain tumor incidence data from the Danish Cancer Registry [5] and the Million Women Study [6], which was also a cohort study using questionnaires from participants in the United Kingdom. With long term follow-up, none of these studies showed a conclusive association between cell phone use and brain tumor development.

14.2 Anatomic considerations

The human nervous system is arranged in two parts: the central nervous system (CNS), which consists of the brain and the spinal cord, and the peripheral nervous system, which connects the central nervous system to the rest of the body. The central nervous system (CNS) is enveloped in three meningeal layers: the dura mater, arachnoid mater, and pia mater, as shown in figure 14.1.

Cerebrospinal fluid (CSF) is contained within the subarachnoid space between the pia and arachnoid layers. CSF surrounds the CNS and circulates within the ventricles and provides immunologic and mechanical protection. Further protection is provided by the skull and vertebral column. Some consider the retina and cranial nerves I (olfactory nerve) and II (optic nerve) part the CNS as they synapse directly with brain tissue [7]. CNS tissue on a cellular level is composed of white and gray matter, which is visible grossly and microscopically. White matter consists of axons and oligodendrocytes and gray matter consists of neurons and unmyelinated fibers and both contain glial cells which provide nutritional and metabolic support to the CNS.

CNS anatomy can be divided into distinct structures that are connected to provide appropriate function: the cerebrum, brain stem, cerebellum, diencephalon, and spinal cord, as illustrated in figure 14.2.

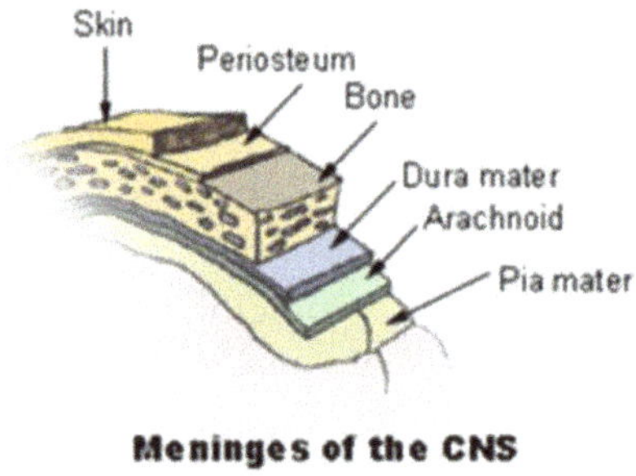

Figure 14.1. Meningeal layers. From: SEER Training Modules. Central Nervous System. U.S. National Institutes of Health, National Cancer Institute. https://training.seer.cancer.gov/anatomy/nervous/organization/cns.html.

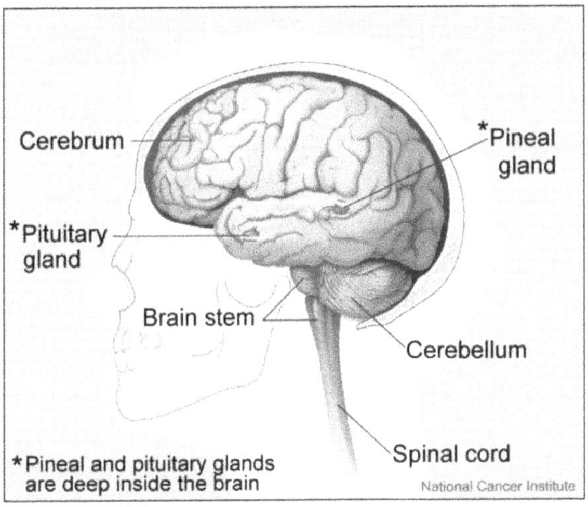

Figure 14.2. Anatomy of the brain, showing the cerebrum, cerebellum, brain stem, and other parts of the brain. From the National Cancer Institute, illustrated by Alan Hoofring.

The cerebrum, composed of two hemispheres, is the largest portion of the human brain. These are formed by the cortex, basal ganglia, amygdala and hippocampus and control a substantial number of brain functions including emotion, memory, perception and motor functions. The brain stem consists of the medulla, the pons, and the midbrain. The medulla is an extension of the spinal cord and has similar functions including control of respiration and blood pressure. Other nuclei also operate balance, taste, hearing and facial muscles. Rostral to the medulla is the pons, which transmits information between the cerebellum and the cerebral cortex. Nuclei in the dorsal pons operate breathing, sleep and taste. The midbrain is above and rostral to the pons, and connects different parts of the motor system including the cerebellum, the basal ganglia and cerebral hemispheres. Parts of the visual and auditory systems are located in the midbrain. The cerebellum is located behind the pons and consists of multiple fissures and lobes. Its chief function is in coordination of movement, but it also has a role in motor functions that have been learned through practice and is also involved in language and cognitive functions [8]. The diencephalon is the posterior portion of the forebrain and includes the epithalamus, thalamus, hypothalamus, and ventral thalamus and the third ventricle. The thalamus sorts out incoming information from the peripheral nervous system on its way to the cerebral hemispheres. The hypothalamus governs many primitive urges such as hunger, thirst and maternal bonding. This is regulated largely by secretion of hormones from the pituitary gland. In addition, the hypothalamus influences many behaviors of the individual. The spinal cord begins at the foramen magnum of the occipital bone and extends to approximately the second lumbar vertebrae. The main function of the spinal cord is to transmit neural signals between the brain and body, thus serving as a pathway from the brain to the peripheral nervous system. However, it also contains neural circuits that can independently control reflexes. Structurally, the spinal cord is divided into 31 segments with 31 corresponding pairs of spinal nerves: 8 cervical segments, 12 thoracic segments, 5 lumbar segments, 5 sacral segments, and 1 coccygeal segment.

14.3 Clinical and diagnostic evaluation

The presenting symptomatology of a primary CNS tumor can be generalized, such as seizure or headache, or focal, with a specific motor or sensory deficit corresponding to a location in the brain or spinal cord. A history and physical examination are critical as they can guide subsequent diagnostic tests. Magnetic resonance imaging (MRI) with gadolinium enhancement is typically the imaging modality of choice for most CNS tumors (figure 14.3). Systemic imaging such as computed tomography (CT) or positron emission tomography (PET) may also be utilized since a new presentation of a brain tumor often represents metastases from another location such as the lung, breast, or gastrointestinal tract. As with other solid tumors, a diagnosis is established by acquisition of tissue for pathologic analysis. This can be in the form of a biopsy or surgical resection, depending on the clinical situation.

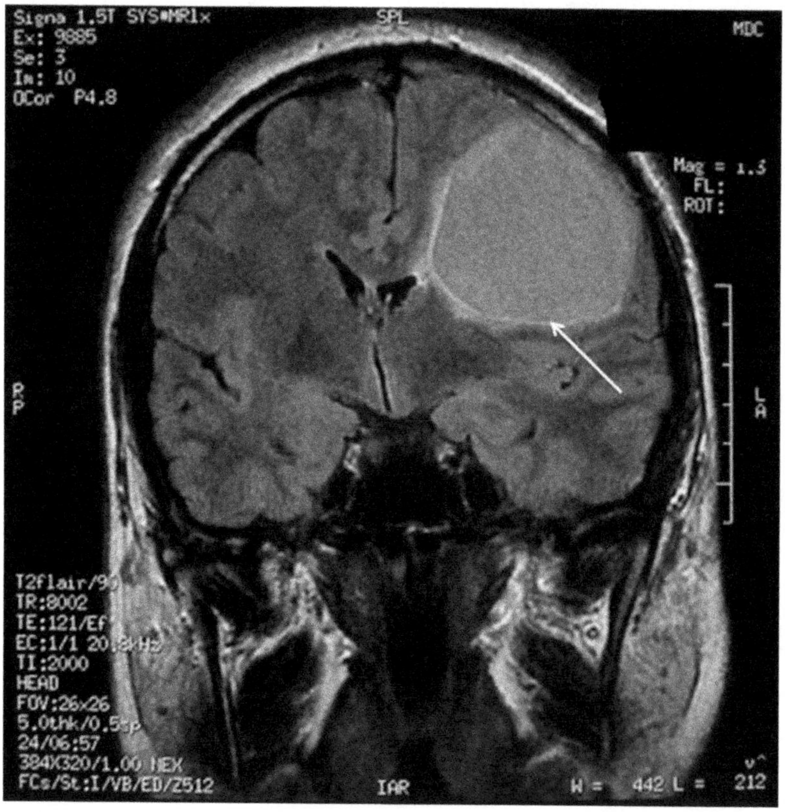

Figure 14.3. Preoperative MRI without enhancement demonstrating left frontal cystic tumor. From [9]. Open access CC BY 3.0.

14.4 Intensity modulated radiation therapy: biologic considerations

Radiation injury to the brain, and other tissues, depends on a number of factors including radiation dose, volume, fraction size, and the type of cell [10]. Some structures, such as the optic chiasm, hypothalamus, and lenses, are relatively more radiosensitive than brain tissue in the cerebrum or cerebellum. This must be taken into account during radiation therapy planning. The mechanism of these injuries is complex, but is believed to involve perturbations of small blood vessels, demyelination, and ultimately necrosis. The clinical manifestations of radiation injury have a highly variable time course from several weeks to months or even years and include motor or sensory deficits, lethargy, and neurocognitive deficiency [11]. The risk of severe radiation injury or 'radiation tolerance dose' (TD) has historically been expressed as the dose required to cause injury at a rate of 5% or 50% at five years or the TD 5/5 or TD 50/5, respectively, with TD 5/5 and 50/5 for whole brain radiation of 60 Gy and 70 Gy, respectively when given at 2 Gy per fraction [12]. Lawrence and colleagues conducted a systematic review of dose–volume effects of brain irradiation [13]. They found for fractionated RT with a fraction size of $<$2.5 Gy given daily, radiation necrosis can be predicted to occur at a rate of 5% and 10% at a biologically effective dose of 120 Gy (range, 100–140) and 150 Gy (range, 140–170), respectively. When twice-daily fractionation is employed, toxicity is substantially increased and necrosis can occur when the biologically effective dose exceeds 80 Gy. For large fraction sizes ($\geqslant$2.5 Gy), the incidence and severity of toxicity is unpredictable. For single-fraction radiosurgery, a correlation between the target size and the risk of adverse events is evident [14]. Cognitive dysfunction in children is often seen when whole brain doses exceed 18 Gy [15]. These dose–volume considerations must be taken into account when planning radiation therapy of any technique. IMRT, however, is even more grounded in dose–volume relationships since the treatment is planned by defining minimum dose to target volumes such as clinical target volume (CTV) and planning target volume (PTV) as well as dose limits to critical structures in close anatomic proximity.

14.5 Intensity modulated radiation therapy: technical considerations

Computed tomography planning and rigid immobilization are critical features of successful delivery of IMRT to patients with CNS tumors. In most cases, the head can be placed in a neutral position so that its major axes are parallel and perpendicular with the table and central axis beam. There are exceptions, however. Tumors of the pituitary gland are well suited to the head in a flexed position so as to avoid the eyes when using rotational techniques. The advent of IMRT may lessen the importance of meticulous head position since avoidance structures can be created with appropriate limitations in dose. However, the optimal dose distribution is achieved most efficiently when the head is properly positioned. Rigid immobilization using thermoplastic masks has been standard practice for decades. These devices have demonstrated reproducibility of 0–3 mm: Bichay and Mayville examined 560 images of five patients being treated for trigeminal neuralgia over a time of 24–64 min [16]. The mean absolute movement in each of longitudinal, lateral or vertical directions was approximately 0.3 mm for the duration of the treatment. The maximum displacement was in the longitudinal direction and reached 2.4 mm compared to the initial setup. The reliability of these devices have allowed clinicians to reduce PTV margins to minute distances, thereby reducing the radiation dose to normal brain. Generally each institution will have internal guidelines on the CTV to PTV margin in accordance with their equipment and experience.

The clinical target volume, while delineated on the planning CT scan with the patient immobilized, is based chiefly on the findings of the diagnostic MRI, which provides better resolution between tumor and normal brain and also shows edema more accurately. Modern software programs allow for co-registration of CT and MRI or PET scan so that contouring can be performed using the MRI on the CT planning workstation [17].

14.6 IMRT for CNS tumors: general considerations

There are numerous advantages of IMRT over more historical 3D planning which can be adapted to different clinical situations [18]. For example, in large tumors or those with complex shape, reasonable dose homogeneity can be achieved. Similarly tumors in locations where the body contour changes abruptly as in the cerebral convexities, can also be treated with relatively homogeneous dose without beam modifying devices or field junctions. Conversely, in clinical situations where inhomogeneity is desired, such as small lesions with roughly spherical shape, IMRT can be used to increase dose within the PTV or CTV, either within a single plan or with a simultaneous integrated boost when variable doses are desired for different anatomic volumes. In this fashion, two phased plans can often be converted to a single plan with a different daily dose to a corresponding target volume. Perhaps most importantly, however, IMRT planning can achieve steep dose gradients that permit dramatic dose escalation to tumors in close proximity to critical structures. As noted previously in this chapter, the brain and spinal cord have numerous anatomic components in close proximity to one another, all of which are critical for humans to function normally (figure 14.4). IMRT allows clinicians to treat aggressive tumors with high-dose radiation without conferring significant risk of neurologic side effects.

In order to create steep dose gradients with dose escalation in target volumes, it is obviously necessary to deliver low-dose radiation to relatively large volumes of normal brain. The precise clinical impact of this is unclear, but it may be of serious concern, particularly in children and young adults since late effects including second malignancy (SM) are more likely with increasing survival [19]. Clinical data on this question are sparse, but investigators have developed risk models to estimate SM after receiving RT using different techniques. Winkfield and colleageus estimated the risk of SM and other toxicities following fractionated RT of pituitary adenoma [20]. A standard case of a patient with a pituitary adenoma was planned using several techniques. Total dose was 50.4 Gy (GyE for proton beam therapy) at daily fractionation of 1.8 Gy (GyE). The excess risk of radiation-associated SM in the brain was calculated using the corresponding dose–volume histograms for the whole

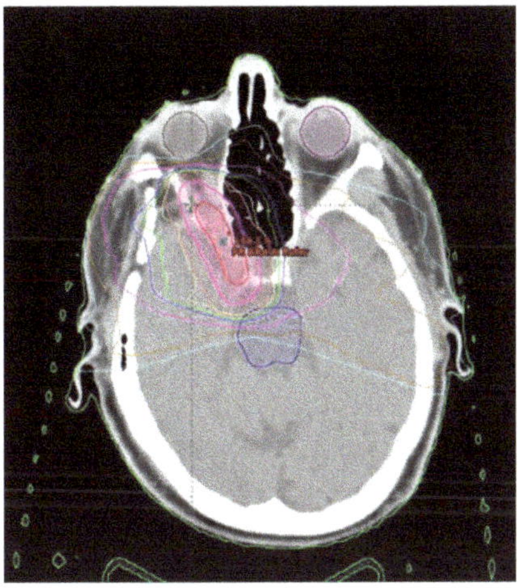

Figure 14.4. Optic nerve glioma treatment with IMRT to total dose 50.4 Gy (yellow isodose line). Note the steep dose gradients to keep the right eye dose less than 30% (blue isodose line). The GTV is noted in red. Courtesy of Joshua Silverman, M.D., Ph.D; New York University School of Medicine.

brain and based on the data published by the United Nation Scientific Committee on the Effects of Atomic Radiation (UNSCEAR) and a risk model proposed by Schneider [21]. Estimates of the excess number of second tumor cases per 10 000 patients per year were 9.8 for 2-field photons, 18.4 with 3-field photons, 20.4 with photon intensity modulated radiation therapy (IMRT), and 25 with photon stereotactic radiotherapy (SRT). Proton radiation resulted in substantially lower risk of SM. Two field plans carried of risk of 5.1, 3-field=12, 4-field=15, and 5-field=16. Temporal lobe toxicity was highest for the 2-field photon plan. Thus, a reduction of temporal lobe toxicity can be achieved with a greater number of fields or IMRT, but this comes at the expense of low-dose irradiation of higher tissue volume and higher risk of radiation-associated SM in this clinical situation. Different conclusions, however, have been reached by other investigators: Hermanto and associates conducted a dosimetric evaluation of 20 patients who received fractionated 3D conformal RT for high grade glioma with attention to the integral dose to normal brain [22]. Patient treatment programs were re-planned for IMRT and compared for target and normal tissue coverage, dose conformity, and normal tissue integral dose. In all 20 patients, IMRT maintained equivalent target coverage, improved target conformity (conformity index [CI] 95% 1.52 versus 1.38, $p < 0.001$), and enabled dose reductions of normal tissues. Mean and maximum brain stem dose were reduced by 19.8% and by 10.7%, respectively, and optic chiasm by 25.3% and 22.6%, respectively. Optic nerve doses were also reduced. More importantly, this was achieved with IMRT while reducing the total non-target integral dose by 7%–10%. Lorentini examined IMRT and 3D conformal plans in 17 patients with brain tumors who received 60 Gy in 30 fractions [23]. The cases were divided into four groups according to how many organs at risk (OAR) overlapped with the PTV: 0, 1, 2 or 3. Plans were compared for target coverage, OAR dose, and exposure to healthy brain tissue. IMRT always provided better target coverage (V95%) than 3DCRT, regardless the clinical group and the difference ranged from 0.82% when no PTV-OAR overlap existed to 7.8% for when PTV overlapped with three OAR. IMRT and 3D conformal RT achieved comparable results in terms of dose homogeneity and conformity and both techniques resulted in similar dose to OAR with a significant dose reduction to the healthy brain in favor of IMRT. The authors found that IMRT seems a superior technique compared to 3DCRT when there are multiple overlaps between OAR and PTV. In this scenario, IMRT allows for a better target coverage while maintaining equivalent OAR sparing and reducing healthy brain irradiation. Thus it appears that the low-dose exposure of normal brain when using IMRT does not always correspond to higher integral dose and those associated risks such as SM and there are clinical situations, such as tumors in close proximity to multiple dose limiting OAR, which can help the clinician select the most appropriate technique. In addition, long term consequences of IMRT are perhaps best analyzed by clinical data as opposed to mathematical estimates, and these will only be discovered as clinical studies mature.

14.7 Clinical experience of IMRT in brain tumors

There are numerous primary tumors of differing cell types that affect the brain. Gliomas, which arise from supporting cells of the nervous system, account for approximately 80% of primary brain tumors [24]. In 2007 the World Health Organization (WHO) categorized gliomas from grade I to grade IV based on pathologic features [25]. The incidence of high grade glioma (WHO grades II and IV) is approximately 5 per 100 000 person-years in Europe and North America and gliobalstoma multiforme (GBM) is the most common subtype [26]. In 2016, the WHO revised their system of classification, mainly to include molecular features in addition to histology in an effort to facilitate clinical and epidemiologic studies that will improve the outcome of these diseases [27].

The current standard of care for glioblastoma multiforme (GBM), is surgical resection followed by radiation therapy and Temazolaide [28]. Even though the addition of Temazolaimde, an oral alkylating agent, improved survival by 2.5 months, the two year progression-free survival is approximately 11% and most patients die of progressive local disease and associated neurologic complications. Given such poor results, increasing the radiation dose is a logical strategy to improve local tumor control and survival. Prior to the advent of IMRT, investigators at the University of Michigan performed a prospective trial in which the radiation dose was escalated to 90 Gy with conventional fractionated 3D conformal RT in which no significant toxicities occurred [29]. The Radiation Therapy Oncology Group conducted a Phase I study escalating dose from 66 to 84 Gy in 2 Gy [30]. Acute and late Grade 3–4 RT-related toxicities did not substantially increase with dose escalation, but neither did the local tumor control or overall survival. Early results of dose escalated IMRT have been encouraging [31]. In a study by Tsien and colleagues, 38 patients received IMRT to doses of 66 Gy to 81 Gy with concurrent daily Temozolomide followed by adjuvant cyclic Temozolomide. IMRT was delivered over 30 fractions (six weeks) even when doses were escalated. This method, termed hypofractionation, increases the biologically effective dose (BED) of radiation by increasing the fractional amount of radiation while maintaining the same number of treatment sessions. In addition to this theoretical advantage, hypofractionation can be more convenient for the patient since the overall treatment time is decreased or at least held constant. Radiation therapy planning was based on gadolinium-enhanced MRI. GTVs were defined as the residual gross tumor or resection cavity, based on the contrast-enhancing T1-weighted MRI and were expanded uniformly by 1.5 cm to form the CTV. CTV and GTV were expanded uniformly by 0.5 cm to generate PTV1 and PTV2, respectively. IMRT plans were generated to deliver 60 Gy in 30 fractions to PTV1 and a simultaneous higher dose (range, 66–81 Gy) to the smaller target, PTV2. T2/FLAIR signal abnormality was not targeted. The maximum dose limits to normal tissue organs at risk were defined as 60 bioGy to the optic nerves and chiasm, and brain stem was limited to 65 bioGy using alpha/beta ratio of 2.5. The investigators also obtained pretreatment (11)C methionone-positron emission tomography (MET-PET) scans to correlate sites of failure with metabolic activity on this specialized imaging study. Late grade ⩾III toxicity was observed at 78 Gy (two of seven patients) and 81 Gy (one of nine patients). None of 22 patients receiving 75 or less Gy developed radiation necrosis. Median overall survival and progression-free survival were 20.1 and 9.0 months, respectively, which were encouraging early results. Twenty-two of 32 patients with pretreatment MET-PET uptake showed uptake beyond the contrast-enhanced MRI and seven of eight patients with suboptimal PET GTV coverage recurred in locations outside the 95% isodose line, which the authors termed non-central failures. Only five of 20 patients with adequate PET GTV coverage developed non-central failures. When analyzed statistically, when treatments did not include the region of increased MET-PET uptake, a significantly increased rate of non-central failure occurred, suggesting the imaging limitations of MRI used alone may be partly responsible for high rates of local failure in GBM. The authors commented that higher doses to volumes of metabolically active regions on MET-PET imaging could further improve response to IMRT.

Chen and colleagues also investigated hypofractionated IMRT in patients with GBM, but with more dramatic dose intensity [32]. Sixteen patients underwent postoperative IMRT with concurrent and adjuvant Temazolamide. All patients received a total dose of 60 Gy to the surgical cavity and residual tumor with a 5 mm margin. Biologic dose intensification was achieved by escalating the daily fraction size from 3 Gy to 6 Gy per fraction in 1 Gy increments. Thus treatment time was reduced from four weeks (20 fractions) in the first group of patients to two weeks in the final group (10 fractions). IMRT with a simultaneous integrated boost was used to deliver a differential radiation dose to different targets. The GTV was defined as the contrast-enhancing residual tumor on the T1-weighted pre-RT brain MRI scan plus the entire surgical cavity. The CTV was defined as the T2-weighted abnormality on the brain MRI. Planning target volume 1 (PTV1) was defined as the GTV plus a 5 mm margin, and PTV2 was defined as the clinical tumor volume plus a 5 mm margin. The investigators optimized IMRT plans to ensure maximal dose conformity and rapid dose falloff toward critical structures. IMRT was delivered with 6 and/or 10 MV photons, using either multiple static beams or modulated dynamic arcs and the dose was prescribed to an isodose line that ensured that ⩾90% of the PTV1 and PTV2 received the prescribed doses. The inhomogeneity across PTV1 was not to be >15% of the prescribed dose. In the final dose group (60 Gy, 10 fractions, two weeks), the recommended maximal dose to the optic chiasm, optic nerves, and the retina of at least one eye was <30 Gy and to the brain stem was <35 Gy. The median survival was 16.2 months (range, 3–33 months). Four patients underwent repeat surgery for suspected tumor recurrence 6–12 months after IMRT and three of these had radio-necrosis. One patient experienced vision loss in the left eye seven months after IMRT. That patient had presented with a tumor in the left inferior frontal lobe and was treated at Level 2 with 60 Gy in 4 Gy/fraction. After treatment with corticosteroids and evaluation with imaging and ophthalmologic evaluation, it was determined that vision loss was caused by radiation-induced optic neuropathy. A review of the IMRT plan showed the maximal dose to the left optic nerve, right optic nerve, and optic chiasm had been 51.6 Gy (3.4 Gy/fraction), 49.2 Gy (3.3 Gy/fraction), and 45 Gy (3 Gy/fraction), respectively. The dose–volume histogram showed that 59% of the left optic nerve had received ⩾30 Gy, 34% ⩾35 Gy, 14% ⩾40 Gy, 3% ⩾45 Gy, and 0.5% ⩾50 Gy. The authors commented that since the study was small, no definitive conclusion could be made regarding the tolerance of those critical structures to hypofractionated RT with Temazolamide and while caution should be exercised for tumors in close proximity to the optic structures, the radiation dose limits should be considered in the clinical context. It may be reasonable to accept a greater risk of toxicity, including blindness, in patients with GBM because without aggressive RT almost all tumors will recur in these locations and result in the same morbidity, except in cases of tumor recurrence there is typically further progression and a fatal outcome.

Thus recent uses of IMRT for the management of brain tumors such as GBM include dose escalation and dose intensification with hypofractionated RT. Given the relatively recent widespread adoption of IMRT in brain tumor management, randomized controlled trials are lacking to show superiority of IMRT over 3D conformal RT, regardless of the fractionation program. A recent Cochrane database of systematic review examined radiation therapy dose escalation for high grade gliomas [33]. The study analyzed several questions that have analyzed the following four questions prospectively in 11 randomized trials: (1) Conventionally fractionated radiation therapy versus no radiation therapy. (2) Hypofractionated RT versus daily conventionally fractionated RT. (3) Hyperfractionated RT versus daily conventionally fractionated RT. (4) Accelerated RT versus daily conventionally fractionated RT. The investigators found that conventionally fractionated RT improved survival for adults with good performance status and HGG as compared to no postoperative RT. Hypofractionation had similar efficacy for survival as compared to conventional fractionation, particularly for individuals aged 60 and older with GBM. There was insufficient data regarding hyperfractionation versus conventionally fractionated RT and for accelerated radiation versus conventionally fractionated.

14.8 Clinical experience of IMRT in spinal and paraspinal tumors

Spinal and paraspinal tumors can generally be categorized as primary tumors, which are quite rare, and metastases, which are extremely common, affecting more than 100 000 patients per year in North America [34]. In either case, the clinical impact is profound, with symptoms that can include pain, motor weakness, paresthesias, and even urinary or bowel incontinence. Patients often have rapid deterioration of performance status and require high doses of narcotic pain medication. Still, there is no broad consensus on optimal management [35]. A single randomized trial was conducted comparing surgical decompression followed by RT versus RT alone in patients with high grade spinal cord compression [36]. The study found that patients in the surgical arm were significantly more likely to regain or retain their ability to walk compared to those treated exclusively with RT. However, for the great number of patients who do not have indications for surgery, such as those without neurologic deficits, or those who are not surgical candidates for medical reasons, RT remains the mainstay of therapy. In cases where radiation treatment must begin emergently, conventional parallel opposed portals are often still used for symptomatic palliation, but result in the anteriorly located normal tissues receiving essentially the same dose as the spine, as shown in figure 14.5.

More importantly, dose to tumor is limited by spinal cord tolerance, thus impacting local tumor control. A 3D technique for limiting spinal cord dose was described by Thambi in 1980 for treating patients with cancer of the thyroid [37]. This technique utilized a centrally blocked moving field which enabled the desired dose to be delivered to the primary, the lymph nodes and the cervical soft tissues while keeping the dose to the spinal cord to acceptable. Still, the dose to surrounding normal structures, including the larynx, could be quite high.

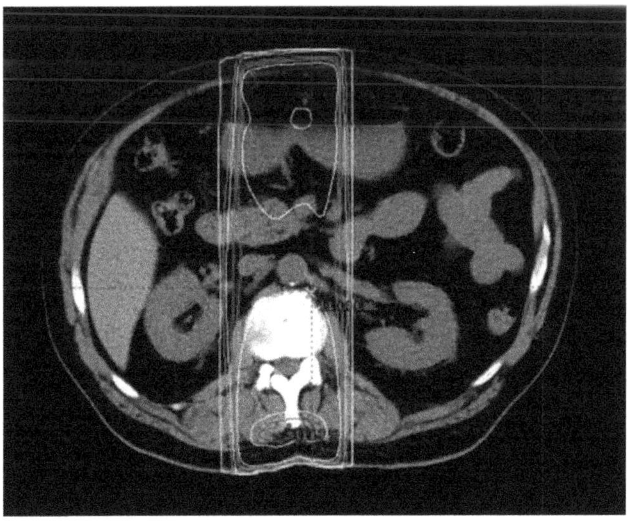

Figure 14.5. Treatment of lumbar spine with parallel opposed portals for relief of pain from spine metastases from prostate cancer. Total dose 30 Gy in 10 fractions. Yellow isodose line notes 100% and magenta line notes 95%. Courtesy of Nicholas Sanfilippo, MD; New York University School of Medicine.

These limitations in treatment planning encouraged investigators to utilize IMRT for spinal tumors. In an early investigation by Leibel at Memorial Sloane-Kettering Cancer Center, 16 paraspinal tumors were treated with IMRT [38]. The series included patients with both metastases and primary tumors. Tumor types varied but they were generally deemed to be radioresistant and/or already received RT to spinal cord tolerance. The most common primary tumors were chondrosarcomas and chordomas and metastases were from renal cell carcinomas and non-small cell lung carcinomas and lesions involved the cervical, thoracic, and lumbar regions. Treatment was accomplished using rigid immobilization with institutionally developed body frame devices. In patients who had prior surgical instrumentation, the metal hardware served as fiducial devices during patient setup. Radiation dose and fractionation varied according to the clinical situation. Patients with primary tumors who did not receive prior were treated with hyperfractionated RT in doses of 1.8 to 2.0 Gy in 33 to 38 fractions. In these cases, median tumor dose was 70 Gy and median maximum dose to the spinal cord was 44 Gy. Two patients who had previous irradiation (45 Gy in 25 fractions) for superior sulcus tumors of the lung were retreated after postoperative local recurrence with 20 Gy in five fractions. In these cases, the maximum spinal cord doses were 2.6 and 4.3 Gy. Patients with spine metastases were generally treated with hypofractionated RT in 4–10 fractions after having received prior palliative RT, usually with 30 Gy in ten fractions. In these cases, median tumor dose with IMRT was 20 Gy (range 20–30 Gy) with median spinal cord dose of 6 Gy. Clinical results were encouraging: In 15 patients who underwent serial post-treatment imaging, 13 had no further growth or a reduction in tumor size with median follow-up of 12 months (range, 2–23 mo). Two patients (one with thoracic chondrosarcoma and one with chordoma) showed tumor progression one year after IMRT. Pain relief was accomplished in 11 of 11 patients, and 4 of 4 patients had improvement in radiculopathy and/or plexopathy. Pain relief was durable in all patients except the two with tumor progression. No patient showed signs or symptoms of radiation-induced myelopathy, radiculopathy, or plexopathy, including 12 patients with a median follow-up of 18 months. These early data were clinically significant because prior to the advent of IMRT, precision in dose delivery for paraspinal was generally limited to proton beam therapy [39]. With IMRT and appropriate imaging and immobilization, patients could receive high-dose RT as initial treatment or be re-irradiated safely.

Perhaps the most common modern adaptation of IMRT in spinal and paraspinal tumors is stereotatic body radiation therapy (SBRT), which is defined by the National Cancer Institute as a type of external radiation therapy that uses special equipment to position a patient and precisely deliver radiation to tumors in the body (except the brain) [40]. Treatment is typically given over three to five fractions, although any number of fractions can be used. From a practical standpoint, SBRT can be thought of as short course hypofractionated RT with meticulous immobilization. In theory, techniques other than IMRT can be employed for SBRT, but IMRT offers the advantage of inverses planning with dose limitations to critical organs, and is therefore most commonly used. Figure 14.6 illustrates these principles in a case of spine SBRT.

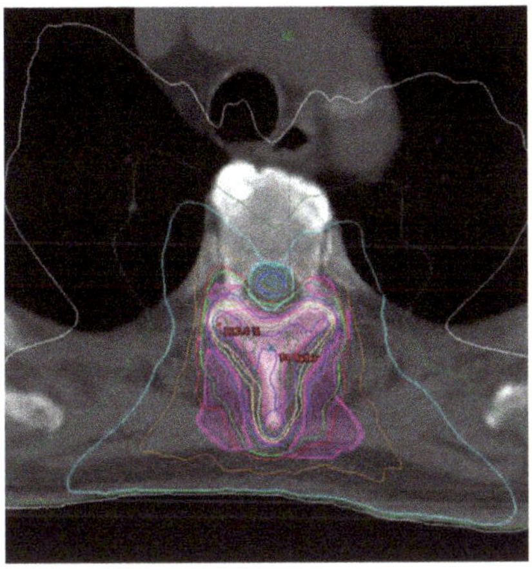

Figure 14.6. SBRT with IMRT in a patient with a history of prostate cancer and an isolated metastasis to the spinous process of T4. The dose delivered was 35 Gy in five fractions and the maximum dose to the spinal cord was 22.5 Gy. Courtesy of Nicholas Sanfilippo, MD; New York University School of Medicine.

Park and associates reported a series of 59 spinal metastatic lesions in 39 patients treated with SBRT using the CyberKnife [41]. Primary tumor sites for these patients were numerous, but 76% did not receive prior RT. Patients were treated with a median radiation dose of 27 Gy (range, 18–35 Gy) in a median of three fractions (range, one to five). With median follow-up period was 7.4 months, only 6.8% lesions demonstrated local progression. Two of four local progressions occurred in re-irradiated tumors after receiving 21 Gy in three fractions. The authors also examined clinical factors that were associated with superior outcome. They found better performance status the absence visceral metastases were associated with significantly improved treatment side specific survival, a measure of neurologic outcome. Better performance status was marginally related to improved overall survival ($p = 0.096$). Regarding complications, two patients developed vertebral compression fractures at 1.2 and 1.4 months after SBRT without evidence of tumor progression and there were no cases of myelopathy. The authors concluded that SBRT should be considered for those patients with a relatively indolent primary tumor, good performance status, and no visceral metastases.

Since SBRT has demonstrated the capacity to control gross paraspinal tumors, the clinical goal in these patients has shifted from mere palliation to durable local control, and SBRT has thus been increasingly utilized in the postoperative setting [42]. In addition, novel surgical techniques combined with SBRT are being developed, designed to minimize morbidity while achieving the traditional goals of stabilization and decompression with durable disease control [43]. The largest series to date by Laufer and colleagues reported on 186 patients treated by spinal decompression and postoperative IMRT either as single-fraction stereotactic radio-gurgery (SRS) (21%) or hypofractionated SBRT given either in high dose (24–30 Gy in three fractions) or low dose (18–38 Gy in 5–6 fractions) [44]. The CTV included gross tumor plus an expansion to account for microscopic disease. In cases of vertebral body lesions, the entire vertebral body was contoured as CTV. Local disease progression was seen in 18% of patients at a median of 4.8 months after IMRT. Patients who received the high-dose hypofractionated SBRT demonstrated one year local progression rates of less than 5%, which were superior to the results of low-dose hypofractionated SRS. The local progression rate after single-fraction SRS was also less than 10%. The authors concluded that patients with high grade spinal cord compression benefit from surgical decompression followed by high dose hypofractionated SBRT or single-fraction SRS. In addition, the long term control of SRS/SBRT favors more limited spinal surgery such as decompression and reconstitution of the CSF space as opposed to more extensive tumor resection.

Guidelines for target definition in spine SBRT were proposed by an International Spine Radiosurgery Constortium, which included radiation oncologists and spine surgeons [45]. The panel determined that the CTV should include abnormal marrow signal suspicious for microscopic invasion and an adjacent normal bony expansion to account for subclinical tumor spread in the marrow space. Preoperative and postoperative imaging should be considered as well as personal communication with the surgeon. No epidural CTV expansion is recommended without epidural disease. Circumferential or 'donut shaped' CTVs that surround the spinal cord should be used only when the vertebral body, bilateral pedicles/lamina, and spinous process are all involved or there is extensive metastatic disease along the circumference of the epidural space. Fusion of diagnostic MRI and treatment planning CT is critical for accurate delineation of tissue at risk. In cases where MRI or MRI-CT fusion is not possible, a CT-myelogram can be used for simulation. There is no consensus on PTV expansion, which likely varies from institution to institution, but a reasonable approach is to add a 1.5 to 2 mm geometric expansion without overlap onto the spinal cord. At present, the ideal dose and fractionation of spine SBRT is unclear. As noted above in the series by Laufer, higher dose per fraction SBRT may be associated with greater rates of local control as compared with lower doses per fraction [44]. Al-Omair reported similar findings: patients receiving 18 to 26 Gy in one to two fractions had better control rates than those receiving 18 to 40 Gy over three to five fractions [46]. Similarly, Puvanesarajah reported better pain outcomes in patients receiving a higher BED [47].

14.9 IMRT for craniospinal irradiation

Central nervous system (CNS) tumors are the most frequently occurring cancers in children and approximately 20% are medulloblastomas [48]. Patients with medulloblastoma are categorized into risk groups and associated treatment protocols. Standard-risk patients are above three years old, with no demonstrable disease outside of the posterior fossa, no post-resection residual tumor larger than 1.5 cm, and no microscopic craniospinal fluid disease [49]. Treatment for standard-risk patients is typically a combination of surgical resection and craniospinal irradiation (CSI), which delivers a dose of 23.4 Gy and *a posterior* fossa boost to a total dose of 54–55.8 Gy with concurrent weekly vincristine. This is followed by maintenance chemotherapy consisting of cisplatin, vincristine, and either cyclophosphamide or

Lomustine (CCNU) for eight cycles and results in progression-free survival rates of 75%–85% [50]. However, with increasing MB patient longevity, the prevalence of late adverse effects is increasing, including neurocognitive deficits, endocrine dysfunction, cardiac toxicity, loss of vision or hearing, and second malignancies [51]. IMRT has the advantage of selective sparing of normal organs, but sometimes at the expense of larger volumes of tissue receiving a low dose, as noted previously in this chapter. Parker and colleagues examined this question specifically for CSI [52]. They found IMRT was superior for PTV coverage and sparing organs at risk. For the heart and liver in particular, the IMRT plans provided considerable sparing in terms of V(10 Gy) and above. In terms of the integral dose, the IMRT plans were superior for liver and heart, but the 3D plan for the body contour. The competing risk that the authors considered most significantly was development of second malignancy due to irradiation of non-target tissue. Radiobiologists have discouraged the use of IMRT in pediatric patients specifically for this reason [53]. The authors commented that the increase in risk for a second cancer is fairly modest when comparing the potential benefits of critical structure sparing using the IMRT technique. Only further clinical investigation will determine if IMRT increases second cancer risk. As pediatric centers are increasingly using proton beam therapy with favorable outcomes, the long term side effects of IMRT may become less relevant [54]. A comparison of IMRT and proton plans for CSI is shown in figure 14.7.

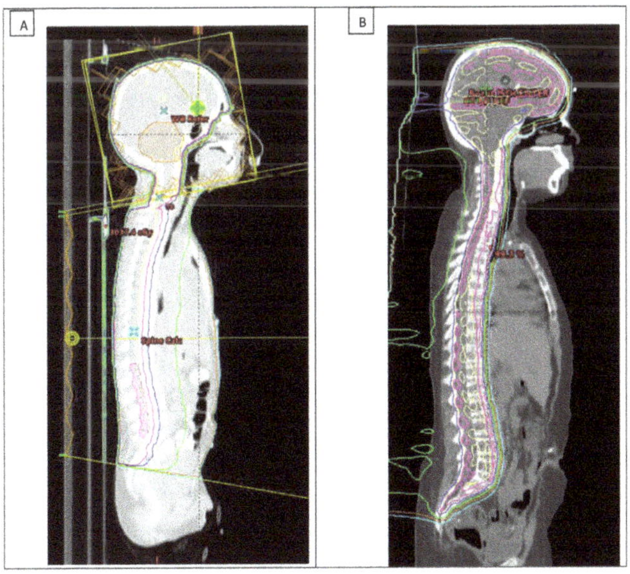

Figure 14.7. A. IMRT plan for CSI where IMRT is used with static posterior field to adjust depth dose and spare anterior organs. The prescription dose (100%) is noted by the yellow line. The green line represents the 70% isodose. B. Proton CSI plan: The 95% isodose line is noted in magenta and the blue line anteriorly represents the 30% isodose. Courtesy of Benjamin Cooper, MD; New York University School of Medicine.

References

[1] http://seer.cancer.gov/statfacts/html/brain.html

[2] Bondy M L *et al* 2008 Brain tumor epidemiology: consensus from the Brain Tumor Epidemiology Consortium *Cancer.* **113** 1953–68

[3] Baan R and Grosse Y *et al* 2011 Carcinogenicity of radiofrequency electromagnetic fields *Lancet Oncol* **12** 624–6

[4] Larjavaara S and Schüz J *et al* 2011 Location of gliomas in relation to mobile telephone use: a case-case and case-specular analysis *Am. J. Epidemiol.* **174** 2–11

[5] Frei P, Poulsen A H, Johansen C, Olsen J H, Steding-Jessen M and Schüz J 2011 Use of mobile phones and risk of brain tumours: update of Danish cohort study *Brit. Med. J.* **343** d6387

[6] Benson V S, Pirie K and Schüz J *et al* 2014 Authors' response to: the case of acoustic neuroma: comment on mobile phone use and risk of brain neoplasms and other cancers *Int. J. Epidemiol.* **43** 275

[7] Estomih Mtui M J 2011 Turlough FitzGerald, Gregory Gruener *Clinical Neuroanatomy and Neuroscience* 6th edn. (Edinburgh: Saunders) p 38

[8] Kandel E R and Schwartz J H 2012 *Principles of Neural Science* 5th edn (New York: McGraw Hill/Appleton & Lange) pp 338–43

[9] Rocka S *et al* 2019 Papillary glioneuronal tumor: a case report *Cureus* **11** e4215

[10] Gondi V and Vogelbaum M *et al* 2011 Primary intracranial neoplasms *Principles and Practice of Radiation Oncology* 6th edn (Philadelphia, PA: Lippincott Williams and Wilkins) p 655

[11] Spiegler B J, Kennedy K, Maze R, Greenberg M L, Weitzman S, Hitzler J K and Nathan P C 2006 Comparison of long-term neurocognitive outcomes in young children with acute lymphoblastic leukemia treated with cranial radiation or high-dose or very high-dose intravenous methotrexate *J. Clin. Oncol.* **24** 3858–64

[12] Emami B, Lyman J, Brown A, Coia L, Goitein M, Munzenrider J E, Shank B, Solin L J and Wesson M 1991 Tolerance of normal tissue to therapeutic irradiation *Int. J. Radiat. Oncol. Biol. Phys.* **21** 109–22

[13] Lawrence Y R, Li X A, el Naqa I, Hahn C A, Marks L B, Merchant T E and Dicker A P 2010 Radiation dose-volume effects in the brain *Int. J. Radiat. Oncol. Biol. Phys.* **76** S20–7

[14] Lax I and Karlsson B 1996 Prediction of complications in gamma knife radiosurgery of arteriovenous malformation *Acta. Oncol.* **35** 49–55

[15] Waber D P *et al* 2007 Neuropsychological outcomes from a randomized trial of triple intrathecal chemotherapy compared with 18 Gy cranial radiation as CNS treatment in acute lymphoblastic leukemia: findings from Dana-Farber Cancer Institute ALL Consortium Protocol 95-01 *J. Clin. Oncol.* **25** 4914–21

[16] Bichay T J and Mayville A 2016 The continuous assessment of cranial motion in thermoplastic masks during cyberknife radiosurgery for trigeminal neuralgia *Cureus.* **8** e607

[17] Paulino A C, Thorstad W L and Fox T 2003 Role of fusion in radiotherapy treatment planning *Semin. Nucl. Med.* **33** 238–43

[18] Burnet N G, Jena R, Burton K E, Tudor G S, Scaife J E, Harris F and Jefferies S J 2014 Clinical and practical considerations for the use of intensity-modulated radiotherapy and image guidance in neuro-oncology *Clin. Oncol. (R Coll. Radiol.)* **26** 395–406

[19] Neglia J P, Friedman D L, Yasui Y, Mertens A C, Hammond S, Stovall M, Donaldson S S, Meadows A T and Robison L L 2001 Second malignant neoplasms in five-year survivors of childhood cancer: childhood cancer survivor study *J. Natl. Cancer Inst.* **93** 618–29

[20] Winkfield K M, Niemierko A, Bussiere M R, Crowley E M, Napolitano B N, Beaudette K P, Loeffler J S and Shih H A 2011 Modeling intracranial second tumor risk and estimates of clinical toxicity with various radiation therapy techniques for patients with pituitary adenoma *Technol. Cancer Res. Treat.* **10** 243–51

[21] Schneider U, Zwahlen D, Ross D and Kaser-Hotz B 2005 Estimation of radiation-induced cancer from three-dimensional dose distributions: Concept of organ equivalent dose *Int. J. Radiat. Oncol. Biol. Phys.* **61** 1510–5

[22] Hermanto U, Frija E K, Lii M J, Chang E L, Mahajan A and Woo S Y 2007 Intensity-modulated radiotherapy (IMRT) and conventional three-dimensional conformal radiotherapy for high-grade gliomas: does IMRT increase the integral dose to normal brain? *Int. J. Radiat. Oncol. Biol. Phys.* **67** 1135–44

[23] Lorentini S, Amelio D, Giri M G, Fellin F, Meliado G, Rizzotti A, Amichetti M and Schwarz M 2013 IMRT or 3D-CRT in glioblastoma? A dosimetric criterion for patient selection *Technol. Cancer Res. Treat.* **12** 411–20

[24] Schwartzbaum J A, Fisher J L, Aldape K D and Wrensch M 2006 Epidemiology and molecular pathology of glioma *Nat. Clin. Pract. Neurol.* **2** 494–503

[25] Louis D N, Ohgaki H, Wiestler O D, Cavenee W K, Burger P C, Jouvet A, Scheithauer B W and Kleihues P 2007 The 2007 WHO classification of tumours of the central nervous system *Acta Neuropathol.* **114** 97–109

[26] Narayanan V, Patel K and Price S 2012 High grade gliomas: pathogenesis, management and prognosis *Adv. Clin. Neurosci. Rehab.* **12** 23–9

[27] Louis D N, Perry A, Reifenberger G, von Deimling A, Figarella-Branger D, Cavenee W K, Ohgaki H, Wiestler O D, Kleihues P and Ellison D W 2016 The 2016 World Health Organization Classification of Tumors of the Central Nervous System: a summary *Acta Neuropathol.* **131** 803–20

[28] Stupp R, Hegi M E and Mason W P *et al* 2009 Effects of radiotherapy with concomitant and adjuvant TMZ versus radiotherapy alone on survival in glioblastoma in a randomised phase III study: 5-Year analysis of the EORTC-NCIC trial *Lancet Oncol.* **10** 459–66

[29] Chan J L, Lee S W and Fraass B A *et al* 2002 Survival and failure patterns of high-grade gliomas after three-dimensional conformal radiotherapy *J. Clin. Oncol.* **20** a635–42

[30] Tsien C, Moughan J and Michalski J M *et al* 2009 Phase I three-dimensional conformal radiation dose escalation study in newly diagnosed glioblastoma: Radiation Therapy Oncology Group trial 98-03 *Int. J. Radiat. Oncol. Biol. Phys.* **73** 699–708

[31] Tsien C I *et al* 2012 Concurrent temozolomide and dose-escalated intensity-modulated radiation therapy in newly diagnosed glioblastoma *Clin. Cancer Res.* **18** 273–9

[32] Chen C, Damek D, Gaspar L E, Waziri A, Lillehei K, Kleinschmidt-DeMasters B K, Robischon M, Stuhr K, Rusthoven K E and Kavanagh B D 2011 Phase I trial of hypofractionated intensity-modulated radiotherapy with temozolomide chemotherapy for patients with newly diagnosed glioblastoma multiforme *Int. J. Radiat. Oncol. Biol. Phys.* **81** 1066–74

[33] Khan L, Soliman H, Sahgal A, Perry J, Xu W and Tsao M N 2016 External beam radiation dose escalation for high grade glioma *Cochrane Database Syst. Rev.* **8** CD011475

[34] Gokaslan Z L, York J E, Walsh G E, McCutcheon I E, Lang F F, Putnam J B, Wildrick D M, Swisher S G, Abi-Said D and Sawaya R 1998 Transthoracic vertebrectomy for metastatic spinal tumors *J. Neurosurg.* **89** 599–609

[35] Yamada Y, Lovelock D M and Bilsky M H 2007 A review of image-guided intensity-modulated radiotherapy for spinal tumors *Neurosurgery.* **61** 226–35

[36] Patchell R A, Tibbs P A, Regine W F, Payne R, Saris S, Kryscop R J, Mohiuddin M and Young B 2005 Direct decompressive surgical resection in the treatment of spinal cord compression caused by metastatic cancer: a randomised trial *Lancet* **366** 643–8

[37] Thambi V, Pedapatti P J, Murthy A and Kartha P K 1980 A radiotherapy technique for thyroid cancer *Int. J. Radiat. Oncol. Biol. Phys.* **6** 239–43

[38] Bilsky M H, Yamada Y, Yenice K M, Lovelock M, Hunt M, Gutin P H and Leibel S A 2004 Intensity-modulated stereotactic radiotherapy of paraspinal tumors: a preliminary report *Neurosurgery.* **54** 823–30

[39] Isacsson U, Hagberg H, Johansson K A, Montelius A, Jung B and Glimelius B 1997 Potential advantages of protons over conventional radiation beams for paraspinal tumours *Radiother. Oncol.* **45** 63–70

[40] http://cancer.gov/publications/dictionaries/cancer-terms?cdrid=386233

[41] Park H J, Kim H J, Won J H, Lee S C and Chang A R 2015 Stereotactic Body Radiotherapy (SBRT) for spinal metastases: who will benefit the most from SBRT? *Technol. Cancer Res. Treat.* **14** 159–67

[42] Sahgal A, Larson D A and Chang E L 2008 Stereotactic body radiosurgery for spinal metastases: a critical review *Int. J. Radiat. Oncol. Biol. Phys.* **71** 652–65

[43] Redmond K J, Lo S S, Fisher C and Sahgal A 2016 Postoperative Stereotactic Body Radiation Therapy (SBRT) for spine metastases: a critical review to guide practice *Int. J. Radiat. Oncol. Biol. Phys.* **95** 1414–28

[44] Laufer I, Iorgulescu J B and Chapman T *et al* 2013 Local disease control for spinal metastases following 'separation surgery' and adjuvant hypofractionated or high-dose single-fraction stereotactic radiosurgery: outcome analysis in 186 patients *J. Neurosurg. Spine* **18** 207–14

[45] Cox B W, Spratt D E and Lovelock M *et al* 2012 International Spine Radiosurgery Consortium consensus guidelines for target volume definition in spinal stereotactic radiosurgery *Int. J. Radiat. Oncol. Biol. Phys.* **83** 597–605

[46] Al-Omair A, Masucci L and Masson-Cote L *et al* 2013 Surgical resection of epidural disease improves local control following postoperative spine stereotactic body radiotherapy *Neuro. Oncol.* **15** 1413–9

[47] Puvanesarajah V, Lo S L and Aygun N *et al* 2015 Prognostic factors associated with pain palliation after spine stereotactic body radiation therapy *J. Neurosurg. Spine* **23** 1–10

[48] Lannering B, Sandstrom P E and Holm S *et al* 2009 Classification, incidence and survival analyses of children with CNS tumours diagnosed in Sweden 1984-2005 *Acta Paediatr.* **98** 1620–7

[49] von Hoff K, Hinkes B and Gerber N U *et al* 2009 Long-term outcome and clinical prognostic factors in children with medulloblastoma treated in the prospective randomised multicentre trial HIT'91 *Eur. J. Cancer* **45** 1209–17

[50] Packer R J, Gajjar A and Vezina G *et al* 2006 Phase III study of craniospinal radiation therapy followed by adjuvant chemotherapy for newly diagnosed average-risk medulloblastoma *J. Clin. Oncol.* **24** 4202–8

[51] Packer R J, Zhou T and Holmes E *et al* 2013 Survival and secondary tumors in children with medulloblastoma receiving radiotherapy and adjuvant chemotherapy: results of Children's Oncology Group trial A9961 *Neuro. Oncol.* **15** 97–103

[52] Parker W, Filion E, Roberge D and Freeman C R 2007 Intensity-modulated radiotherapy for craniospinal irradiation: target volume considerations, dose constraints, and competing risks *Int. J. Radiat. Oncol. Biol. Phys.* **69** 251–7

[53] Hall E J 2006 Intensity-modulated radiation therapy, protons, and the risk of second cancers *Int. J. Radiat. Oncol. Biol. Phys.* **65** 1–7

[54] Yock T I *et al* 2016 Long-term toxic effects of proton radiotherapy for pediatric medulloblastoma: a phase 2 single-arm study *Lancet Oncol.* **17** 287–98

Indra J Das, Nicholas J Sanfilippo, Antonella Fogliata and Luca Cozzi

Chapter 15

Head and neck cancer

15.1 Epidemiology

Cancers of the head and neck account for 3% of all malignancies in the United States with approximately 62 000 new cases and 13 000 deaths [1]. There are approximately 500 000 cases worldwide with males affected more than females in most countries [2]. According to the Surveillance, Epidemiology, and End Results (SEER) Program, overall mortality rates for head and neck cancers in the United States have declined since 2001 and the incidence of head and neck cancers in African Americans has declined over the past two decades and is now lower than that in whites [3]. The mortality rate also has decreased among African Americans but is still higher than that in whites. Tobacco use is probably the most important risk factor for head and neck cancer development with heavy smokers having a greater than 5-fold increased risk of cancer compared with non-smokers [4]. There also appears to be a relationship between quantity of tobacco use and head and neck cancer development. In a case control study by Andre, individuals who smoked more than one pack of cigarettes per day had a 13-fold increase in risk of head and neck cancer [5]. The age of smoking onset (under 18 years of age) and duration of smoking (over 35 years) were high-risk factors while stopping smoking reduced risk, but only for those who smoked less than seven cigarettes per day. Other tobacco products, such as chewing tobacco and snuff, associated with an increased risk of cancer of the oral cavity and pharynx [6]. Alcohol consumption is another independent risk factor, although its influence is difficult to separate from that of tobacco since both are often present in the same individuals [7]. Investigators have found that tobacco smoking appears to have an interactive and multiplicative effect on the risk of developing head and neck cancer [8].

Viral infections are also risk factors for head and neck cancer. Human papilloma virus, primarily type 16, is associated with cancers of the base of the tongue and the tonsils and is generally seen in younger men who are not tobacco and alcohol users [9]. The Epstein–Barr virus plays a causal role in nasopharyngeal cancer as evidenced by

doi:10.1088/978-0-7503-1335-3ch15

EBV DNA detection in tumor cells and expression of EBV-dependent proteins [10]. Immunodeficiency also increases risk of head and neck cancer: in a series of 2817 organ transplant patients, 175 developed 391 head and neck malignancies [11]. Most, however, were cutaneous tumors, with 51% being squamous cell carcinoma and 42% basal cell carcinomas. An additional 2% were papillary thyroid cancer, 1% squamous cell carcinoma of the tongue, and 3% miscellaneous mucosal sites including larynx, oral cavity, nasal cavity, oropharynx, nasopharynx, and salivary duct. There is also a 2–3-fold increase in the incidence of squamous cell carcinoma of the head and neck (and other cancers) for individuals infected with human immunodeficiency virus (HIV) [12].

15.2 Anatomy

Anatomy of the head and neck is complex and a detailed description is beyond the scope of this text. Generally, cancers of the head and neck are classified into a number of anatomic sites including the oral cavity, larynx, pharynx, salivary glands, nasal cavity, paranasal sinuses, orbit, and the ear. Some of these sites can be further divided into subsites. The pharynx, for example, consists of the nasopharynx, oropharynx, and hypopharynx and the larynx includes the supraglottis, glottis, and subglottis. Lymph node stations in the neck have historically been described in different ways. A general schematic of head and neck sites is illustrated in figure 15.1.

However, a consensus statement from the American Head and Neck Society and American Academy of Otolaryngology-Head and Neck Surgery has recommended they be grouped into six numerical levels, illustrated in figure 15.2: Level I, submental and submandibular group; Level II, upper jugular group; Level III,

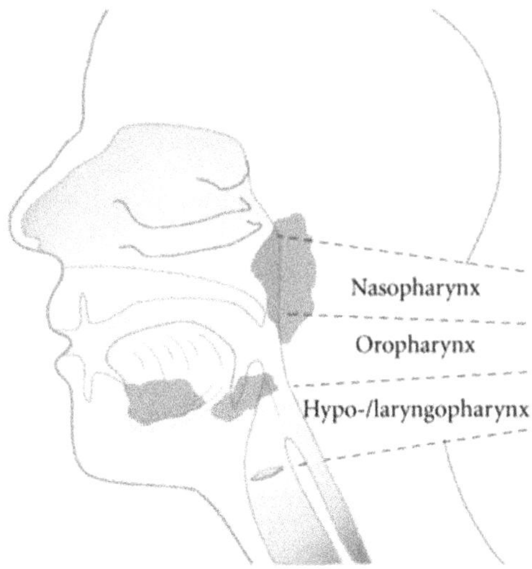

Figure 15.1. Schematic anatomy of the head and neck region. Reproduced from [13], copyright Shirley K Knauer. Open access CC BY 3.0.

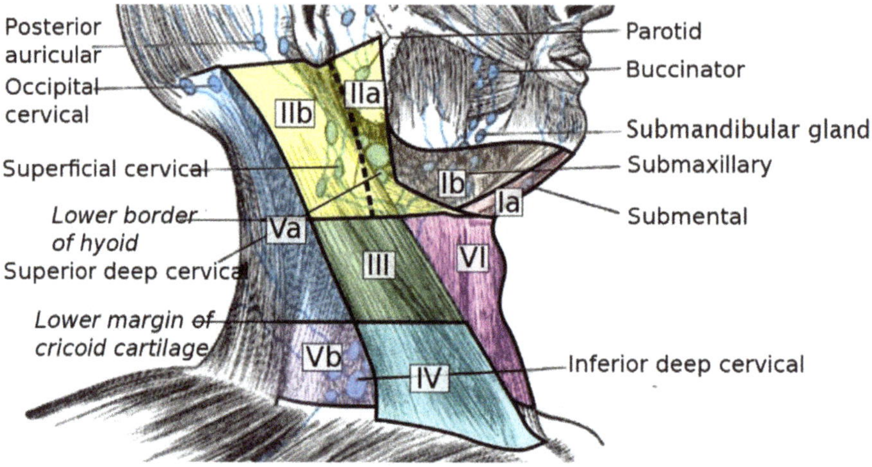

Figure 15.2. Topography of the cervical lymph node regions with description of the neck muscles relevant for the classification. In the preauricular region the parotid gland and in level I the submandibular gland is revealed. The accessory nerve delineates the limit between the levels IIA and B and is part of the level V. This image has been obtained from the Wikimedia website [https://commons.wikimedia.org/wiki/File:Cervical_lymph_nodes_and_levels.svg], where it is stated to have been released into the public domain. It is included within this article on that basis.

middle jugular group; Level IV, lower jugular group; Level V, posterior triangle group; Level VI, anterior compartment [14].

These levels provide an important frame of reference both for surgeons when performing neck dissections and radiation oncologists when defining target volumes. Retropharyngeal nodes, which are located just anterior to the cervical vertebral bodies and can be found as low as T4, are not included in this numerical system, but are nonetheless important for the radiation oncologist in certain disease sites.

15.3 Nasopharyngeal carcinoma: general considerations

The nasoparhynx is bounded superiorly by the skull base (cribiform plate and sphenoid sinus), inferiorly by the space posterior to the soft palate, laterally by the Eustachian tube opening and the Fossa of Rosenmuller, posteriorly by the mucosa overlying the first and second vertebral bodies, and anteriorly by the opening to the nasal cavity. Nasopharynx tumors have a variety of pathways of spread including direct local invasion and along the cranial nerves that traverse the cavernous sinus (II, IV, V1, V2, and VI), which must be accounted for in radiation treatment planning [15]. In addition, the nasopharynx has a rich bilateral lymphatic network, and studies have shown that approximately 85% of patients present with clinical lymphadenopathy [16]. Ho and colleagues found that the most commonly involved regions include retropharyngeal (69%) and level II lymph nodes (70%) [17]. The overall probability of levels III, IV, and V nodal involvement are 45%, 11%, and 27%, respectively. Low-risk node groups included the supraclavicular, levels IA/IB and VI nodes, and parotid nodes with involvement rates at 3%, 0%, 3%, 0%, and 1%, respectively. Nodal metastases followed an orderly pattern and the probability of skip metastasis between levels varied between 0.5%–7.9%.

Pre treatment clinical evaluation of patients with nasopharyngeal carcinoma (NPC) includes a thorough history and attention to nationality since the tumor is common in southern China and southeast Asia [18]. Physical examination should include neck lymph nodes, a neurologic exam since cranial nerves can be affected, and fiber-optic nasolaryngoscopy for assessment of primary tumor extent. As with almost all cancers, diagnosis is made by biopsy which can usually be performed in an office with local anesthetic. Pathologically, these tumors have been classified into four subtypes by the World Health Organization: Type 1 (keratinizing carcinoma), type 2.1 (non-keratinizing differentiated carcinoma, type 2.2 non-keratinizing undifferentiated carcinoma, and type 3 (basaloid squamous cell carcinoma [19]. These have some epidemiologic and prognostic significance. Tumors in the Asian population are approximately 90% types 2–3 but much lower in Western nations [20]. Type 3 tumors also tend to have more favorable prognosis [21]. Disease extent is evaluated by a number of diagnostic imaging studies. Magnetic resonance imaging (MRI) is the preferred study for assessment of local disease as it is more sensitive in detecting bony involvement of the skull base, specifically the petrous apex, clivus and the sphenoid wing [22]. An example of locally advanced nasopharyngeal cancer is illustrated in figure 15.3].

Evaluation of systemic metastases is commonly done with positron emission tomography (PET), in which radioactive glucose is injected intravenously and selectively taken up by metabolically active tumor cells. PET scan, which is often performed concurrently with CT (PET-CT) has the advantage of providing a full

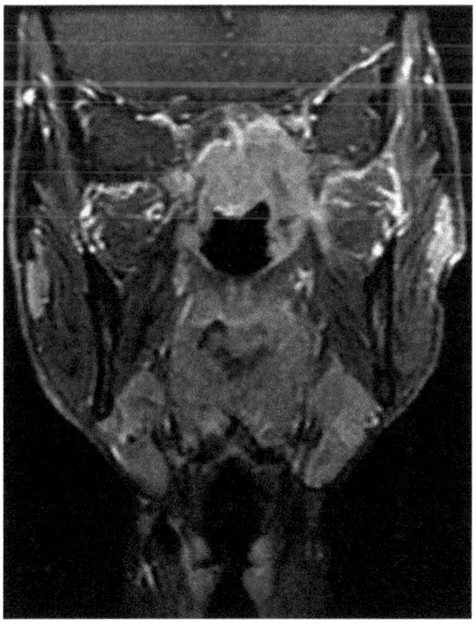

Figure 15.3. Image of tumor invasion into the sphenoid sinus in patient with NPC. A contrast enhanced coronal T1-weighted MR image revealed that the primary nasopharyngeal lesion invaded into the sphenoid sinus and that the floor of the sphenoid sinus was destroyed. Reproduced from [23]. Copyright 2014 Tian *et al.* Open access CC BY 4.0.

body study (except brain) in one procedure. Blood chemistries are also part of the standard pre-treatment workup to evaluate fitness for cancer treatment. These include renal and liver function tests, a complete blood count with differential, and a test to check for antibodies to the Epstein–Barr virus. Lastly, since treatment can affect dentition or hearing, a dental evaluation and hearing test should be done.

The current standard of care for nasopharyngeal carcinoma is typically combined RT and chemotherapy (RCT). Surgery is rarely done due to the difficult approach, proximity of critical structures, and difficulty in obtaining negative margins [24]. In selected patients with limited primary tumors and no neck disease, RT alone may be sufficient. However, since lymphadenopathy in the neck is a common presenting symptom, most patients will benefit from the addition of chemotherapy, which was established in a landmark study by Al-Sarraf [25]. In this trial, 147 patients were randomly assigned to receive RT alone (70 Gy in 35–39 fractions) or the same RT plus cisplatin (100 mg m^{-2} on days 1, 22, and 43) during RT and three courses of cisplatin (80 mg m^{-2}) and 5-fluorouracil (1000 mg m^{-2} d^{-1} days 1–4) every four weeks. The median progression-free survival (PFS) time was 15 months for eligible patients on the radiotherapy arm and was not reached for the CRT group. The three year PFS rate was significantly improved in the CRT group (24% versus 69%) and the median survival time was 34 months for the RT group and not reached for the CRT group. Most importantly, the three year survival rate was 47% versus 78%, which reached statistical significance. The authors concluded that CRT was superior to RT alone in patients with locally advanced nasopharyngeal carcinoma. While CRT is now the widely established standard for nasopharyngeal carcinoma, the role of chemotherapy after CRT is the subject of some debate. Chen and colleagues conducted a study where 308 patients were randomized to CRT alone or CRT followed by adjuvant chemotherapy and found no difference in survival outcomes [26]. However, since median follow-up was only 38 months this regimen has not been widely adopted as a new standard. Other strategies, particularly for high-risk patients, include induction chemotherapy followed by CRT. These have shown promising early results and are the subject of ongoing investigation [27].

15.4 IMRT for nasopharyngeal carcinoma

Due to the complex anatomy of the neck and skull base, management of nasopharyngeal carcinoma illustrates, perhaps better than any other tumor sites, how advances in radiation therapy such as IMRT can improve clinical care. Structures including the brain, brainstem, spinal cord, pituitary gland, optic nerve, optic chiasm, eyes, cochlea, salivary glands, and larynx must all be considered in treatment planning. As most of these structures are in close proximity to one another, rigid immobilization is required and accomplished with a heat-moldable thermoplastic mask at simulation. This is comparable to how brain tumor simulation is performed. Since the neck is essentially always irradiated for clinical or subclinical lymphadenopathy, the immobilization device must include either shoulder retractors or extended thermoplastic to cover the low neck and superior aspect of the shoulders. Both of these systems are commercially available. CT simulation is performed using thin cuts (less than 5 mm) from the

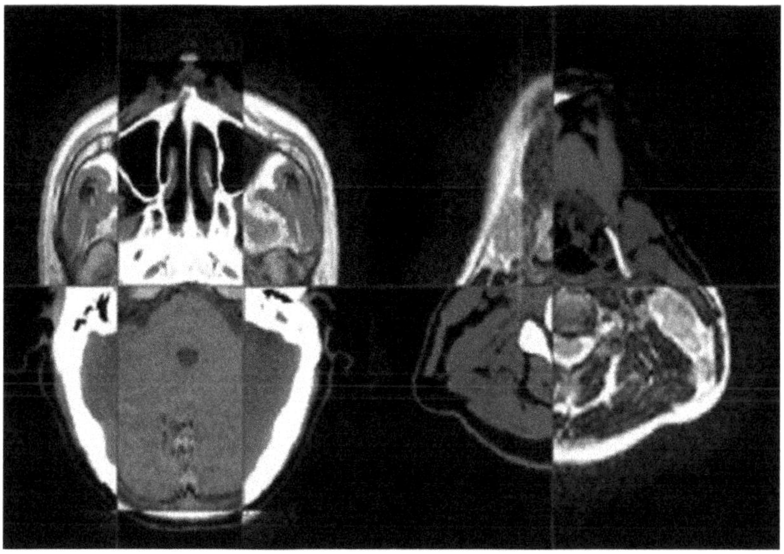

Figure 15.4. Successful fusion of MRI onto the CT planning images for IMRT, obtained by performing the MRI scan with the patient inside the radiotherapy cast. From [28]. Copyright 2007 International Cancer Imaging Society. Open access CC BY 4.0.

vertex through the upper mediastinum. Iodinated contrast may be used, but in any case co-registration of the planning CT and diagnostic MRI usually provides the most accurate assessment of disease and should be used for contouring target structures, as shown in figure 15.4.

Emami and colleagues examined the influence of MRI-based contouring on target and normal organ dosimetry in IMRT for nasopharyngeal carcinoma [29]. Eight patients with nasopharyngeal carcinoma had plans calculated using either CT only or CT/MRI fusion using a planned PTV dose of 57.6 Gy and 70.2 Gy for initial treatment and boost, respectively. They found MRI targets were 74% larger and more irregularly shaped, which resulted in PTV dose (D95) of approximately 60 Gy (14% under-dosing) when MRI volumes were not used for planning. Fusion of the two modalities, by contrast, yielded an average PTV dose (D95) of 69.3 Gy while keeping brainstem, spinal cord, cochlea, and parotid glands within tolerance limits.

As noted previously, nasopharyngeal tumors can spread via direct extension, along cranial nerve pathways, or to draining lymph nodes. Clinical target volumes for subclinical disease must therefore include these areas. For most cases of nasopharyngeal carcinoma, the initial volume includes (in addition to the nasopharynx and primary tumor extension) the sphenoid sinus, orbital apex, posterior one-third of maxillary sinuses and nasal cavity, and regional lymph nodes (figure 15.5).

Regarding lymph node delineation, a number of cooperative organizations including the European Organization for Research and Treatment of Cancer and the Radiation Therapy Oncology Group, have published consensus guidelines for lymph node contouring in head and neck tumors [30]. For nasopharyngeal carcinoma, nodal basins for elective treatment include retropharyngeal nodes and levels II-V. Just as

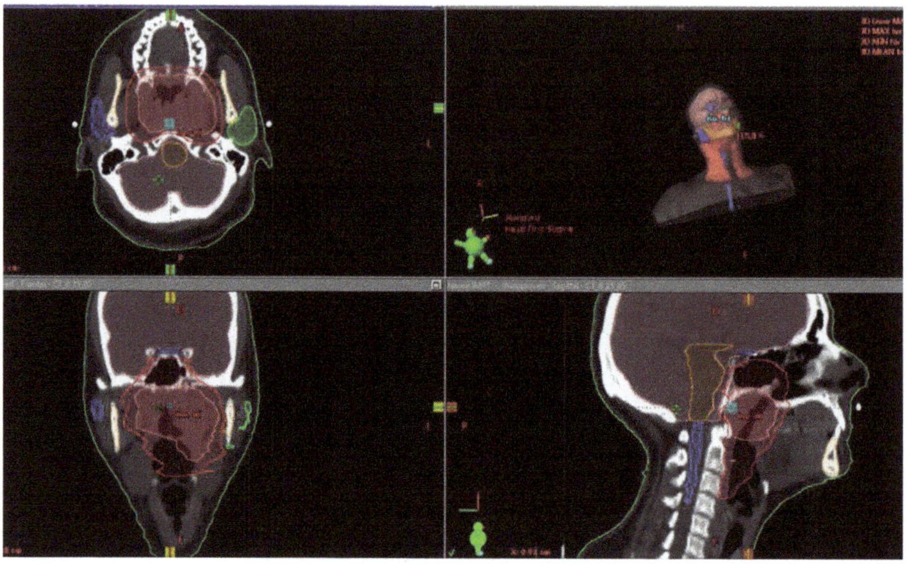

Figure 15.5. Axial, coronal, and sagittal images showing contours of a patient with NPC being planned for IMRT. The gross tumor is outlined in pink and the volume containing subclinical disease is in red, which includes lymph node stations and potential areas of direct tumor extension. Courtesy of Nicholas J Sanfilippo, M.D., New York University School of Medicine.

critical as PTV delineation is normal organ contouring with assignment of associated dose constraints since many structures with critical function, as noted previously, are irradiated in the curative management of this tumor. It should be noted that radiation tolerance limits may vary in any individual based on a number of factors including medical co-morbidities, genetic factors, prior history of RT, as well as radiation fractionation. While radiation dose parameters may vary slightly among institutions, Merlotti and colleagues from an Italian IMRT working group published a comprehensive list of dose constraints that can be applied when using standard fractionation RT of approximately 2 Gy per day (table 1) [31]. The authors recommend that certain critical structures, such as the spinal cord, brainstem, and optic structures, be expanded by up to 5 mm to form a planning reference volume (PRV) for added safety.

RT dose and fractionation when using IMRT offers the clinician the possibility of delivering a higher dose per day to gross tumor, for example, than uninvolved nodal basins in the neck. Lee and colleagues employed this fractionation program in one of the early investigations of IMRT for nasopharyngeal carcinoma from the University of California at San Francisco [32]. Sixty seven patients received IMRT to a prescribed dose of 65–70 Gy in 6–6.5 weeks to the GTV (2.12–2.25 Gy per day) while receiving 60 Gy in the same number of fractions to a CTV of surrounding tissue. Uninvolved lymph node regions of the neck received 50–60 Gy in fractions of 1.8–2 Gy. Twenty six patients also underwent an intra-cavitary brachytherapy boost of 5–7 Gy in two fractions. Cancer control was excellent with four year estimates of local and regional control greater than 95% and four year estimated survival of 88%. This study also described the evolution of IMRT: in their initial experience, IMRT

Table 1. Organs at risk (OAR) and associated radiation dose parameters. PRV = planning reference volume, PRIM = primary, SEC = secondary.

OAR	Priority	Endpoint	Goal	Minor variation	Comment
Cord	PRIM	0.1 c.c.	$D_{max} \leqslant 44$–45 Gy	D_{max} 46 Gy	
Cord (PRV)	PRIM	0.1 c.c.	D_{max} 44–48 Gy	D_{max} 48–50 Gy	
Brain	PRIM	1 c.c.	D_{max} 60 Gy	D_{max} 63 Gy	
Temporal lobes	PRIM	1 c.c.	D_{max} 60 Gy	D_{max} 65 Gy	
Brainstem (PRV)	PRIM	0.1 c.c.	D_{max} 54 Gy	D_{max} 60 Gy	
Chiasm (PRV)	PRIM	0.1 c.c.	D_{max} 54 Gy	D_{max} 60 Gy	
Optic nerve (PRV)	PRIM	0.1 c.c.	D_{max} 54 Gy	D_{max} 60 Gy	
Larynx	PRIM	1 c.c.	D_{max} 73.5 Gy	D_{max} 77 Gy	
Mandible	PRIM	1 c.c.	D_{max} 70–73.5 Gy	D_{max} 75–77 Gy	
Inner ear	SEC	D_{mean}	<50 Gy	<52.5 Gy	
Larynx (without cartilaginous framework)	SEC	V50	<25%	<30%	Oedema
Larynx (supraglottis)	SEC	D_{max}	<66 Gy		Dysphonia
Larynx (whole organ)	SEC	D_{max}	<50 Gy		Aspiration
Mandible	SEC	V55	<20%		
Esophagus	SEC	1 c.c.	D_{max} 45 Gy	D_{max} 55 Gy	
Parotid gland	SEC	V30	<50%	<60%	At least one
	SEC	D_{mean}	$\leqslant$26 Gy		At least one
	SEC	V40	<33% (contralat)		
Upper GI mucosa (outside PTV)	SEC	1 c.c.	<30 Gy	<36 Gy	
Upper GI mucosa (whole volume)	SEC	V66.5	D_{max} 64 Gy (<3%?)	D_{max} 70 Gy (<5%)	
Brachial plexus	PRIM	0.1 c.c.	D_{max} 60 Gy	D_{max} 66 Gy	SEC in selected
Thyroid Gland	SEC	V45	<50%		
Submandibular gl	SEC	D_{mean}	<35 Gy		
Constrictor pharyngeal mm	SEC	D_{mean}	<50 Gy		
Lacrimal gland	PRIM	D_{mean}	26 Gy		SEC in selected cases
Lens	PRIM	D_{max}	<4 Gy	<6 Gy	SEC in selected cases
Retina	PRIM	0.1 c.c.	D_{max} 54 Gy	D_{max} 60 Gy	
Pituitary gland	SEC	D_{max}	<50 Gy		
TM joints	PRIM	0.1 c.c.	<70 Gy		

was used for the primary tumor while the upper neck was treated with opposed lateral fields and the low neck nodes were treated with a low anterior neck anterior field. This was replaced by utilization of IMRT for the primary tumor and upper nodes matched to a low anterior neck field at the level of the larynx with a split beam technique. Finally, the most recent technique used was 'extended field' IMRT which treated the entire neck without the need for any matching. Most centers currently use one of the two latter techniques and there is some debate over the superiority of one technique over another. Proponents of extended field IMRT point to the lack of match line and ease of treatment setup while advocates of the mixed IMRT/low anterior neck illustrate that there is less laryngeal irradiation when a midline block I placed [33].

Long term toxicity outcomes for IMRT in nasopharyngeal carcinoma also exemplify the value of this technique since, as described previously, so many normal structures in close proximity to target volumes. Xiao and associates described late toxicities in 68 patients treated with IMRT with at least four years of follow-up [34]. The investigators utilized simultaneous modulated accelerated radiation therapy (SMART) whereby gross tumor receives higher dose than subclinical target volumes, as described previously. The five year local control was 94.9%. They reported no cases of Grade 3–4 complications except one case of Grade 3 subcutaneous fibrosis. Significant xerostomia, which was ubiquitous in head and neck cancer RT prior to advent of IMRT, was dramatically reduced, with only 4.4% $\geqslant$ Grade 2 and 38% having none at all. Temporal lobe necrosis was seen in only 11 patients (16%) and at Grade 1–2 levels. Low grade (Grade 1–2) hearing loss was the most common late side effect, occurring in 91% of patients. This can be partly attributed to IMRT, but also to cisplatin-based chemotherapy, which is ototixic [35]. There were no reported cases of mandibular necrosis or chronic dysphagia. This study illustrates that long term toxicity rates are reasonably favorable when IMRT is employed.

15.5 Oropharyngeal carcinoma: general considerations

The oropharynx consists of the tonsils, base of tongue, soft palate, and pharyngeal walls. Overall management may involve surgery, radiation therapy, chemotherapy, or some combination thereof depending on tumor location, disease extent, expected functional morbidity, and institutional practice. Surgery may be preferred in localized lesions with absent or minimal lymphadenopathy in an effort to avoid RT completely if no adverse pathologic features such as positive margins are found [36]. Alternatively, patients with locally advanced tumors where it is thought RT would not result in local control may also benefit from primary surgical treatment followed by adjuvant therapy [37]. As there is no broad consensus on the optimal primary management, cases are best discussed in a multidisciplinary forum so that all risks and benefits are considered.

Perhaps the greatest addition to our knowledge of the behavior of OPC is the impact of human papilloma virus (HPV). HPV positive OPC, which tends to affect younger individuals, has a 58% lower risk of mortality compared with HPV negative cases [38]. Prognosis on HPV positive OPC can also be affected by smoking status, involvement of regional lymph nodes, and the patient's co-morbidities [39]. Given the difference in prognosis from HPV negative OPC, investigators from the International

Collaboration on Oropharyngeal cancer Network for Staging (ICON-S) recently proposed a new staging classification specific to HPV+ OPC, which offers some refinement in the tumor and nodal categories to more accurately reflect prognosis [40]. All of these prognostic considerations have inspired investigators to examine new ways to treat HPV positive OPC, with attention to reduction in treatment intensity [41]. However, while this is a subject of active research, a recent Cochrane Database Review found insufficient high quality evidence for (or against) de-escalation of therapy for HPV positive OPC [42].

When RT is employed as the primary local treatment chemotherapy may be delivered concurrently in patients with large primary tumors (stage T3 or T4) or clinically involved lymph nodes in an effort to improve outcome. Pignon and colleagues reported a meta-analysis of 93 randomized studies examining the benefit of concurrent chemotherapy found an absolute survival benefit of 6.2% when compared with RT alone [43]. The investigators also found that chemotherapy delivered concurrently provided greater benefit than when it was used for induction (prior to RT). RT alone, therefore, is reserved primarily for early stage tumors.

15.6 IMRT for oropharyngeal carcinoma

Pretreatment IMRT evaluation is comparable to that of nasopharyngeal carcinoma and includes axial imaging of the neck with CT, MRI, or PET-CT although MRI for evaluation of local disease is not required. Systemic staging must include a minimum of a chest x-ray but many use PET-CT as a full body study for disease assessment. When PET-CT is unavailable, chest CT may be used for locally advanced cases to rule out pulmonary metastases. Patients should have a swallowing evaluation and dental examination with appropriate preventative measures. Routine blood tests to evaluate renal, liver, and bone marrow function are also indicated. Technical preparation for RT is essentially the same as for NPC and most other tumors of the head and neck with a heat-moldable mask and CT planning with thin slices (less than 5 mm). As in other tumors, contouring of target volumes follows disease extent. Oropharyngeal tumors can spread via local extension and particularly along the submucosa which is often better appreciated on clinical examination than on imaging studies [44]. Lymphatic spread is common and typically involves levels II-V, although risk of microscopic disease in the low neck (levels IV and Va) are uncommon when pathologic nodes in the upper neck are absent.

Studies of IMRT for OPC have also utilized altered fractionation with a simultaneous boost. In a multi-institutional trial by the Radiation Therapy Oncology Group (RTOG), 69 patients with early stage OPC were treated with IMRT alone (no chemotherapy) to a primary tumor PTV dose of 66 Gy in 30 fractions (2.2 Gy per day) while sites of potential subclinical disease received 54–60 Gy at 1.8–2 Gy per fraction [45]. All patients received bilateral neck irradiation. With median follow-up of 2.8 years, the two year probability of loco-regional recurrence was 9% and all cases of recurrence or second cancers were in patients with a history of smoking. The most common acute local toxicities (Grade ⩾2) were cutaneuous erythema (21%), dysphagia (52%), mucositis (57%), mouth dryness (49%) and thick sticky saliva (42%). Late toxicities that were Grade 2 or higher occurred in the skin (12%), mucosa (24%), salivary glands (67%), esophagus (19%), and bone (6% osteoradionecrosis). Longer follow-up showed a reduction late toxicity in all categories. For example, late Grade⩾2 xerostomia was observed in 55% of patients at six months but 25% and 16% at 12 and 24 months, respectively. Interestingly, improvements in xerostomia did not correspond to a significant recovery of salivary flow after IMRT. Still, the authors noted that these results compared favorably, with lower salivary toxicity, to previous RTOG studies where 3D conformal techniques were used.

Perhaps the most debilitating long term side effect of RT is mouth dryness or xerostomia. Irradiation of salivary tissue, namely the major salivary glands, causes changes in the volume, consistency and pH of saliva [46]. In an analysis of long term survivors of head and neck cancer treated from 1965–1995 without IMRT, 64% of survivors suffered from moderate to severe xerostomia with associated difficulties in speech, swallowing, and dental decay [47]. As IMRT came into greater use, investigators saw the possibility of mitigating this side effect. In an early study by Chao, salivary flow and quality of life was assessed in 41 patients who underwent RT to the head and neck, 27 of which received IMRT and 14 3D conformal RT [48]. The investigators observed a correlation between parotid mean dose and salivary flow when tested six months after RT and quality of life metrics such as eating and speaking significantly correlated with the amount of salivary flow. Interestingly, the radiation technique did not significantly influence the functional outcome. The radiation dose was the most important predictive factor for xerostomia, suggesting that any technique that can lower parotid gland dose will improve quality of life. More importantly, the study group developed a dose-response model and found that saliva is reduced exponentially (for each gland independently) at a rate of approximately 4% per Gy of mean parotid dose. Subsequent studies further characterized the effects of radiation on saliva in an effort to establish a dose tolerance. Investigators from Amsterdam studied xerostomia using a questionnaire based assessment in 192 patients who received IMRT or conventional RT between 1999 and 2003 [49]. Patients treated with IMRT encountered significantly less swallowing difficulty and required less water during the day, night or with meals. They also experienced fewer problems speaking and eating in public. The authors also noted that xerostomia scores were better in patients who had a mean parotid dose to the spared parotid below 26 Gy. Thus, while parotid dose should be kept as low as possible without risking tumor recurrence, a mean dose of approximately 26 Gy is recognized as an approximate tolerance level. An example of parotid sparing with IMRT is illustrated in figure 15.6.

These data prompted the initiation of larger clinical trials and the capability of IMRT to improve quality of life through parotid gland sparing was demonstrated in a phase 3 trial in the United Kingdom [50]. In this study, 94 patients with pharyngeal carcinoma, 85% of which were oropharynx, were randomly assigned to IMRT or conventional RT and received a mean dose of 60–65 Gy in 30 fractions (50–54 Gy to elective nodal volumes). Groups were similar with respect to age, gender, primary site, tumor stage, RT dose, and chemotherapy use. Statistically significant differences ($p < 0.001$) were noted, however, in mean parotid dose. In the conventional

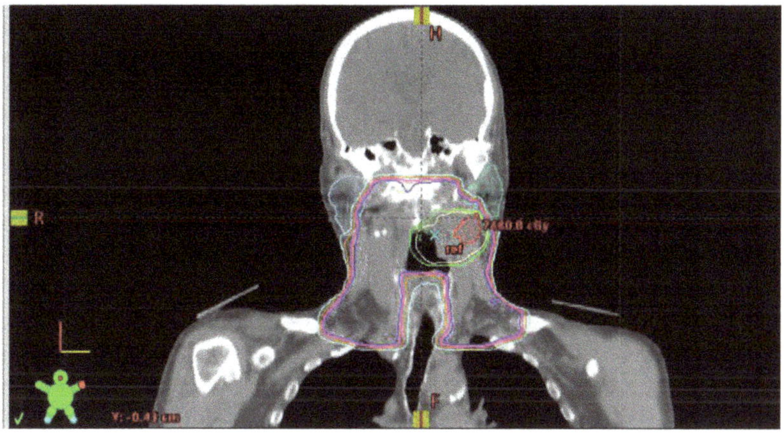

Figure 15.6. IMRT dose plan for T2N1M0 base of tongue carcinoma. Note the 70 Gy isodose line (yellow) encompassing the primary tumor and pathologic lymph node while the superior aspect of the parotid glands are being largely spared. From: Nicholas J Sanfilippo, M.D., New York University School of Medicine.

RT group, mean doses to the ipsilateral and contralateral parotid glands were both 61 Gy. In patients who received IMRT, mean doses to the ipsilateral and contralateral parotid glands were 47.6 Gy and 25.4 Gy, respectively. Late toxicity was assessed primarily by the Late Effects of Normal Tissues Subjective-Objective Management Analytic (LENT-SOMA) scoring systems at numerous time points after RT [51, 52]. Quantitative saliva assessments were also performed. At each time point (3 to 24 months), fewer patients in the IMRT group reported Grade ⩾2 lENT-SOMA xerostomia compared with conventional radiotherapy. In addition, the degree of disparity increased over time, indicating some gland recovery following IMRT. At three months, the absolute reduction in Grade ⩾2 xerostomia from IMRT was 11% (87% in the conventional radiotherapy group versus 76% in the IMRT group). At 12 months, the absolute reduction was 35% (73% versus 38%) and at 24 months, it was 54% (83% versus 29%). Salivary flow, both stimulated and un-stimulated, was also greater in the IMRT group and there was a strong correlation between contralateral saliva flow and xerostomia. Regarding non-xerstomia toxicities, no significant differences were observed, and both groups had similar loco-regional control and overall survival. This study, primarily of OPC, conclusively demonstrated that parotid gland sparing with IMRT significantly reduced the incidence of xerostomia resulted in improved quality of life. The role of IMRT was thus firmly established in the radiotherapeutic management of head and neck malignancies.

Dysphagia is another long term side effect of patients who receive RT for head and neck cancer. This is particularly true for OPC given that primary management often entails RT that is intensified with altered fractionation or concurrent chemotherapy. Caudell and colleagues found that the long term dysphagia rate in patients who received neck RT was 38.5% [53]. Factors that increased the probability were tumor location, including the tongue base and pharyngeal wall (also larynx and hypopharynx) as well as increasing age and the use of concurrent chemotherapy. These patients were more likely to require a long term gastrostomy tube, have aspiration, or need dilatation of a pharyngeal stricture. The same investigators subsequently sought to identify dosimetric factors that were associated with severe dysphagia in patients treated with IMRT [54]. They examined at three specific as surrogates for severe dysphagia endpoints in patients who underwent IMRT: gastrostomy dependence at one year, requirement of pharyngeal dilatation, or aspiration on modified barium swallow. After excluding patients who were re-irradiated, treated post-operatively, had local recurrence or follow-up less than 12 months, 83 patients were eligible for analysis. They observed that a mean dose greater than 41 Gy and volume receiving 60 Gy (V(60)) greater than 24% to the larynx were significantly associated with gastrostomy tube dependence and aspiration. A V(60) greater than 12% to the inferior pharyngeal constrictor was associated with increased PEG tube dependence and aspiration and V(65) greater than 33% to the superior pharyngeal constrictor or greater than 75% to the middle pharyngeal constrictor was associated with stricture. While a precise 'safe' dose to prevent long term severe dysphagia has not been identified, a review by Duprez that examined seven studies of patients who underwent RT found that reduction in the mean dose to the constrictor muscles (all groups) from 61–64 Gy to 52–55 Gy resulted in less swallowing morbidity [55]

Perhaps the most effective way to avoid morbidity when delivering RT, regardless of technique, is to reduce target volume. Oropharyngeal tumors, specifically tumors of the tonsil, are unique in that they are often amenable to unilateral treatment since contralateral lymph node metastases are primarily related to the size, extent of the primary tumor [56]. In a landmark study by O'Sullivan, 228 patients with early tonsillar cancers who underwent ipsilateral RT, typically with a wedged-pair technique, were analyzed for patterns of disease recurrence [57]. Most were early stage (T1 or T2; less than 4 cm) and had no clinically evident neck disease. Recurrence in the opposite neck was seen in only 3.5% of cases. An example of ipsilateral irradiation for tonsillar cancer is shown if figure 15.7.

A series of 102 patients treated at the MD Anderson Cancer Center reported a disease free survival rate of 96% using ipsilateral RT [58]. Tumors were well lateralized with less than 1 cm of soft palate invasion, no tongue base involvement, and no N3 neck disease (node greater than 6 cm), and no low neck disease (level IV). IMRT offers further refinement in dose delivery. Cerezo reported 5 year local control of 100% in 20 well lateralized cases of OPC and oral cavity carcinoma treated with IMRT with no contralateral failures [59]. Mean dose to the contralateral parotid and submandibular glands were 4.72 Gy and 15.3 Gy, respectively. No xerostomia symptoms were reported by 56% and 31.2% reported Grade 1 xerostomia (dry or thick saliva). However, only 12.5% had Grade 2 xerostomia, defined as requiring dietary alteration and no Grade 3 events were observed. Thus in selected cases of cancer of the tonsil, ipsilateral irradiation with IMRT can produce outstanding tumor control rates with very low long term toxicity.

15.7 Carcinoma of the oral cavity: general considerations

The oral cavity consists of numerous structures located anterior to the oropharynx, including the oral tongue (anterior two-thirds), floor of mouth, hard palate, gingivae,

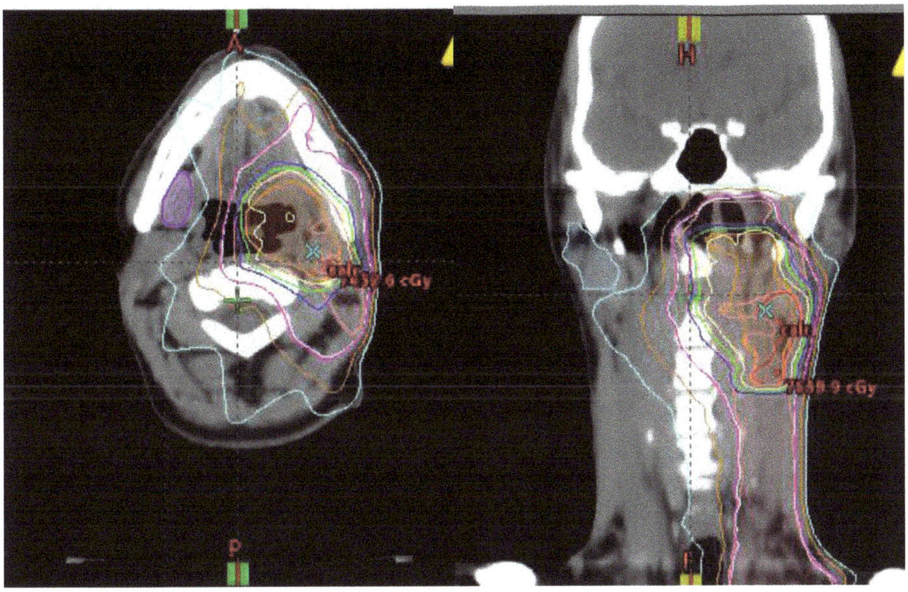

Figure 15.7. Axial and coronal images of a patient undergoing ipsilateral RT for a left tonsillar cancer, stage T1N0M0. Note the right submandibular gland (purple) and the right parotid gland (blue) and are well outside of the 21 Gy isodose line (light blue). From: Nicholas J Sanfilippo, M.D., New York University School of Medicine.

lips, buccal mucosa, retromolar trigone, and the upper and lower alveolar ridges. Cancers of the oral cavity can spread by local invasion through lymph node channels, but distant metastases are uncommon at presentation. Pretreatment evaluation is similar to that of cancers described earlier with attention to depth of invasion. Primary management can be with surgery or RT, but in most centers surgery is initial treatment of choice as it may be associated with less morbidity. When primary RT is selected, intra-oral cone or interstitial brachytherapy can be used for dose escalation (figure 15.8).

Wendt and colleagues reported on 103 patients with oral tongue cancer who had definitive RT with either external beam alone or in combination with interstitial brachytherapy [60]. The authors found that outcome was inversely related to the proportion of dose delivered by external beam: local control was 65% when the external beam dose was greater than 40 Gy and 92% when less than 40 Gy, thus favoring a higher proportion of dose delivered by brachytherapy. Still, toxicity was quite high with 13% having severe late complications mainly related to mandibular necrosis, and authors commented that a general policy of primary surgical treatment with adjuvant RT for adverse pathologic risk factors should be adopted. Definitive RT thus tends to be reserved for patients who cannot tolerate surgery or in cases where functional impairment would be overwhelming [61].

Pathologic factors associated with local recurrence after surgery include, generally, close or positive surgical margins, deeply invasive tumors, pathologically involved lymph nodes, and perineural invasion [62, 63]. Patients with these tumor features should be considered for postoperative RT. In addition, some patients

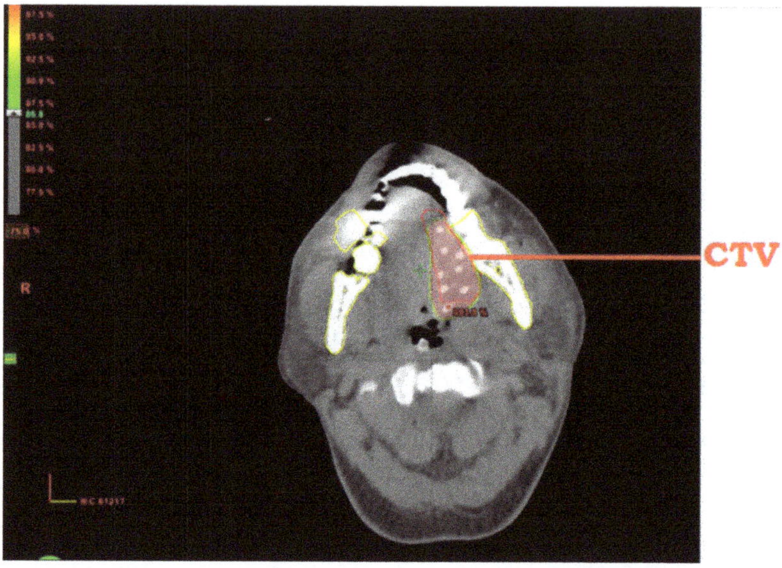

Figure 15.8. Tongue brachytherapy clinical target volume and dose color wash in the left lateral side of the anterior two-thirds of the tongue showing adequate target volume coverage. From [64]. Open access CC BY 4.0.

benefit the addition of concurrent chemotherapy to RT. In an analysis of two prospective randomized trials that tested RT alone or chemotherapy plus RT in the postoperative setting, Bernier reported that patients with extracapsular nodal extension and positive surgical margins derived the greatest benefit from the addition of chemotherapy to RT [65]. Optimal management of the neck was historically the subject of some debate, particularly when no clinical nodal metastases were present [66]. However, a recently published randomized trial favored elective neck dissection in early stage cases of oral cavity carcinoma, 85% of which were oral tongue tumors [67]. The benefit was mainly in cases where depth of invasion was greater than 3 mm. Since depth of invasion is difficult to determine preoperatively, a selective neck dissection is performed at the time of primary tumor resection in most cases. Decisions can then be made on re-resection or adjuvant therapy based on full pathologic analysis.

15.8 IMRT for oral cavity carcinoma

The primary advantage of IMRT in the postoperative treatment of oral cavity carcinoma is, as in other cancers of the head and neck, preservation of saliva. Since there is no GTV, special attention when contouring is critical to avoid marginal failures, especially when perineural invasion is present. This concern was illustrated in some of the early reports of IMRT in the postoperative setting. Daly and colleagues examined patterns of failure in 37 patients with oral cavity carcinoma, 30 of whom were treated after surgery [68]. Among postoperative patients, three year actuarial estimates of local control and local-regional control were 67% and 53%, respectively. The authors observed two marginal failures and one failure completely outside the target volume which emphasized the importance of target definition since opposed lateral fields would have probably encompassed these locations. They also noted that the interval from surgery to RT, when greater than six weeks, predicted for a higher rate of local failure, which has been corroborated in other reports [69]. Toxicity rates were generally favorable with only three patients (8%), two of whom also received chemotherapy, requiring a treatment break of greater than three days. Grade 2–3 mucositis and Grade 1–2 dermatitis were common but only one case of Grade 4 dermatitis was observed in patient who also received concurrent cetuximab, suggesting a multifactorial etiology. Long term xerostomia rates were not reported. Thus, when considering IMRT in the postoperative setting, clinicians must weigh the benefit of parotid sparing versus the risk of recurrence, particularly since planning time may be longer than with conventional planning. Every effort should be made to begin adjuvant RT less than six weeks after surgery. A clinical consideration when using IMRT post-operatively is time of treatment delivery. A known problem in patients who have undergone extensive oral surgery is difficulty in managing secretions, and longer treatment durations with IMRT may exacerbate this problem. In most cases, however, pre-treatment suction and experience of the therapy staff can mitigate this issue.

Regarding dose and fractionation, the absence of gross tumor usually allows clinicians to reduce the total dose to 60–66 Gy for high-risk volumes, such as the primary tumor bed or any location of extracapsular nodal extension. Still, a second lower risk volume is typically treated to 50–60 Gy and includes all relevant draining lymphatic levels and potential perineural spread. Some clinicians may even contour a third volume and designate three risk levels depending on pathologic features. In selected well lateralized tumors of the oral cavity (greater than 1.5 cm from midline), ipilateral treatment with IMRT can be used like in cancer of the tonsil. Lymph node drainage is generally to levels I–IV although level Ia can be omitted in certain tumors, such as those that originate in the buccal mucosa. Level V nodes should be included on the side of the neck where clinically evident nodes are present. Oral tongue cancers, particularly those with ⩾4 mm of invasion or those that have clinically positive nodes at presentation, often require bilateral neck irradiation. A multi-institutional retrospective study by Ganly found that even in 'low-risk' oral tongue cancer, classified as less than 4 cm without lymph node metastases (T1–T2N0), regional recurrence rate was 5.7% for tumors with less than 4 mm of invasion and 24% for tumors ⩾4 mm [70]. In addition, regional recurrence was ipsilateral to the primary tumor in 61% and 39% contralateral, suggesting that bilateral irradiation may be indicated in cases with deep invasion. Tumors of the floor of mouth or tip of the oral tongue require bilateral neck irradiation since these structures are essentially midline.

15.9 Cancer of the larynx and hypopharynx: general considerations

The hypopharynx consists of the pyriform sinuses, post-cricoid area and posterior pharyngeal wall while the larynx is divided into three sections: the supraglottis, glottis, and subglottis. Both of these tumors can spread by direct extension and larynx tumors have access to spaces, namely the para-glottic and pre-epiglottic spaces for tumor spread which must be taken into account when planning treatment.

These locations are often discussed together as their management principles are similar. Surgery or RT can be used as primary treatment depending on factors such as tumor extent, anticipated local control and functional morbidity, medical co-morbidities of the patient and the potential need or avoidance of adjuvant treatment. In small lesions where a larynx-sparing operation can be performed, primary surgery may be an excellent treatment choice. With careful patient selection, this may allow the patient to avoid postoperative RT and its attendant side effects completely. In these cases where adverse pathologic features are found, such as close or positive margins, multiple involved lymph nodes, or extracapsular nodal extension, RT is delivered post-operatively. Dose and fractionation schedules as described for oral cavity are used with 'high-risk' locations usually receiving 60–66 Gy over 6–7 weeks. One caveat to total dose in this setting is in cases when the laryngeal remnant (after conservative surgery) requires RT, some investigators have observed higher rates of complications with dose escalation. Spriano and colleagues noted laryngeal edema was more than twice as common when total dose to the laryngeal remnant exceeded 50 Gy [70].

Many patients with larynx and hypopharynx cancers, however, fall into a category where surgery alone is not a feasible treatment choice but where organ preservation is realistic. RT and more recently IMRT plays a key role in these patients. As described previously for other tumors of the head and neck, cases of locally advanced primary tumors or involved lymph nodes often require concurrent chemotherapy and RT. In a three-arm randomized study of stage III and IV patients with laryngeal cancer, over 1000 patients were treated with either induction chemotherapy followed by RT, concurrent chemotherapy and RT, or RT alone [71]. The investigators found no difference in overall survival, but larynx preservation was significantly higher in the concurrent chemotherapy/RT arm. Target delineation for larynx tumors includes, in addition to the primary lesion and adjacent spaces described above, lymph node levels II-IV. If the pharyngeal wall is also affected by tumor, then retropharyngeal nodes should be encompassed. For subglottic tumors, the elective volume includes paratracheal lymphatics and may extend to the upper mediastinum. For hypopharynx cancer, target volumes for subclinical disease include, in addition to the primary tumor with margin, lymph node levels II-IV and retropharyngeal nodes. Level V and upper mediastinal nodes may be contoured in advanced cases, as shown in figure 15.9.

Dose and fractionation are comparable to those utilized for oropharynx carcinoma, with total dose to gross tumor of 66–70 Gy in fraction sizes of 2–2.4 Gy per day and subclinical disease generally receiving at least 50 Gy. Clinicians may use two or three volumes according to level of risk. Clinical outcomes of IMRT for tumors of the larynx and pharynx have been reported with favorable results. Gujral and associates reported five year outcomes in 60 patients with stage III–IV tumors of the laryngopharynx [72]. Patients were treated initially with doses of 63 Gy and 51.8 Gy in 28 fractions to PTVs of gross and microscopic tumor, respectively. Later, the dose was escalated to 67.2 Gy and 56 Gy, respectively. All patients received

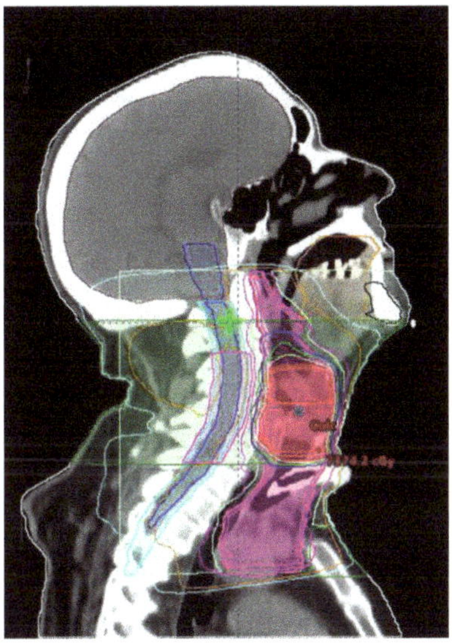

Figure 15.9. Sagittal image of patient with locally advanced hypopharynx cancer undergoing IMRT. Node the volume of subclinical disease receiving 50 Gy (shaded in magenta) extends from retropharyngeal nodes superiorly to the upper mediastinum inferiorly. The gross primary tumor (shaded in red) is receiving 70 Gy. From: Nicholas J. Sanfilippo, M.D., New York University School of Medicine.

induction chemotherapy with cisplatin and 5-flurouracil followed by IMRT with concurrent cisplatin. Five year local control was 68% and 75% for the low and high dose levels, respectively, and only three cases of late toxicity (pharyngeal stricture) were reported. With median follow-up of approximately six years, these data establish IMRT as effective treatment for tumors of the larynx and pharynx.

References

[1] Siegel R L, Miller K D and Jemal A 2016 Cancer statistics *CA Cancer J. Clin.* **66** 7–30

[2] Jemal A, Bray F, Center M M, Ferlay J, Ward E and Forman D 2011 Global cancer statistics *CA Cancer J. Clin.* **61** 69–90

[3] http://seer.cancer.gov/statfacts/html/oralcav.html

[4] Wyss A and Hashibe M *et al* 2013 Cigarette, cigar, and pipe smoking and the risk of head and neck cancers: pooled analysis in the International Head and Neck Cancer Epidemiology Consortium *Am. J. Epidemiol.* **178** 679–90

[5] Andre K, Schraub S, Mercier M and Bontemps P 1995 Role of alcohol and tobacco in the aetiology of head and neck cancer: a case-control study in the Doubs region of France *Eur. J. Cancer B. Oral Oncol.* **31B** 301–9

[6] Sapkota A, Gajalakshmi V, Jetly D H, Roychowdhury S, Dikshit R P, Brennan P, Hashibe M and Boffetta P 2007 Smokeless tobacco and increased risk of hypopharyngeal and laryngeal cancers: a multicentric case-control study from India *Int. J. Cancer* **121** 1793–8

[7] Hashibe M, Brennan P, Benhamou S, Castellsague X, Chen C, Curado M P, Dal Maso L, Daudt A W and Fabianova E *et al* 2007 Alcohol drinking in never users of tobacco, cigarette smoking in never drinkers, and the risk of head and neck cancer: pooled analysis in the International Head and Neck Cancer Epidemiology Consortium *J. Natl. Cancer Inst.* **99** 777–89

[8] Murata M, Takayama K, Choi B C and Pak A W 1996 A nested case-control study on alcohol drinking, tobacco smoking, and cancer *Cancer Detect. Prev.* **20** 557–65

[9] Gillison M L, D'Souza G, Westra W, Sugar E, Xiao W, Begum S and Viscidi R 2008 Distinct risk factor profiles for human papillomavirus type 16-positive and human papillomavirus type 16-negative head and neck cancers *J. Natl Cancer Inst.* **100** 407–20

[10] Raghupathy R, Hui E P and Chan A T 2014 Epstein-Barr virus as a paradigm in nasopharyngeal cancer: from lab to clinic *Am. Soc. Clin. Oncol. Educ. Book* **34** 149–53

[11] Rabinovics N, Mizrachi A, Hadar T, Ad-El D, Feinmesser R, Guttman D, Shpitzer T and Bachar G 2014 Cancer of the head and neck region in solid organ transplant recipients *Head Neck* **36** 181–6

[12] Patel P, Hanson D L, Sullivan P S, Novak R M, Moorman A C, Tong T C, Holmberg S D, Brooks J T and Adult and Adolescent Spectrum of Disease Project and HIV Outpatient Study Investigators 2008 Incidence of types of cancer among HIV-infected persons compared with the general population in the United States, 1992-2003 *Ann. Intern. Med.* **148** 728–36

[13] Knauer S K 2009 Prognostic and therapeutic potential of nuclear receptors in head and neck squamous cell carcinomas *J Oncol* **2009** 349205

[14] Robbins K T, Clayman G, Levine P A, Medina J, Sessions R, Shaha A and Wolf G T *et al* 2002 Neck dissection classification update: revisions proposed by the American Head and Neck Society and the American Academy of Otolaryngology-Head and Neck Surgery *Arch Otolaryngol Head Neck Surg.* **128** 751–8

[15] Lok B H and Setton J *et al* 2013 *Nasopharynx. In: Principles and Practice of Radiation Oncology* 6th edn (Philadelphia, PA: Lippincott Williams and Wilkins)

[16] Perez C A, Devineni V R, Marcial-Vega V, Marks J E, Simpson J R and Kucik N 1992 Carcinoma of the nasopharynx: factors affecting prognosis *Int. J. Radiat. Oncol. Biol. Phys.* **23** 271–80

[17] Ho F C, Tham I W, Earnest A, Lee K M and Lu J J 2012 Patterns of regional lymph node metastasis of nasopharyngeal carcinoma: a meta-analysis of clinical evidence *BMC Cancer* **21** 98

[18] Cao S M, Simons M J and Qian C N 2011 The prevalence and prevention of nasopharyngeal carcinoma in China *Chin. J. Cancer.* **30** 114–9

[19] Chan J, Bray F and McCarron P 2005 Nasopharyngeal carcinoma *Pathology and Genetics of Head and Neck Tumours. World Health Organization Classification of Tumours* ed L Barnes, J W Eveson, P A Reichart and S D Lyon (Lyon: IARC Press) pp 85–97

[20] Tse L A, Yu I T, Mang O W and Wong S L 2006 Incidence rate trends of histological subtypes of nasopharyngeal carcinoma in Hong Kong *Br. J. Cancer* **95** 1269–73

[21] Lee J T and Ko C Y 2005 Has survival improved for nasopharyngeal carcinoma in the United States? *Otolaryngol. Head Neck Surg.* **132** 303–8

[22] Chong V F and Fan Y F 1996 Skull base erosion in nasopharyngeal carcinoma: detection by CT and MRI *Clin. Radiol.* **51** 625–31

[23] Tian L *et al* 2014 Nasopharyngeal carcinoma with paranasal sinus invasion: the prognostic significance and the evidence-based study basis of its T-staging category according to the AJCC staging system *BMC Cancer* **14** 832

[24] Wilson C P 1951 The approach to the nasopharynx *Proc. R Soc. Med.* **44** 353–8

[25] Al-Sarraf M *et al* 1998 Chemoradiotherapy versus radiotherapy in patients with advanced nasopharyngeal cancer: phase III randomized Intergroup study 0099 *J. Clin. Oncol.* **16** 1310–7

[26] Chen L and Hu C S *et al* 2012 Concurrent chemoradiotherapy plus adjuvant chemotherapy versus concurrent chemoradiotherapy alone in patients with locoregionally advanced nasopharyngeal carcinoma: a phase 3 multicentre randomised controlled trial *Lancet Oncol.* **13** 163–71
[27] Lan X W, Zou X B, Xiao Y, Tang J, OuYang P Y, Su Z and Xie F Y 2016 Retrospective analysis of the survival benefit of induction chemotherapy in stage IVa-b nasopharyngeal carcinoma *PLoS One* **11** e0160758
[28] King A D 2007 Multimodality imaging of head and neck cancer *Cancer Imag.* **7** S37–46
[29] Emami B, Sethi A and Petruzzelli G J 2003 Influence of MRI on target volume delineation and IMRT planning in nasopharyngeal carcinoma *Int. J. Radiat. Oncol. Biol. Phys.* **57** 481–8
[30] Grégoire V *et al* Delineation of the neck node levels for head and neck tumors: a 2013 update. DAHANCA, EORTC, HKNPCSG, NCIC CTG, NCRI, RTOG, TROG consensus guidelines *Radiother. Oncol.* **110** 172–81
[31] Merlotti A and Alterio E *et al* 2014 Technical guidelines for head and neck cancer IMRT on behalf of the Italian association of radiation oncology – head and neck working group *Radiat. Oncol.* **9** 264
[32] Lee N, Xia P, Quivey J M, Sultanem K, Poon I, Akazawa C, Akazawa P, Weinberg V and Fu K K 2002 Intensity-modulated radiotherapy in the treatment of nasopharyngeal carcinoma: an update of the UCSF experience *Int. J. Radiat. Oncol. Biol. Phys.* **53** 12–22
[33] Amdur R J, Li J G, Liu C, Hinerman R W and Mendenhall W M 2004 Unnecessary laryngeal irradiation in the IMRT era *Head Neck* **26** 257–64
[34] Xiao W W, Huang S M, Han F, Wu S X, Lu L X, Lin C G, Deng X W, Lu T X, Cui N J and Zhao C 2011 Local control, survival, and late toxicities of locally advanced nasopharyngeal carcinoma treated by simultaneous modulated accelerated radiotherapy combined with cisplatin concurrent chemotherapy: long-term results of a phase 2 study *Cancer.* **117** 1874–83
[35] Dille M F, Wilmington D, McMillan G P, Helt W, Fausti S A and Konrad-Martin D 2012 Development and validation of a cisplatin dose-ototoxicity model *J. Am. Acad. Audiol.* **23** 510–21
[36] Monnier Y and Simon C 2015 Surgery versus radiotherapy for early oropharyngeal tumors: a never-ending debate *Curr. Treat. Options Oncol.* **16** 42
[37] Lybak S, Liavaag P G, Monge O R and Olofsson J 2011 Surgery and postoperative radiotherapy a valid treatment for advanced oropharyngeal carcinoma *Eur. Arch. Otorhinolaryngol.* **268** 449–56
[38] Ang K K *et al* 2010 Human papillomavirus and survival of patients with oropharyngeal cancer *N. Engl. J. Med.* **363** 24–35
[39] Huang S H and Xu W *et al* 2015 Refining American Joint Committee on Cancer/Union for International Cancer Control TNM stage and prognostic groups for human papillomavirus-related oropharyngeal carcinomas *J. Clin. Oncol.* **33** 836–45
[40] O'Sullivan B and Huang S H *et al* 2016 Development and validation of a staging system for HPV-related oropharyngeal cancer by the International Collaboration on Oropharyngeal cancer Network for Staging (ICON-S): a multicentre cohort study *Lancet Oncol.* **17** 440–51
[41] Owadally W *et al* 2015 PATHOS: a phase II/III trial of risk-stratified, reduced intensity adjuvant treatment in patients undergoing transoral surgery for Human papillomavirus (HPV) positive oropharyngeal cancer *BMC Cancer* **27** 602
[42] Masterson L, Moualed D, Masood A, Dwivedi R C, Benson R, Sterling J C, Rhodes K M, Sudhoff H, Jani P and Goon P 2014 De-escalation treatment protocols for human papillomavirus-associated oropharyngeal squamous cell carcinoma *Cochrane Database Syst. Rev.* CD010271

[43] Pignon J P, le Maître A, Maillard E, Bourhis J and MACH-NC Collaborative Group 2009 Meta-analysis of chemotherapy in head and neck cancer (MACH-NC): an update on 93 randomised trials and 17,346 patients *Radiother. Oncol.* **92** 4–14

[44] Slama J, Gilleson M and Brizel D 2013 Oropharynx *Principles and Practice of Radiation Oncology* 6th edn (Philadelphia, PA: Lippincott Williams and Wilkins) p 819

[45] Eisbruch A, Harris J, Garden A S, Chao C K, Straube W, Harari P M, Sanguineti G, Jones C U, Bosch W R and Ang K K 2010 Multi-institutional trial of accelerated hypofractionated intensity-modulated radiation therapy for early-stage oropharyngeal cancer (RTOG 00-22) *Int. J. Radiat. Oncol. Biol. Phys.* **76** 1333–8

[46] Dirix P, Nuyts S and Van den Bogaert W 2006 Radiation-induced xerostomia in patients with head and neck cancer: a literature review *Cancer* **107** 2525–34

[47] Wijers O B, Levendag P C, Braaksma M M, Boonzaaijer M, Visch L L and Schmitz P I 2002 Patients with head and neck cancer cured by radiation therapy: a survey of the dry mouth syndrome in long-term survivors *Head Neck* **24** 737–47

[48] Chao K S, Deasy J O, Markman J, Haynie J, Perez C A, Purdy J A and Low D A 2001 A prospective study of salivary function sparing in patients with head-and-neck cancers receiving intensity-modulated or three-dimensional radiation therapy: initial results *Int. J. Radiat. Oncol. Biol. Phys.* **49** 907–16

[49] van Rij C M, Oughlane-Heemsbergen W D, Ackerstaff A H, Lamers E A, Balm A J and Rasch C R 2008 Parotid gland sparing IMRT for head and neck cancer improves xerostomia related quality of life *Radiat. Oncol.* **9** 41

[50] Nutting C M *et al* 2011 PARSPORT trial management group. Parotid-sparing intensity modulated versus conventional radiotherapy in head and neck cancer (PARSPORT): a phase 3 multicentre randomised controlled trial *Lancet Oncol.* **12** 127–36

[51] Rubin P, Constine L S, Fajardo L F, Phillips T L and Wasserman T H 1995 RTOG Late Effects Working Group—overview: late effects of normal tissues (LENT) scoring system *Int. J. Radiat. Oncol. Biol. Phys.* **31** 1041–2

[52] Pavy J J, Denekamp J and Letschert J *et al* 1995 EORTC Late Effects Working Group—late effects toxicity scoring: the SOMA scale *Int. J. Radiat. Oncol. Biol. Phys.* **31** 1043–7

[53] Caudell J J, Schaner P E, Meredith R F, Locher J L, Nabell L M, Carroll W R, Magnuson J S, Spencer S A and Bonner J A 2009 Factors associated with long-term dysphagia after definitive radiotherapy for locally advanced head-and-neck cancer *Int. J. Radiat. Oncol. Biol. Phys.* **73** 410–5

[54] Caudell J J, Schaner P E, Desmond R A, Meredith R F, Spencer S A and Bonner J A 2010 Dosimetric factors associated with long-term dysphagia after definitive radiotherapy for squamous cell carcinoma of the head and neck *Int. J. Radiat. Oncol. Biol. Phys.* **76** 403–9

[55] Duprez F, Madani I, De Potter B, Boterberg T and De Neve W 2013 Systematic review of dose–volume correlates for structures related to late swallowing disturbances after radiotherapy for head and neck cancer *Dysphagia* **28** 337–49

[56] Lim Y C, Koo B S, Lee J S, Lim J Y and Choi E C 2006 Distributions of cervical lymph node metastases in oropharyngeal carcinoma: therapeutic implications for the N0 neck *Laryngoscope* **116** 1148–52

[57] O'Sullivan B *et al* 2001 The benefits and pitfalls of ipsilateral radiotherapy in carcinoma of the tonsillar region *Int. J. Radiat. Oncol. Biol. Phys.* **51** 332–43

[58] Chronowski G M, Garden A S and Morrison W H *et al* 2012 Unilateral radiotherapy for the treatment of tonsil cancer *Int. J. Radiat. Oncol. Biol. Phys.* **83** 204–9

[59] Cerezo L, Martín M, López M, Marín A and Gómez A 2009 Ipsilateral irradiation for well lateralized carcinomas of the oral cavity and oropharynx: results on tumor control and xerostomia *Radiat. Oncol.* **4** 33
[60] Wendt C D, Peters L J, Delclos L, Ang K K, Morrison W H, Maor M H, Robbins K T, Byers R M, Carlson L S and Oswald M J 1990 Primary radiotherapy in the treatment of stage I and II oral tongue cancers: importance of the proportion of therapy delivered with interstitial therapy *Int. J. Radiat. Oncol. Biol. Phys.* **18** 1287–92
[61] Sykes A J, Allan E and Irwin C 1996 Squamous cell carcinoma of the lip: the role of electron treatment *Clin. Oncol. (R Coll. Radiol.)* **8** 384–6
[62] Ganly I, Goldstein D, Carlson D L, Patel S G, O'Sullivan B, Lee N, Gullane P and Shah J P 2013 Long-term regional control and survival in patients with 'low-risk,' early stage oral tongue cancer managed by partial glossectomy and neck dissection without postoperative radiation: the importance of tumor thickness *Cancer* **119** 1168–76
[63] Hinerman R W, Mendenhall W M, Morris C G, Amdur R J, Werning J W and Villaret D B 2004 Postoperative irradiation for squamous cell carcinoma of the oral cavity: 35-year experience *Head Neck* **26** 984–94
[64] Vedasoundaram P *et al* 2020 The effect of high dose rate interstitial implant on early and locally advanced oral cavity cancers: update and long-term follow-up study *Cureus* **12** e7910
[65] Bernier J *et al* 2005 Defining risk levels in locally advanced head and neck cancers: a comparative analysis of concurrent postoperative radiation plus chemotherapy trials of the EORTC (#22931) and RTOG (# 9501) *Head Neck* **27** 843–50
[66] Bessell A, Glenny A M, Furness S, Clarkson J E, Oliver R, Conway D I, Macluskey M, Pavitt S, Sloan P and Worthington H V 2011 Interventions for the treatment of oral and oropharyngeal cancers: surgical treatment *Cochrane Database Syst. Rev.* **9** CD006205
[67] D'Cruz A K *et al* 2015 Elective versus therapeutic neck dissection in node-negative oral cancer *N. Engl. J. Med.* **373** 521–9
[68] Daly M E, Le Q T, Kozak M M, Maxim P G, Murphy J D, Hsu A, Loo B W Jr, Kaplan M J, Fischbein N J and Chang D T 2011 Intensity-modulated radiotherapy for oral cavity squamous cell carcinoma: patterns of failure and predictors of local control *Int. J. Radiat. Oncol. Biol. Phys.* **80** 1412–22
[69] Huang J, Barbera L, Brouwers M, Browman G and Mackillop W J 2003 Does delay in starting treatment affect the outcomes of radiotherapy? A systematic review *J. Clin. Oncol.* **1** 555–63
[70] Spriano G *et al* 2000 Laryngeal long-term morbidity after supraglottic laryngectomy and postoperative radiation therapy *Am. J. Otolaryngol.* **21** 14–21
[71] Forastiere A A *et al* 2003 Concurrent chemotherapy and radiotherapy for organ preservation in advanced laryngeal cancer *N. Engl. J. Med.* **349** 2091–8
[72] Gujral D M *et al* 2014 Final long-term results of a phase I/II study of dose-escalated intensity-modulated radiotherapy for locally advanced laryngo-hypopharyngeal cancers *Oral Oncol.* **50** 1089–97

IOP Publishing

Intensity Modulated Radiation Therapy

A clinical overview

Indra J Das, Nicholas J Sanfilippo, Antonella Fogliata and Luca Cozzi

Chapter 16

Lung cancer

16.1 Epidemiology

There were predicted to be an estimated 224 390 new cases of lung cancer in the United States in 2016 according to the American Cancer Society [1]. Lung cancers can be generally divided into two types: small cell and non-small cell, although some may consider carcinoid tumors a third type. Approximately 85% of lung cancers are caused by tobacco smoking, but about 10% occur in individuals who have never smoked [2]. Cigarette smoke contains at least 73 carcinogens including benzo[a] pyrene, NNK, and 1,3 butadiene [3]. Radon gas, which is found in the Earth's crust and varies by locality, is the second leading risk factor for developing lung cancer in the United States [4]. Its decay products ionize respiratory tissue after being inhaled, thereby increasing cancer risk. Asbestos exposure can also cause lung cancer and when combined with tobacco exposure, there is a 45-fold increase in risk compared to the general population [5]. Outdoor air pollution is believed to account for 1%–2% of lung cancers and is related to fine particulates, sulfate aerosols from traffic exhaust, and nitrogen dioxide [6]. The role of indoor air pollution on lung cancer development is controversial, but early reports suggest that burning of certain fuels (charcoal, dung, crop residue) for heating and cooking may account for up to 1.5% of lung cancer deaths globally [7]. Approximately 8% of lung cancers are caused by inherited factors and patients with family history are twice as likely to develop lung cancer than those who do not [8]. Lastly, the International Agency for Research on Cancer has published a list of substances with sufficient evidence to characterize them as carcinogenic [9]. These include certain metals, such as cadmium, chromium, beryllium, and nickel; combustion products such as diesel exhaust and coal gasification; certain toxic gases such as methyl ether and sulfur mustard; and rubber production and crystalline silica dust. They also determined that ionizing radiation elevated risk of lung cancer.

The prognosis of lung cancer is generally poor, with only 17.5% of individuals diagnosed in the United States surviving five years according to the Surveillance,

doi:10.1088/978-0-7503-1335-3ch16

Epidemiology, and End Results Program of the National Institutes of Health [10]. Given the generally poor prognosis and high correlation with tobacco smoking as a causative factor, many nations, including the United States, France, Italy, Ireland, Malta, the Netherlands, Sweden, Scotland, Spain, and England, have introduced policies to limit exposure to environmental tobacco smoke [11]. These policy efforts, in early analysis, appear to have reduced the prevalence of smoking. In Ireland, there was a reduction in smoking prevalence from 27% prior to a ban on public smoking in 2004 which declined to 23.6% in March of 2008 [11]. Individuals who have a substantial smoking history are also eligible for screening. Although the subject of screening has been controversial due the possibility of false positive results on screening tests that may lead to unnecessary procedures, the US Preventative Services Task Force issued guidelines for lung cancer screening in 2014 [12]. They concluded that annual screening for lung cancer should be performed with low-dose computed tomography in individuals 55 to 80 years old who have a 30 pack per year smoking history and currently smoke or have quit within the past 15 years. Screening should be discontinued once a person has not smoked for 15 years or develops a health problem that substantially limits life expectancy or the capacity to have curative lung surgery.

16.2 Anatomy

The lungs are the primary organs of respiration and lie within the thorax. Both lungs have a central recess called the hilum where major airways and blood vessels enter the lung. The hilum also contains lymph nodes. The lungs are lined by two membranes called pleurae which assist with expansion. The parietal pleura is the outer membrane and visceral pleura is the inner membrane. The right lung is the larger of the two and has three lobes: upper, middle, and lower. Figure 16.1 illustrates the basic thoracic anatomy.

The horizontal fissure separates the upper and middle lobe and the oblique fissure separates the middle and lower lobe. The left lung shares space on the left side of the chest with the heart and the mediastinal surface of the left lung has a large cardiac impression. The left lung has two lobes (upper and lower) separated by the oblique fissure. The mediastinum is the central compartment of the thorax that separates the right and left lung. The mediastinum contains the heart and its vessels, the esophagus, trachea, phrenic and cardiac nerves, the thoracic duct, thymus and lymph nodes of the central chest. Lymph node stations in the thorax can be intrapulmonary, referring to lymph nodes that lie within the lungs. These can be peripheral nodes, which are located in the outer regions of the lungs, or hilar lymph nodes, which are more central. Mediastinal lymph nodes are always a concern in lung cancer and these may be ipsilateral or contralateral. The International Association for the Study of Lung Cancer has issued anatomic guidelines for mediastinal lymph nodes, which include a total of 14 stations, all of which have a left and right designation except for subcarinal nodes (level 7), which are centrally located [13]. Locations of lymph nodes in the chest are illustrated in figure 16.2.

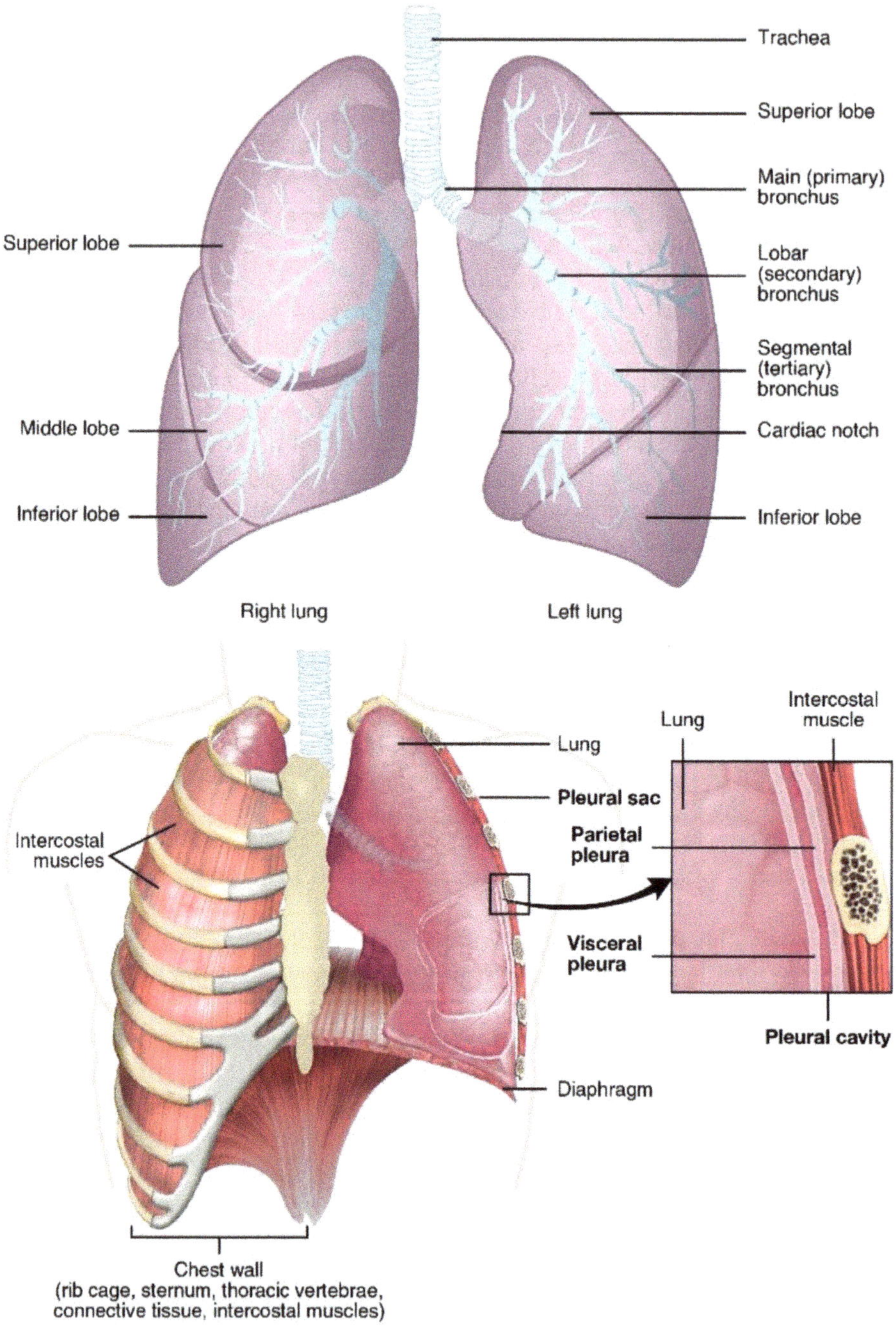

Figure 16.1. Basic thoracic anatomy. Reproduced from [14]. CC BY 4.0. Access for free at https://openstax.org/books/anatomy-and-physiology/pages/1-introduction

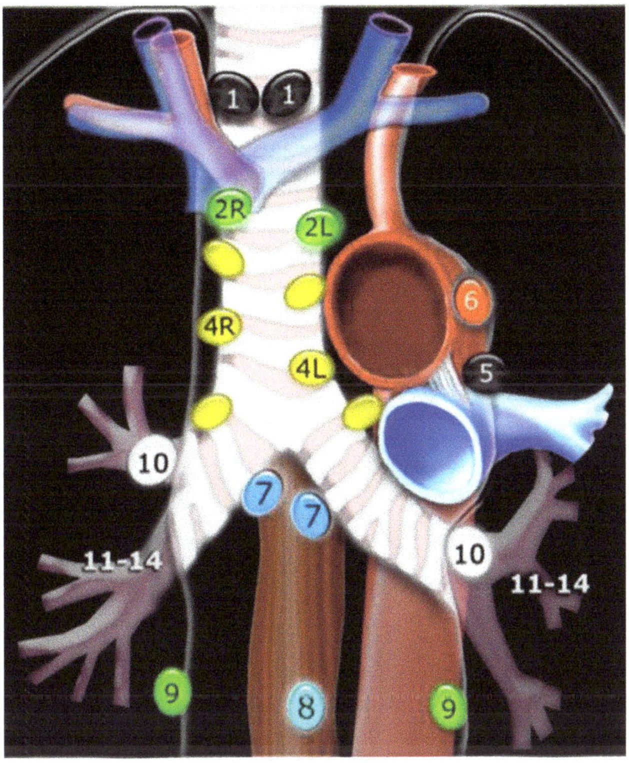

Figure 16.2. Lymph node stations in the mediastinum. Lymph node stations 3a and b are only visible on side views and not accessible by endobronchial ultrasound (EBUS) or endoscopic ultrasound (EUS). Reproduced from [15]. Copyright 2011 European Society of Radiology. Open access CC BY 4.0.

Lastly, extra-thoracic lymph nodes may also be involved in lung cancer and these include supraclavicular lymph nodes, located in the area just above the collar bone; and scalene lymph nodes, which are in the neck, near the uppermost rib.

16.3 Lung cancer: general considerations

The clinical presentation of lung cancer can be manifested in a variety of ways since symptoms can arise from problems related to local disease, metastatic disease, or paraneoplastic syndromes. Symptoms related to the primary mass include cough, shortness of breath, hemoptysis, or pain in cases where there is chest wall or vertebral column invasion. Symptoms related to metastases may involve pain, particularly for osseous metastases; neurologic symptoms such as weakness, loss of balance, or seizure, in cases of central nervous symptoms involvement; or weight loss or generally declining performance status from metastatic disease. Paraneoplastic syndromes associated with lung cancer include hypercalcemia with nausea, constipation, and abdominal pain. Patients may have a syndrome of inappropriate anti-diuretic hormone (SIADH) which can manifest with varied symptoms such as nausea, confusion, muscle weakness or

Lamber–Eaton Myesthenic Syndrome (LEMS) which generally presents with weakness of the proximal muscles. Tumors in the apex of the lung, often termed Pancoast Tumors, may cause Horner's Syndrome, which is cause by damage of the sympathetic trunk in the chest. The triad of this syndrome is by miosis (pupillary contriction), ptosis (droopy eyelid), and anhidrosis (decreased sweating), all of which occur on the involved side of the lung lesion. In addition, approximately 10% of patients have no symptoms at all and a lesion is detected incidentally on chest radiography [16]. A clinical example of Horner's Syndrome is illustrated in figure 16.3.

After evaluation of symptoms and signs with history and physical examination, a chest radiograph is usually obtained to evaluate for lung cancer or other cause of pulmonary symptoms. Imaging studies directed to other organ symptoms may also be

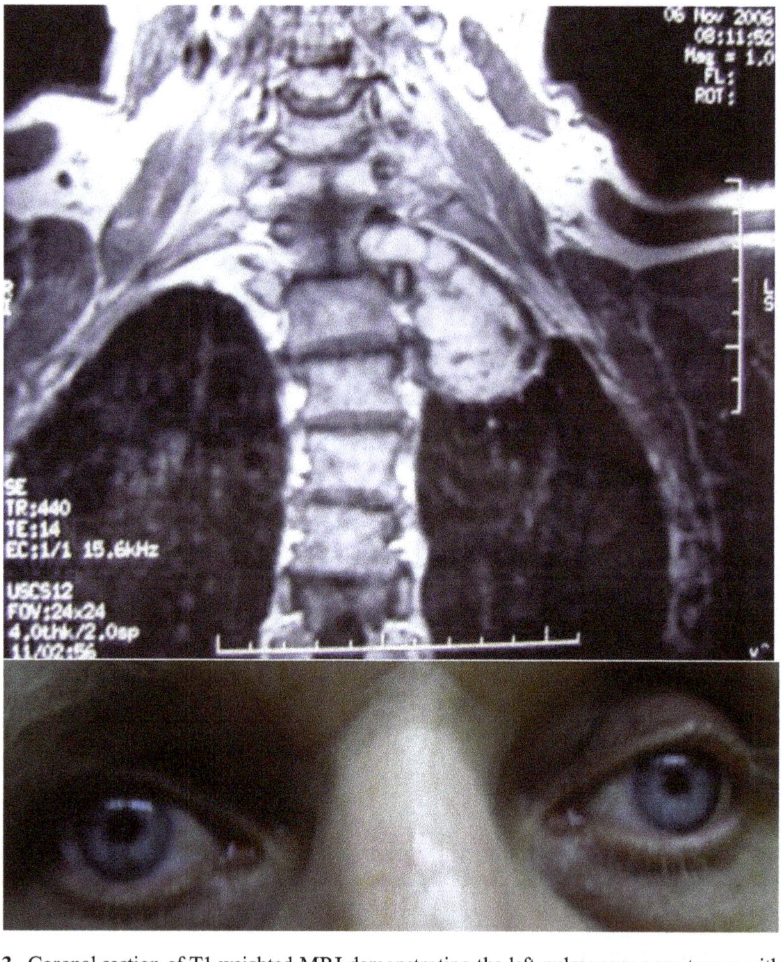

Figure 16.3. Coronal section of T1 weighted MRI demonstrating the left pulmonary apex tumor with extension into T1–2 intervertebral foramen (top image). Left sided miosis due to T1 lesion—incomplete Horner's syndrome (bottom image). Reproduced from [17]. Copyright 2007 Bošnjak *et al.* Open access CC BY 2.0.

obtained as guided by symptoms. Since the chest x-ray provides useful information for a variety of pathologies, it is commonly performed early in the evaluation. When a mass is present, chest CT is performed to provide greater anatomic information and guide the next step in diagnosis which may be bronchoscopy or CT-guided biopsy depending on the location of the tumor and risks of each procedure [16]. Like other solid tumors, lung cancer is definitively diagnosed by histopathologic examination [18]. As described previously, lung cancers are generally divided into two categories: small cell lung cancer (SCLC) and non-small cell lung cancer (NSCLC), the latter comprising about 80% of lung cancers [19]. The two main subtypes of NSCLC are adenocarcinoma and squamous cell carcinoma. While both are associated with smoking in most cases, there is a subtype of adenocarcinoma called bronchioalveolar carcinoma which occurs in females that do not have a smoking history and this entity may have overall better prognosis [20]. Squamous cell carcinoma and large cell carcinoma are other subtypes of NSCLC. Small cell lung cancers, when examined under a microscope contain neuro-secretory granules which contain hormones that may cause paraneoplastic syndromes [21]. Small cell lung cancers are highly aggressive with approximately 60%–70% presenting with extensive stage disease, defined as disease that cannot be safely encompassed in a radiation therapy plan [18]. Due to the propensity for lung cancers of either type to metastasize, staging evaluation is thorough. Chest x-ray and/or chest CT are usually done prior to tissue diagnosis, thus subsequent staging is directed to rule out systemic metastases. Full body PET/CT is commonly used as it can accurately stage lymph nodes in the chest as well as metastases outside the chest cavity. PET/CT staging of mediastinal lymph nodes for the purpose of selecting therapy must be done carefully. Bille and colleagues reported on 1001 nodal stations evaluated by PET/CT and subsequently by pathologic evaluation and found that the overall sensitivity, specificity, positive and negative predictive values, and accuracy of PET/CT for detecting metastatic lymph nodes were 54.2%, 91.9%, 74.3%, 82.3% and 80.5% on a per-patient basis, and 57.7%, 98.5%, 74.5%, 96.8% and 95.6% on per-nodal-station basis [22]. The authors concluded that the high specificity but low sensitivity warranted continued surgical staging in patients considered for definitive surgical therapy. Patients with locally advanced disease or any neurologic symptoms should also have brain imaging, ideally with MRI. Other tests to complete the evaluation of a patient with lung cancer include complete blood count and basic metabolic panel and pulmonary function tests since these will assess fitness for treatment. The staging system for lung cancer depends on the tumor type. NSCLC is staged according the tumor, lymph nodes and metastases while SCLC is either limited stage or extensive stage, depending on if it can be safely encompassed in an RT portal, as noted above.

The management of lung cancer depends on numerous factors such as cell type (SCLC versus NSCLC), extent of disease, and the patient's fitness for treatment. Non-small cell lung cancer may be treated surgically or with primary radiation or chemo-radiation. Early stage disease with no evidence of lymph node metastases may be managed surgically or by RT. According to the National Comprehensive Cancer Network, surgery, which typically involves tumor resection and lymph node sampling is preferred in patients who are medically operable [23]. In these cases, pathologic assessment of margin status and lymph nodes may result in the need for postoperative RT. Patients with positive surgical margins are routinely treated with RT. Regarding lymph nodes, patients who have N2 disease, defined as positive ipsilateral mediastinal lymph nodes, benefit from postoperative RT [24]. In early stage cases with negative lymph nodes where surgery is not done for medical reasons or patient refusal, sterotactic radiation may be performed, and early results have been promising [25]. Chang and colleagues examined data from two prospective randomized trials of surgery versus stereotactic RT that closed due to slow accrual [26]. Estimated overall survival at three years was 95% in the RT group compared with 79% in the surgery group ($p = 0.037$). Three (10%) patients in the RT group had grade 3 treatment-related adverse events and no patients had grade 4 events or treatment-related death. In the surgery group, one (4%) patient died of surgical complications and 12 (44%) patients had grade 3–4 treatment-related adverse events. The authors concluded that due to short follow-up, stereotactic RT should not be considered standard practice, but results were encouraging and further studies were warranted. In locally advanced cases, such as stage III tumors, primary RT, usually with concurrent chemotherapy is the mainstay of treatment [27].

Small cell lung cancer differs in management since the likelihood of metastases is very high. Surgery is therefore used only in selected cases with small tumors and negative mediastinal nodes that are ideally assessed by mediastinoscopy prior to definitive resection. If these cases are node negative at final pathology, then postoperative chemotherapy alone may be used; if positive, chemotherapy and thoracic RT are indicated [28]. The majority of SCLC cases are managed by chemotherapy with or without RT, and this decision is first guided by the patient's stage. As noted previously, SCLC is staged as either limited or extensive depending on if the disease can be safely encompassed in an RT portal. If so, it is limited stage and if not then it is extensive stage. Limited stage cases are generally managed with concurrent chemotherapy and RT with RT starting at cycle 1 or 2 [29]. The optimal dose and fractionation for limited stage SCLC is the subject of some debate. Twice daily fractionation to 45 Gy has been shown to be superior to once daily fractionation to the same dose. A prospective trial by Turrisi tested these to fractionation schedules with concurrent cisplatin and etopiside [30]. The survival rates for patients receiving once daily radiotherapy were 41% at two years and 16% at five years and for patients receiving twice daily radiotherapy, the survival rates were 47% at two years and 26% at five years. Rates of grade 3 esophagitis were significantly greater in patients receiving twice daily treatment. More recent studies have examined once daily treatment, albeit at higher total dose levels, to determine if sufficient local control can be achieved [31]. While a comparison of twice daily and once daily treatment is the subject of ongoing investigation, current guidelines suggest that once daily treatment may be used, but to doses of 60–70 Gy [32].

16.4 IMRT for lung cancer

As in other solid tumors, the rationale for IMRT in lung cancer reflects a need for adequate dose delivery to control local disease without causing undue toxicity.

Retrospective studies have examined RT dose escalation and some have concluded that treatment beyond doses of approximately 60 Gy may improve local control and survival. In the pre-IMRT era, Kong and colleagues reported on 106 patients with stage I-III NSCLC who received 63–103 Gy in 2.1 Gy fractions [33]. Treatment volume included primary tumor and lymph nodes larger than 1 cm and 19% also received neo-adjuvant chemotherapy. Median survival was 19 months and five year overall survival (OS) was 13%. The five year OS was 4%, 22%, and 28% for patients receiving 63–69, 74–84, and 92–103 Gy, respectively. Although presence of nodal disease was negatively associated with locoregional control on univariate analysis, radiation dose was the only significant predictor when multiple variables were included ($p = 0.015$). The five year control rate was 12%, 35%, and 49% for 63–69, 74–84, and 92–103 Gy, respectively. The authors concluded that for each additional 1 Gy in dose, there was a 1.25% increase in local control and 3% reduction in risk of death. Rengan and colleagues from Memorial Sloane-Kettering Cancer Center found similar results in a group of 72 patients with tumors larger than 100 cc treated with 3DCRT [34]. Patients were divided into two groups: those treated to less than 64 Gy (37 patients) and those treated to 64 Gy or higher (35 patients). The one year and two year local failure rates were 27% and 47%, respectively, for stage III patients treated to 64 Gy or higher, and 61% and 76%, respectively, for those treated to less than 64 Gy ($p = 0.024$). The median survival time for patients treated to 64 Gy or higher was 20 months versus 15 months for those treated to less than 64 Gy ($p = 0.068$). Multivariate analysis revealed that dose and GTV were predictors of local failure-free survival with a 10 Gy increase in dose resulting in a 36.4% reduction in local failure. Thus, from retrospective reports it seemed that dose escalation could improve outcome in NSCLC. However, a large prospective phase III study reported by Bradley cast some doubt on this hypopthesis [35]. This landmark study from the Radiation Therapy Oncology Group (study number 0617) examined 544 patients who were randomly assigned to receive 60 Gy or 74 Gy of RT with concurrent chemotherapy with or without cetuximab. Approximately 52% received 3DCRT and 48% underwent IMRT. Median overall survival was 28.7 months for patients who received standard-dose RT and 20.3 months for those who received high-dose RT and there was no significant difference in grade 3 or greater toxicity between the two groups. The use of cetuximab, however, was associated with higher rate of grade 3 or greater adverse events (86 versus 70%). The authors concluded that dose escalation to 74 Gy from 60 Gy was not beneficial and potentially harmful and that cetuximab provided no benefit to patients with locally advanced non-small cell lung cancer. Despite negative results in terms of tumor control or overall survival with dose escalation, IMRT did reduce the risk of high grade pneumonitis by 60% in RTOG 0617 despite larger treatment volumes (median 427 ml versus 486 ml, $p = 0.005$) and a greater proportion of patients with stage IIIB disease [36]. IMRT also produced lower heart doses in this study. Thus, there is still a role for IMRT in the definitive management of locally advanced NSCLC, and National Comprehensive Cancer Network has recognized its superiority to 3DCRT in their updated guidelines [37]. Figure 16.4 illustrates an IMRT for locally advanced NSCLC.

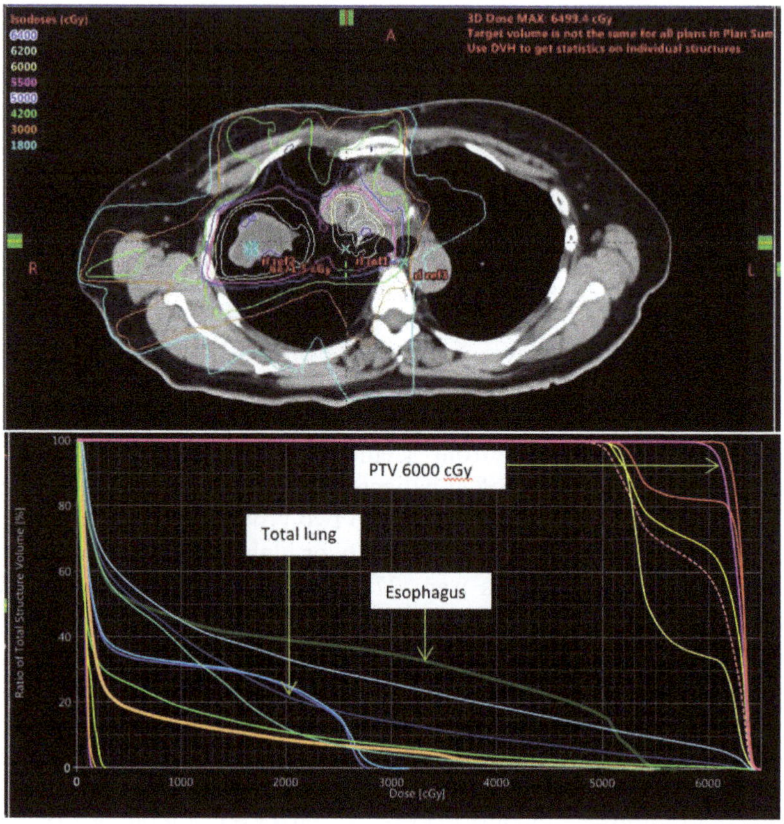

Figure 16.4. Dosimetry plan (above) and dose–volume histogram (DVH, below) for a patient with stage IIIA NSCLC. A dose of 6000cGy as noted by the yellow line is being delivered to the right side primary mass and lymph node station 4. Note on the DVH that total lung V20 is approximately 22%. From Nicholas J Sanfilippo, M.D., New York University School of Medicine.

A similar rationale can be adopted for management of SCLC. As noted previously, hyper-fractionated RT to a dose of 45 Gy in 30 fractions with concurrent chemotherapy was established as superior once daily RT to the same dose by Turrisi in a prospective study [30]. However, given the practical difficulties of twice daily treatment, recent efforts in SCLC have focused on dose escalation using once daily treatment. Retrospective studies using have illustrated differences in outcome. Tomita and associates reviewed the outcome in 127 patients with limited stage SCLC who received one of three dose regimens: 45 Gy with accelerated hyper-fractionation (1.5 Gy twice daily), <54 Gy with standard fractionation (1.8–2 Gy once daily), or greater than or equal to 54 Gy with standard fractionation [38]. The highest dose in the standard fractionation group was 66 Gy. Fifty-five patients (43%) were alive at the time of this analysis, and the median follow-up time of the surviving patients was 33 months. The median survival times were 30.0 months for the hyper-fractionation group, 14.0 months for the low-dose standard fractionation group, and 41.0 months for the high-dose standard fractionation group. As for the local control rates, and the overall and progression-free survival rates, all outcomes were significantly lower in the group that received <54 Gy once daily than in the other two groups, although no significant difference was found between the hyper-fractionated or high-dose groups. There were only two treatment-related deaths from radiation pneumonitis: one in the standard fractionation (<54 Gy) group and the other in the standard fractionation (⩾54 Gy) group. Five patients developed grade 2 radiation pneumonitis, four in the once daily <54 Gy group and one in the once daily ⩾54 Gy group. No other toxicities were reported. The authors did not describe RT technique in detail, but did note that fluoroscopy was often used for the initial portion of treatment, implying that advanced techniques were not likely used. Based on these and similar data, cooperative groups have launched studies testing hyper-fractionated RT with conventionally fractionated high-dose RT. The Radiation Therapy Oncology group is currently accruing subjects to a three arm study (Number 0538) which randomly assigns patients to receive either (1) 45 Gy in 30 fractions given twice daily; (2) 70 Gy in 35 fractions given once daily; or (3) 61.2 Gy in 34 fractions (1.8 Gy) given initially once daily for 16 days and then twice daily for nine days. All patients will receive concurrent chemotherapy with either cisplatin or carboplatin and etopiside. An example of high-dose IMRT for SCLC is illustrated in figure 16.5.

As noted earlier in this chapter, stereotactic body radiation therapy is more commonly being used for early stage NSCLC, and there is no consensus on the optimal technique for SBRT. Proponents of using 3DCRT for SBRT will cite the ability to more accurately track tumor motion during the respiratory cycle. Li and colleagues described a system whereby cine MV imaging can be used to track tumor during treatment to verify position as well as corroborate that dose planned was actually dose delivered [39]. Such verification is not possible with IMRT since the MLC leaves are in motion and this blocks the field of view. Proponents of IMRT-based SBRT will cite the rate of complications in the early SBRT experience when 3DCRT was exclusively used. Fakiris reported grade 3–5 toxicity rates of 10.4% in patients with peripheral tumors and 27.3% in patients with central tumors [40]. Patients in this study received SBRT to doses of 60–66 Gy in 3 fractions with 3DCRT. Timmerman reported 12.7% grade 3 toxicities in patients who received 60 Gy in three fractions which was done is less than 14 days [25] Heterogeneity corrections were not used and subsequent analysis showed that actual planning target volume dose was approximately 54 Gy in 3 fractions [41]. In this study, eligibility required that tumors be greater than 2 cm from the proximal tracheo-bronchial tree. Rib fractures have also been noted in SBRT series. Pettersson reported 13 rib fractures in seven patients among 33 patients who received SBRT with 3DCRT (45 Gy in three fractions) [42]. The investigators examined the dose–volume relationship and determined that if the dose to 2 cm^3 was less than 7 Gy per fraction, the risk of rib fracture was close to zero while dose of 9.1 Gy and 16.6 Gy resulted in fracture risks of 5% and 50%, respectively, with follow-up of 29 months. With IMRT, constraints like these can be placed to reduce the possibility of complications.

Treatment time is also a consideration in SBRT since added time may increase dose variability from tumor motion. One of the more recent developments in

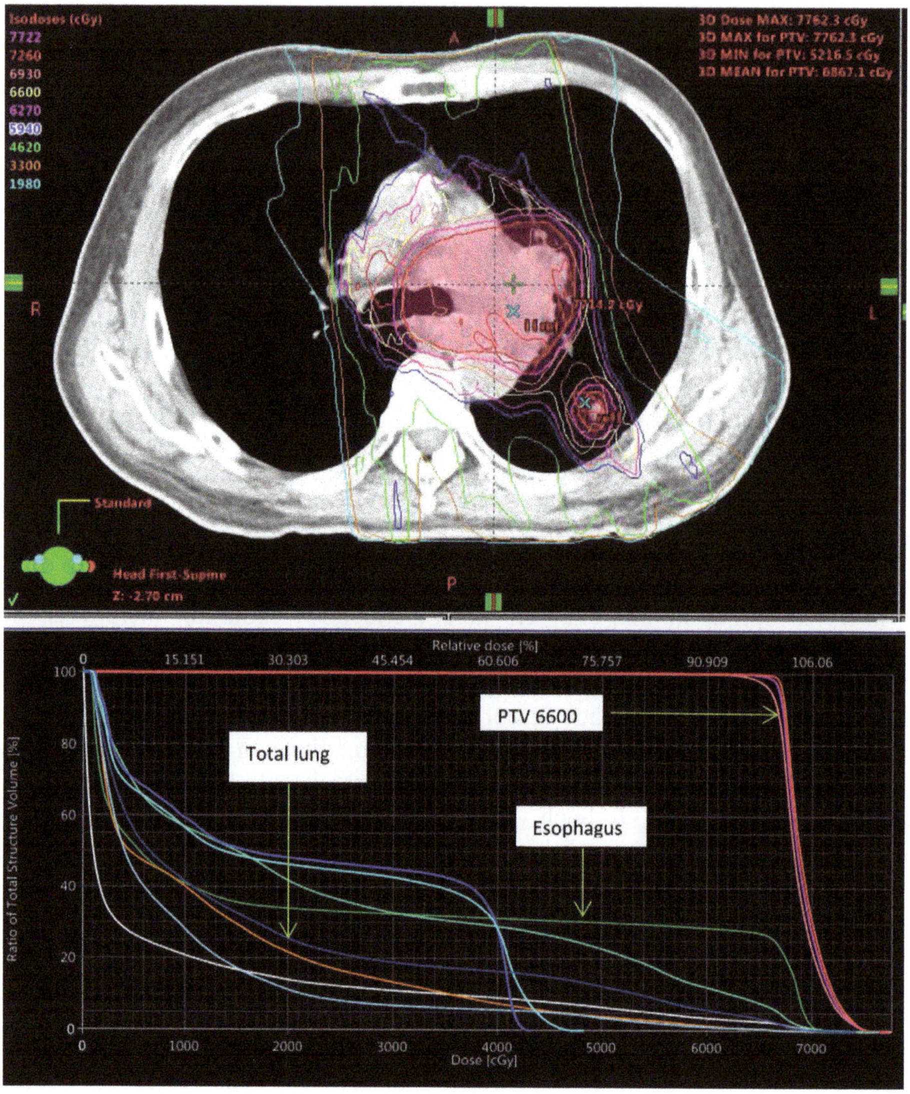

Figure 16.5. Dosimetry plan (top image) and dose–volume histogram (DVH, bottom image) for a patient with limited stage SCLC treated with IMRT to total dose 66 Gy. Note massive mediastinal disease with relatively small left sided primary tumor. Total lung V20 is 25%. From Nicholas J Sanfilippo, M.D., New York University School of Medicine.

treatment delivery is volumetric modulated arc therapy with an un-flattened beam, also called flattening free filter (FFF) mode. Navarria and colleagues examined 132 patients who underwent SBRT: 86 by 3DCRT with flattened beams and 46 with VMAT un-flattened beams (FFF) [43]. All patients were treated with 48 Gy in four fractions of 12 Gy each. Both techniques achieved adequate dose conformity to the target but with a statistically significant reduction of ipsilateral lung doses in VMAT plans (V_{5Gy}, V_{10Gy}, and V_{20Gy}) and also of beam-on-time with FFF mode. 3DCRT treatments lasted on average 1.5 min versus 8.3 min for VMAT-FFF. The median follow-up was 16 months (range 2–24 months). At one year, local control rate was 100% with FFF beams compared with 92.5% with FF beams ($p = 0.03$). Thus, favorable clinical endpoints were achieved with superior lung dosimetry and shortened treatment time. An example of VMAT-FFF for lung SBRT is shown in figure 16.6.

IMRT therefore has numerous roles in the management of lung cancer. In NSCLC, the main effort is toxicity reduction as dose escalation has not been shown to improve outcome. In SCLC, dose escalation studies for limited stage disease are in progress and IMRT may show improved patient tolerance. Lastly, SBRT has

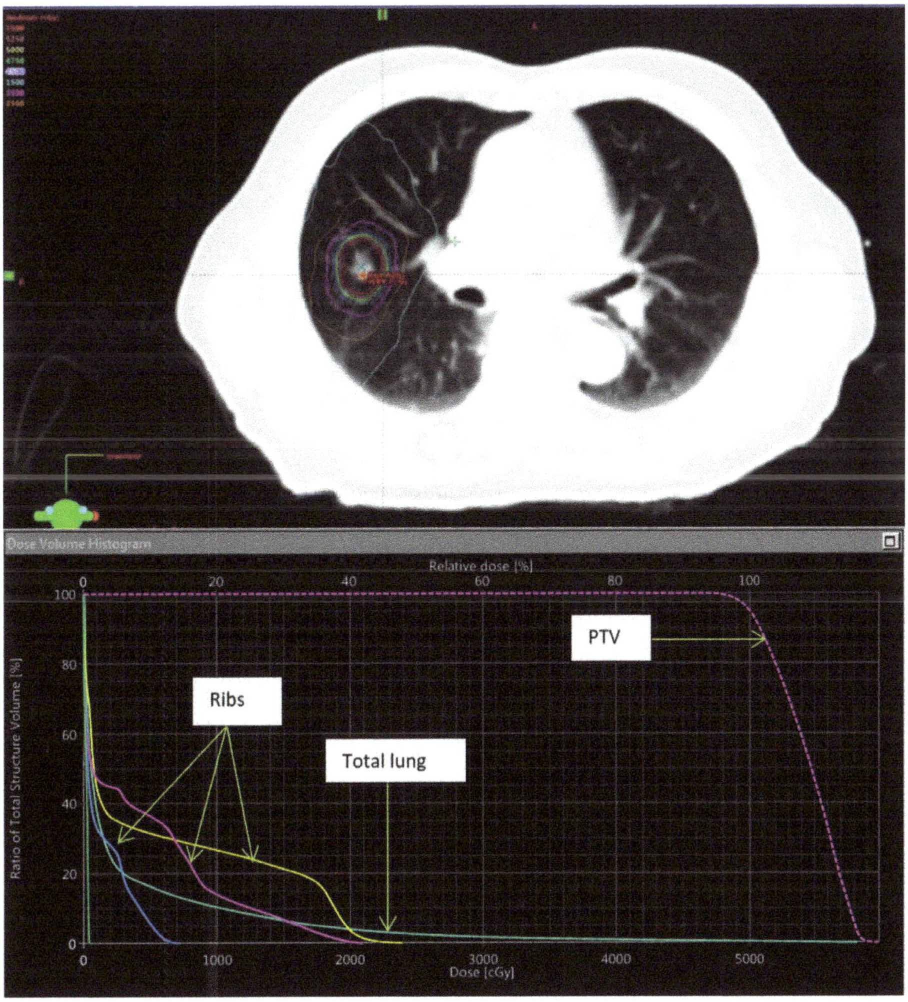

Figure 16.6. Dosimetry plan (top image) dose–volume histogram (DV, bottom image) of SBRT using WMAT-FFF in a patient with stage I NSCLC receiving 5000 cGy in five fractions. Note that lung dose is extremely low with V20 of 5%. From Benjamin Cooper, M.D., New York University School of Medicine.

become increasingly popular as an alternative to surgery in early stage tumors, and IMRT has the advantage of constraining dose to certain structures, such as ribs in peripheral lesions, to avoid rib fracture when doses in excess of 10 Gy per fraction are frequently used.

References

[1] http://www.cancer.org/acs/groups/content/@research/documents/document/acspc-047079.pdf

[2] Thun M J and Hannan M L *et al* 2008 Lung cancer occurrence in never-smokers: an analysis of 13 cohorts and 22 cancer registry studies *PLoS Med.* **5** e185

[3] Hecht S S 2012 Lung carcinogenesis by tobacco smoke *Int. J. Cancer* **131** 2724–32

[4] Choi H and Mazzone P 2014 Radon and lung cancer: assessing and mitigating the risk *Cleve. Clin. J. Med.* **81** 567–75

[5] O'Reilly K M, Mclaughlin A M, Beckett W S and Sime P J 2007 Asbestos-related lung disease *Am. Fam. Physician* **75** 683–8

[6] Chen H, Goldberg M S and Villeneuve P J 2008 A systematic review of the relation between long-term exposure to ambient air pollution and chronic diseases *Rev. Environ. Health* **23** 243–97

[7] Lim W Y and Seow A 2012 Biomass fuels and lung cancer *Respirology* **17** 20–31

[8] Yang I A, Holloway J W and Fong K M 2013 Genetic susceptibility to lung cancer and co-morbidities *J. Thorac. Dis.* **5** S454–62

[9] Cogliano V J *et al* 2011 Preventable exposures associated with human cancers *J. Natl Cancer Inst.* **103** 1827–39

[10] http://seer.cancer.gov/statfacts/html/lungb.html

[11] McNabola A and Gill L W 2009 The control of environmental tobacco smoke: a policy review *Int. J. Environ. Res. Public Health* **6** 741–58

[12] Moyer V A and U.S. Preventive Services Task Force 2014 Screening for lung cancer: U.S. Preventive Services Task Force recommendation statement *Ann. Intern. Med.* **160** 330–8

[13] El-Sherief A H, Lau C T, Wu C C, Drake R L, Abbott G F and Rice T W 2014 International association for the study of lung cancer (IASLC) lymph node map: radiologic review with CT illustration *Radiographics* **34** 1680–91

[14] Gordon Betts J *et al* 2013 *Anatomy and Physiology* (OpenStax)

[15] Schuhmann M, Eberhardt R and Herth F J 2011 Direct nodal sampling by echoendoscopy in lung cancer: the clinician's expectations: Direct nodal sampling by echoendoscopy in lung cancer *Insights Imag.* **2** 133–40

[16] Collins L G, Haines C, Perkel R and Enck R E 2007 Lung cancer: diagnosis and management *Am. Fam. Physician* **75** 56–63

[17] Bošnjak R, Bacovnik U, Podnar S and Benedicic M 2007 T1-nerve root neuroma presenting with apical mass and Horner's syndrome *J. Brachial Plex. Peripher. Nerve Inj.* **19** 7

[18] Horn L, Lovly C M and Johnson D H 2015 Chapter 107: neoplasms of the lung ed D L Kasper, S L Hauser, J L Jameson, A S Fauci, D L Longo and J Loscalzo *Harrison's Principles of Internal Medicine* 19th edn (New York: McGraw-Hill)

[19] Lu C, Onn A and Vaporciyan A A *et al* 2010 78: cancer of the Lung *Holland-Frei Cancer Medicine* 8th edn (Hamilton, ON: BC Decker)

[20] Raz D J, He B, Rosell R and Jablons D M 2006 Bronchioloalveolar carcinoma: a review *Clin. Lung Cancer* **7** 313–22

[21] Rosti G, Bevilacqua G, Bidoli P, Portalone L, Santo A and Genestreti G 2006 Small cell lung cancer *Ann. Oncol.* **17** ii5–10

[22] Billé A, Pelosi E, Skanjeti A, Arena V, Errico L, Borasio P, Mancini M and Ardissone F 2009 Preoperative intrathoracic lymph node staging in patients with non-small-cell lung cancer: accuracy of integrated positron emission tomography and computed tomography *Eur. J. Cardiothorac. Surg.* **36** 440–5

[23] https://www.nccn.org/professionals/physician_gls/pdf/nscl.pdf

[24] Douillard J Y, Rosell R, De Lena M, Riggi M, Hurteloup P and Mahe M A 2008 Impact of postoperative radiation therapy on survival in patients with complete resection and stage I, II, or IIIA non-small-cell lung cancer treated with adjuvant chemotherapy: the Adjuvant Navelbine International Trialist Association (ANITA) randomized trial *Int. J. Radiat. Oncol. Biol. Phys.* **72** 695–701

[25] Timmerman R *et al* 2010 Stereotactic body radiation therapy for inoperable early stage lung cancer *JAMA* **303** 1070–6

[26] Chang J Y *et al* 2015 Stereotactic ablative radiotherapy versus lobectomy for operable stage I non-small-cell lung cancer: a pooled analysis of two randomised trials *Lancet Oncol.* **16** 630–7

[27] Dillman R O, Seagren S L, Propert K J, Guerra J, Eaton W L, Perry M C, Carey R W, Frei E F 3rd and Green M 1990 A randomized trial of induction chemotherapy plus high-dose radiation versus radiation alone in stage III non-small-cell lung cancer *N. Engl. J. Med.* **323** 940–5

[28] https://www.nccn.org/professionals/physician_gls/pdf/sclc.pdf

[29] Govindan R, Page N, Morgensztern D, Read W, Tierney R, Vlahiotis A, Spitznagel E L and Piccirillo J 2006 Changing epidemiology of small-cell lung cancer in the United States over the last 30 years: analysis of the surveillance, epidemiologic, and end results database *J. Clin. Oncol.* **24** 4539–44

[30] Turrisi A T 3rd, Kim K, Blum R, Sause W T, Livingston R B, Komaki R, Wagner H, Aisner S and Johnson D H 1999 Twice-daily compared with once-daily thoracic radiotherapy in limited small-cell lung cancer treated concurrently with cisplatin and etoposide *N. Engl. J. Med.* **340** 265–71

[31] Roof K S, Fidias P, Lynch T J, Ancukiewicz M and Choi N C 2003 Radiation dose escalation in limited-stage small-cell lung cancer *Int. J. Radiat. Oncol. Biol. Phys.* **57** 701–8

[32] https://www.nccn.org/professionals/physician_gls/pdf/sclc.pdf

[33] Kong F M, Ten Haken R K, Schipper M J, Sullivan M A, Chen M, Lopez C, Kalemkerian G P and Hayman J A 2005 High-dose radiation improved local tumor control and overall survival in patients with inoperable/unresectable non-small-cell lung cancer: long-term results of a radiation dose escalation study *Int. J. Radiat. Oncol. Biol. Phys.* **63** 324–33

[34] Rengan R *et al* 2004 Improved local control with higher doses of radiation in large-volume stage III non-small-cell lung cancer *Int. J. Radiat. Oncol. Biol. Phys.* **60** 741–7

[35] Bradley J D *et al* 2015 Standard-dose versus high-dose conformal radiotherapy with concurrent and consolidation carboplatin plus paclitaxel with or without cetuximab for patients with stage IIIA or IIIB non-small-cell lung cancer (RTOG 0617): a randomised, two-by-two factorial phase 3 study *Lancet Oncol.* **16** 187–99

[36] Chun S G *et al* 2017 Impact of Intensity-modulated radiation therapy technique for locally advanced non-small-cell lung cancer: a secondary analysis of the NRG oncology RTOG 0617 randomized clinical trial *J. Clin. Oncol.* **35** 56–62

[37] https://www.nccn.org/professionals/physician_gls/pdf/nscl.pdf

[38] Tomita N, Kodaira T, Hida T, Tachibana H, Nakamura T, Nakahara R and Inokuchi H 2010 The impact of radiation dose and fractionation on outcomes for limited-stage small-cell lung cancer *Int. J. Radiat. Oncol. Biol. Phys.* **76** 1121–6

[39] Li G, Cohen P, Xie H, Low D, Li D and Rimner A 2012 A novel four-dimensional radiotherapy planning strategy from a tumor-tracking beam's eye view *Phys. Med. Biol.* **57** 7579–98

[40] Fakiris A J, McGarry R C, Yiannoutsos C T, Papiez L, Williams M, Henderson M A and Timmerman R 2009 Stereotactic body radiation therapy for early-stage non-small-cell lung carcinoma: four-year results of a prospective phase II study *Int. J. Radiat. Oncol. Biol. Phys.* **75** 677–82

[41] Xiao Y, Papiez L and Paulus R *et al* 2009 Dosimetric evaluation of heterogeneity corrections for RTOG 0236: stereotactic body radiotherapy of inoperable stage I-II non-small-cell lung cancer *Int. J. Radiat. Oncol. Biol. Phys.* **73** 1235–42

[42] Pettersson N, Nyman J and Johansson K A 2009 Radiation-induced rib fractures after hypofractionated stereotactic body radiation therapy of non-small cell lung cancer: a dose- and volume-response analysis *Radiother. Oncol.* **91** 360–8

[43] Navarria P *et al* 2013 Volumetric modulated arc therapy with flattening filter free (FFF) beams for stereotactic body radiation therapy (SBRT) in patients with medically inoperable early stage non small cell lung cancer (NSCLC) *Radiother. Oncol.* **107** 414–8

Chapter 17

Breast cancer

17.1 Epidemiology

An estimated 231 840 new breast cancer cases occurred in the United States with an additional 60 290 cases of *in situ* carcinoma [1]. Over 40 000 women die per year with only lung cancer accounting for more deaths in women [1]. A woman living in the United States has an approximately one in eight lifetime risk of developing this disease. While there are a myriad of factors that increase the likelihood of developing breast cancer, they can generally be divided into modifiable and non-modifiable factors [1]. Age, family history, early menarche and late menopause, for example, are non-modifiable factors while post-menopausal obesity, use of combined estrogen/progestin hormones, alcohol consumption, and not breast feeding are modifiable [1]. Lifestyle habits that can reduce a woman's chance of developing breast cancer include engaging in regular exercise, avoiding weight gain, and minimizing alcohol intake [2]. Reproductive factors also play a role. Having children later in life or not at all places a woman at increased risk, particularly for tumors that are estrogen receptor positive [3]. Breast feeding has a protective effect against breast cancer, particularly if done for longer than one year. In a study of almost 150 000 women from 30 countries by the Collaborative Group on Hormonal Factors in Breast Cancer, the results indicated that the relative risk of breast cancer decreased by 4.3% for every 12 months of breast feeding [4]. Recent use of hormonal contraceptives, specifically combined estrogen/progestin preparations, also appears to increase risk in women who begin taking them before age 20 or prior to their first pregnancy [5]. Similarly, the use of hormone replacement therapy after menopause, also with combined estrogen/progestin medications, increases risk of breast cancer. A study of over one million women in the United Kingdom illustrated that there was greater risk associated with longer exposure, such as those who began treatment shortly after menopause than those who started later [6].

A history of radiation exposure will increase risk of breast cancer. This has been observed in survivors of the atomic bomb where younger age at exposure and higher

doi:10.1088/978-0-7503-1335-3ch17

radiation dose were related to development of disease (with slight downturn at higher doses) [7]. In addition, girls treated for Hodgkin's Disease with RT between ages 10 and 20 have higher risk of breast cancer, with median time to diagnosis of approximately 15 years after RT [8]. This often occurs when these women are between 30 and 40 years old, which is before routine breast cancer screening is implemented. Travis and colleagues found that breast cancer risk increased with doses greater than 4 Gy and risk remains elevated for more than 25 years [9]. The same study also found, however, that there was some risk reduction in women who had ovarian RT to doses greater than 5 Gy or chemotherapy with alkylating agents which reduce ovarian hormone production, suggesting that there is a hormonal mechanism at work even in radiation induced breast cancer. In either case, the authors recommended lifelong surveillance for women who received RT to the breast during childhood or adolescence.

17.2 Anatomy

The breast is a mass of glandular and fatty tissue with connective tissue support. It consists of a number of components designed to produce and carry milk to the nipple. These include lobules, which are the glands that produce milk; ducts, which are the tubes that carry milk from the lobules to the nipple; the nipple, which acts as the final conduit for milk; the areola, which contains secretory tissue to release sweat for lubrication during breast feeding. There is also surrounding fatty and connective tissue which supports and protects the lobules and ducts so as to optimize milk production and secretion. This mass of tissue overlies the chest wall and pectoralis muscle. Breast anatomy is illustrated in figure 17.1.

The primary difference in right and left sided tumors when RT is considered is obviously the left sided location of the heart. Patterns of spread of breast tumors may be local, although given the size of the breast, invasion of adjacent organs is unlikely; lymphatic, primarily to the axillary nodes, or blood born. From a standpoint of the radiation oncologist, knowledge of lymph node anatomy is critical for RT planning. The axillary lymph nodes are divided into three levels based on their relationship to the pectoralis minor muscle. Level I nodes are inferior and lateral to the muscle, level II are beneath the muscle, and level III are superior and medial to the pectoralis minor (figure 17.2).

Breast tumors are capable of lymph node metastases beyond the axilla to the infraclavicular nodes, which are deep the clavicle and the supraclavicular nodes which are superior to the clavicle at the base of the neck. Lastly, breast cancers can spread to the internal mammary lymph nodes which are medial to the breast where the ribs meet the sternum. Any or all of these nodal basins may be involved or at risk when planning RT for breast cancer depending on the clinical situation.

17.3 Breast cancer: general considerations

Breast cancer can be detected in a number of ways including systematic self-examination, examination by physician, screening mammography, and even by accident (found by partner/spouse or accidentally by the patient). In a study of 361

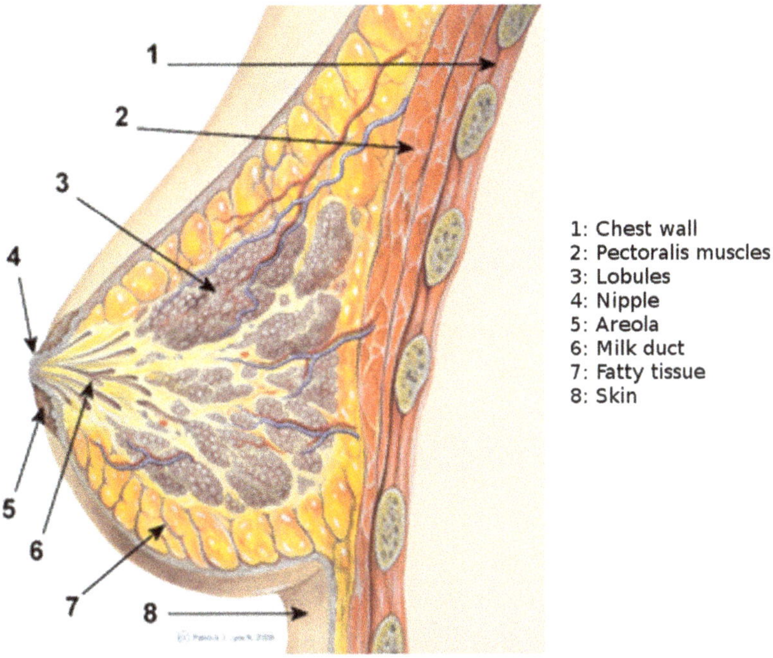

Figure 17.1. Breast anatomy. From: A B Rivard, L Galarza-Paez, D C Peterson 2020 Anatomy thorax, breast *StatPearls* [Internet] (Treasure Island, FL: StatPearls Publishing). Open access publication. Illustration contributed by Patrick J Lynch, medical illustrator. Open access CC BY 3.0 https://creativecommons.org/licenses/by/3.0/deed.en Image courtesy: https://commons.wikimedia.org/wiki/File:Breast_anatomy_normal_scheme.png.

long-term female breast cancer survivors, Roth and colleagues found that 56% of cancers were found by methods other than screening mammography [10]. Still, 43% were detected by mammography and there has been controversy over the value of this screening tool. The questionable value was noted in a 2013 Cochrane Database Review [11]. The investigators analyzed eight trials of over 600 000 women and found that in trials with adequate randomization, there was no significant difference in breast cancer mortality in women who had screening versus those who did not. In four trials with inadequate randomization, there was a reduction in breast cancer mortality with a relative risk of 0.75. The number of surgeries and RT treatments was high in those that had screening mammography. The authors concluded that it was unclear if mammographic screening was beneficial from a population standpoint. In contrast, a report from the US Preventative Services Taskforce found that mammography screening reduced breast cancer mortality by 15% for women age 39–49 and for women age 50–59 years [12]. Impact on mortality was less compelling for women 60–70 and data were insufficient for women older than 70. Current guidelines from the American Cancer Society recommend that women with an average risk of breast cancer should undergo regular screening mammography starting at age 45 years [13]. Women aged 45 to 54 years should be screened annually (qualified recommendation) and those older than 55 should have biennial screening or have the opportunity to continue screening annually (qualified recommendation).

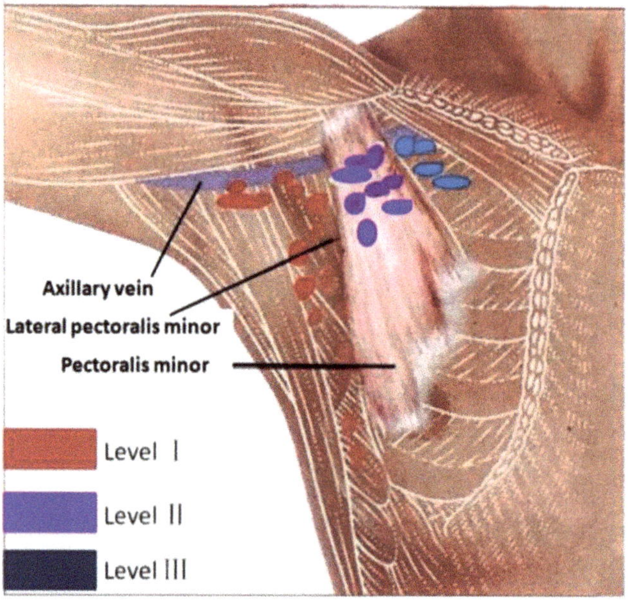

Figure 17.2. Diagrammatic representation of axillary lymph node levels. Lymph nodes were classified as level 1, level 2, or level 3 based on anatomic location. Level I: latissimus dorsi to lateral pectoralis minor; level II: posterior to pectoralis minor; level III: medial pectoralis minor to thoracic inlet. Reproduced from [14]. Copyright 2013 Lu *et al.* Open access CC BY 3.0.

Women should have the opportunity to begin annual screening between the ages of 40 and 44 years and should continue screening mammography as long as their overall health is good and they have a life expectancy of ten years or longer (both qualified recommendations). The American Cancer Society does not recommend clinical breast examination for breast cancer screening among average-risk women at any age. Diagnosis of breast cancer is made by biopsy which may include fine needle aspiration, particularly for palpable lesions, vacuum assisted core biopsy or other image guided procedures [15]. In many cases an excisional biopsy or lumpectomy may serve simultaneously as a diagnostic and therapeutic procedure. Evaluation of the extent of disease depends on the clinical presentation. According to the National Comprehensive Cancer Network, in early stage tumors additional diagnostic studies (after bilateral mammogram) should be considered only if directed by signs or symptoms [16]. Thus, procedures such as bone scan or chest CT scan should be performed in the context of skeletal or pulmonary symptoms, respectively. The use of breast MRI has been the subject of some debate. Investigators have noted that MRI detects subclinical disease in an additional 16% of patients over conventional imaging alone [17]. However, while this changes surgical management in a number of cases, leading to more extensive surgery, there has been no demonstrated impact on recurrence [18]. The indications of MRI in the initial evaluation breast cancer therefore remain undefined.

The general management of breast cancer, as in other cancers, is ideally done in a multidisciplinary setting with surgeons, radiation oncologists, medical oncologists, radiologists, and pathologists. More often than not, treatment involves a combination of modalities depending on several factors. Patients with stage I (less than 2 cm) and II tumors (2–5 cm) are generally candidates for breast conservation therapy (BCT) which includes an operation to remove the gross tumor, often called a partial mastectomy or lumpectomy, followed by RT to eradicate microscopic disease. Alternatively removal of all breast tissue or mastectomy can be performed. Several randomized controlled trials have shown that BCT and mastectomy result in equivalent rates of survival while allowing women to retain their breast [19–22]. Most patients with early stage breast cancer are candidates for BCT, but certain contraindications exist including pregnancy, previous RT to the breast, multiple tumors in different quadrants of the breast or diffuse calcifications on mammogram, cases where negative margins cannot be achieved with conservative surgery, and perhaps certain collagen vascular diseases [23]. In addition to breast tumor removal, the lymph nodes of the axilla are surgically assessed in most cases. This may include a sentinel lymph node biopsy where the tumor location in the breast is injected with blue dye or radioactive material which then drains to the first or 'sentinel' lymph node (figure 17.3).

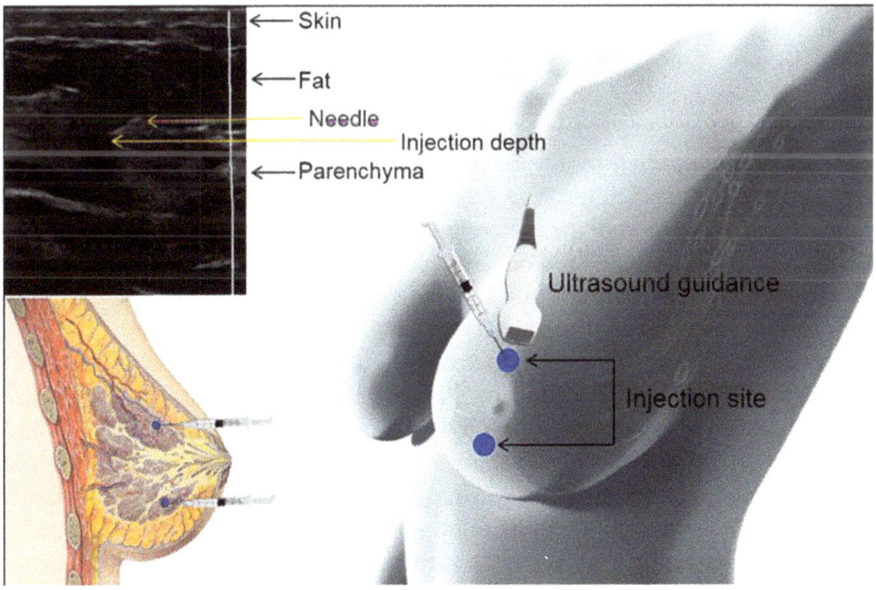

Figure 17.3. Schematic of sentinel lymph node biopsy of the breast. The injection is done under ultrasound guidance and then drains to the sentinel node. Reproduced from [24]. Available from: https://www.intechopen.com/books/breast-cancer-from-biology-to-medicine/internal-mammary-sentinel-lymph-node-biopsy. Open access: http://creativecommons.org/licenses/by/3.0

This procedure has gained popularity because when the sentinel node is negative, the likelihood of other nodes harboring disease is very small, and patients can avoid more extensive surgery. In a study of 163 patients, Veronesi reported that the sentinel lymph node procedure accurately predicted lymph node status in 97.5% of cases [25]. When lymph nodes are enlarged at presentation, however, usually axillary lymph node dissection is indicated with removal of a greater amount of lymphatic tissue, which then may guide RT techniques. RT volume for BCT generally includes whole breast RT to a total dose of approximately 50 Gy over five weeks with or without a boost to the primary tumor bed. In the National Surgical Adjuvant Breast and Bowel Project (NSABP) B-06 trial, for example, RT was delivered to the entire breast to 50 Gy without a boost [26]. However, other trials have utilized a tumor bed boost, usually with an electron beam, to a total dose of approximately 60 Gy using 2 Gy per day [17]. In any case, opposed tangential fields were used for breast treatment with additional supraclavicular and/or axillary portals in cases where risk of nodal involvement to these areas was sufficiently high.

RT is commonly used in cases of locally advanced breast cancer, which can be broadly defined when the primary tumor is greater than 5 cm, is fixed to the chest wall, has significant skin infiltration, or when pathologically enlarged lymph nodes are present. In most cases, patients with locally advanced breast cancer receive chemotherapy as initial or 'neoadjuvant' treatment followed by surgery and and RT [27]. Surgical considerations are similar to those for early breast cancer, although a larger proportion of patients may require mastectomy. When breast conservation can be achieved, RT is indicated in all cases. If mastectomy is performed, pathologic features guide the decision to use postoperative RT, but it is used in most cases, especially when lymph nodes were involved or there was extensive skin infiltration. The value of RT after mastectomy has been widely established in patients with certain risk features. In a randomized study reported by Overgaard, 1375 women with high risk breast cancer, defined as node positive, tumor size greater than 5 cm, invasion to skin or pectoral fascia, or any combination of these characteristics, underwent treatment with adjuvant endocrine therapy with tamoxifen or tamoxifen plus RT [28]. RT volume included the chest wall with surgical scar and all regional lymph nodes (supraclavicular, infraclavicular, axillary, and internal mammary nodes in the four upper intercostal spaces). The intended dose was either a median absorbed dose in the target volume of 50 Gy in 25 fractions in 35 days, or 48 Gy in 22 fractions in 38 days. The recommended procedure was to use an anterior photon field against the supraclavicular and axillary region, and an anterior electron field against the internal mammary nodes and the chest wall. *A posterior* axillary boost field was recommended for patients with large anterior to posterior diameter to limit the maximum absorbed dose to 55 Gy in 25 fractions, or 52.8 Gy in 22 fractions. Locoregional recurrence occurred in 8% of patients who received RT plus tamoxifen and 35% in those who received of the tamoxifen alone ($p < 0.001$). Disease-free survival was 36% in the RT plus tamoxifen group and 24% in the tamoxifen alone group ($p < 0.001$). Overall survival was also higher in the group that underwent RT (45 vs 36% at 10 years, $p = 0.03$).

While RT for breast cancer has allowed many patients to retain their breast and improve survival in high risk cases, there is concern over long-term toxicity,

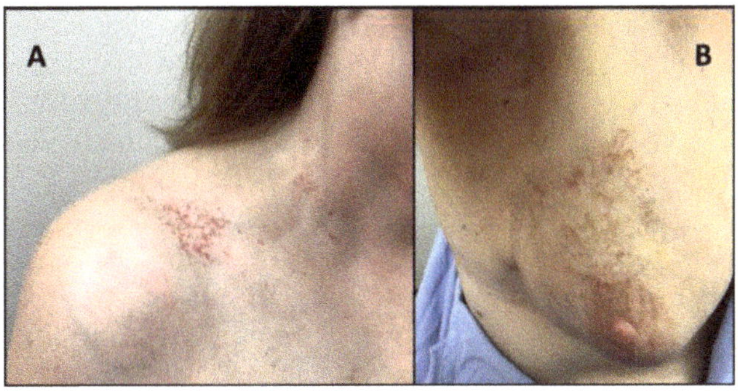

Figure 17.4. Late radiation injury after breasts radiation therapy, including fibrosus and telengiectasia. Reproduced from [29]. Open access CC BY 3.0.

especially as patients are living longer. Complications, while uncommon, can include breast fibrosis, breast shrinkage, telangiectasia, and overall poor cosmesis which can contribute to psychological morbidity (figure 17.4) [30].

Perhaps the main concern that has had recent exposure is cardiac toxicity. Bouillon and colleagues analyzed 4456 women treated for breast cancer with RT between 1954 and 1984 who had a minimum of five years of follow-up [31]. They found that women who received RT had a 1.76-fold higher risk of dying of cardiac disease and a 1.33-fold higher risk of dying of vascular disease than those who did not receive RT. Those treated for left sided breast cancer had a 1.56-fold higher risk of cardiac mortality than those treated for right-sided tumors. A similar study by Hooning in the United States confirmed these findings in 4414 patients treated between 1970 and 1986 [32]. With a median follow-up of 18 years, the investigators observed 942 cardiac events, which corresponded to an additional 62.9 cases per 10 000 patient years. They also noted that smoking and RT together were associated with more than an additive risk on myocardial infarction. However, a study by Darby which analyzed over 300 000 SEER registrants in the United States indicated that patients treated in more recent years may have less cardiac mortality [33]. Results from this study showed that for women treated between 1973 and 1982, the cardiac mortality ratio (left versus right tumor laterality) was 1.20 less than 10 years afterwards, 1.42 10–14 years afterwards, and 1.58 after 15 years or more. For women treated between 1983 and 1992, the cardiac mortality ratio was 1.04 less than ten years afterwards and 1.27 (0.99–1.63) ten or more years afterwards. However, for those treated from 1993 to 2001, the cardiac mortality ratio was 0.96, with none yet followed for ten years. Thus a declining trend was noted as study periods became more recent.

17.4 IMRT for breast cancer

The rationale for IMRT use in breast cancer is slightly different than in other tumors since local control rates in breast conservation, for example, are typically in the 90% range for early stage tumors [34]. The intent therefore is not primarily for improved tumor control, but rather reduction of side effects or to shorten overall treatment duration with hypofractionation. Early experiences of IMRT focused on improving dose homogeneity in the breast: Kestin and colleagues from the William Beaumont Hospital reported ten patients with breast cancer where multiple static multileaf collimator segments were used to reduce hotspots [35]. A total of 6–8 segments or 'fields within fields' were used in most cases. The investigators found that a median of only 0.1% of the treatment volume received greater than or equal to 110% of the prescribed dose when using IMRT versus 10% with standard wedged techniques. An example of this IMRT technique is shown in figure 17.5.

Note that IMRT in this example is not as complex as in other tumors where numerous organs at risk must be avoided. A more complex version of IMRT may be necessary in larger and deeper tumors where heart and lung dose may be elevated. However, in most cases of breast cancer, this simple version of IMRT may be most appropriate. Vicini and associates later reported clinical outcomes of breast IMRT from the same institution [36]. A total of 281 patients with stage 0, I and II breast cancer were treated after breast conserving surgery with IMRT. The median percentage of the treatment given with open fields was 83% (range 38%–96%) and the median treatment time was <10 min The median volume of breast receiving 105% of the prescribed dose was 11% (range 0%–67.6%) and the median breast volume receiving 110% of the prescribed dose was 0% (range 0%–39%). All patients were prescribed a whole breast dose of 45 Gy in 25 fractions, followed by a boost to the tumor bed of 16 Gy in eight fractions using an electron beam. No patient received axillary or supraclavicular fossa RT since all patients were node negative. A total of 157 patients (56%) experienced Radiation Therapy Oncology Group Grade 0 or I acute skin toxicity; 102 patients (43%) developed Grade II acute skin toxicity and only 3 (1%) experienced Grade III toxicity. The cosmetic results at 12 months (with 95 patients eligible for analysis) were rated as excellent/good in 94

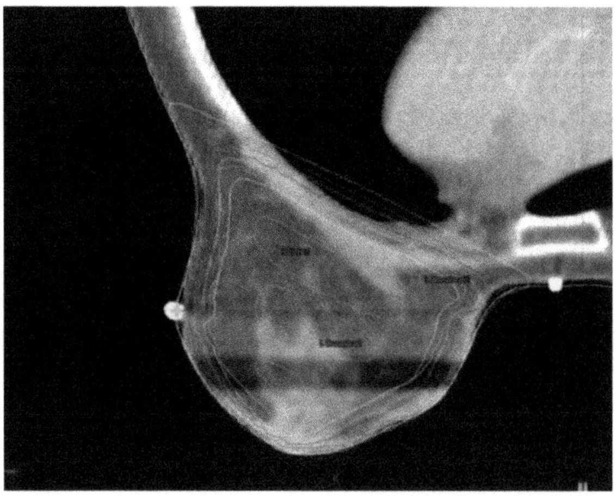

Figure 17.5. Left sided breast cancer treated in the prone position with field within field IMRT technique. Note excellent homogeneity with 100% line (yellow) encompassing the entire breast with maximum point dose of only 105.8%. Courtesy of Carmen Perez, M.D., New York University School of Medicine.

patients (99%). No skin telengiectasias, significant fibrosis, or persistent breast pain were reported.

Promising early experience of IMRT prompted the launching of randomized trials comparing IMRT to more conventional techniques. The Cambridge Breast IMRT Trial, reported by Mukesh, examined tangential plans of 1145 patients undergoing whole breast irradiation [37]. A total of 815 patients had inhomogeneous plans, defined as $\geqslant 2\ cm^3$ receiving 107% of prescribed dose (40 Gy in 15 fractions). These were randomly assigned to standard RT or re-planned with simple IMRT. The remaining 330 patients with satisfactory dose homogeneity were treated with standard RT and underwent the same follow-up as the randomly assigned patients. Breast tissue toxicities were assessed at five years using photographic assessment for overall cosmesis and breast shrinkage as well as clinical assessment for telangiectasia, induration, edema, and pigmentation. The investigators found that on univariate analysis, compared with standard RT, fewer patients in the simple IMRT group developed suboptimal overall cosmesis and skin telangiectasia. No evidence of difference was seen for breast shrinkage, breast edema, tumor bed induration, or pigmentation. The benefit of IMRT was maintained on multivariate analysis for both overall cosmesis and skin telangiectasia and the authors concluded that centers should be encouraged to implement simple breast IMRT. However, other studies have not corroborated the benefit of IMRT. A recently published Canadian multicenter trial examined the benefit of breast IMRT in patients with median follow-up time of 9.8 years [38]. A total of 358 patients were enrolled in the trial which randomized women to receive 50 Gy in 25 fractions with standard wedge technique or IMRT. IMRT could be either forward planned or inverse planned and randomization was blocked 1:1 according to breast size and the delivery of an additional boost to the surgical bed. There were no significant differences in tumor or treatment characteristics or breast size between the groups. Dose homogeneity was significantly better with IMRT with average maximum dose 110% in the standard arm and 105% in the IMRT arm. Improvements in dose distribution, however, did not translate into improved clinical outcome as there were no differences in grade I or II chronic pain or global breast cosmetic outcome. There were no significant differences in the rates of telangiectasia and fibrosis between the two groups, although the investigators commented that this may have been due to the study's small sample size. Quality of life, as measured by two self-assessment questionnaires, was similar for both techniques. As expected, there were no differences in local-recurrence or overall survival. The authors thus concluded that IMRT could not be recommended for all patients to reduce long-term side effects but that it could be used for selected patients. Thus the routine use of IMRT for standard fractionation RT remains controversial, but may be beneficial in patients where there is substantial inhomogeneity using standard techniques.

In addition to analyzing dose distribution and toxicity, investigators have also examined the use of hypofractionated RT to shorten treatment time. Since standard fractionation RT for breast conservation, for example, requires 6–7 weeks of daily treatment, hypofractionated RT offers the potential benefit of improve convenience and access to treatment so long as tumor control or cosmetic outcome is not compromised. James and colleagues analyzed two trials with a total of 2644 women treated with hypofractionated RT defined as greater than 2 Gy per day [39]. Specific characteristics were required: node negative tumors, negative margins, less than 5 cm, and small separation (46% less than 25 cm). Hypofractionation did not appear to affect local-recurrence free survival, breast appearance, survival at five years, late skin toxicity at five years, or late radiation toxicity in sub-cutaneous tissue. Similarly, Ishihara and colleagues reported long-term results in 237 women treated to the whole breast with after breast conserving surgery median follow-up of five years (minimum three years) [40]. The whole breast was irradiated with a total dose of 42.56 Gy/16 fx with a boost if positive margins were present. The investigators reported overall survival, cause-specific survival, relapse-free survival, and local control rates of 96.0, 97.5, 95.3, and 99.7% respectively. Grade 2 radiation pneumonitis occurred in five patients and grade 2 radiation dermatitis occurred in 17 patients. No severe late complications were observed. An example of whole breast hypofractionated RT is shown in figure 17.6.

Based on these promising results with whole breast RT and an effort to limit toxicity, investigators began using hypofractionated IMRT in selected patients to irradiate only the tumor bed and adjacent tissue, a termed accelerated partial breast irradiation (APBI, figure 17.7).

In a subgroup analysis of a randomized trial comparing whole breast IMRT (WBI) to APBI with IMRT, Meattini reported on 117 patients aged 70 years or older [41]. WBI treatment was 50 Gy in 25 fractions with a tumor bed boost and APBI was 30 Gy in five fractions over two weeks without a boost. At a median follow-up of five years, the ipsilateral breast tumor recurrence was 1.9% in both groups. The five year disease-free survival (DFS) rates in the WBI group and APBI group were 6.1 and 1.9%, respectively ($p = 0.33$). However, the APBI group was superior in terms of acute skin toxicity, considering both any grade ($p = 0.0001$) and

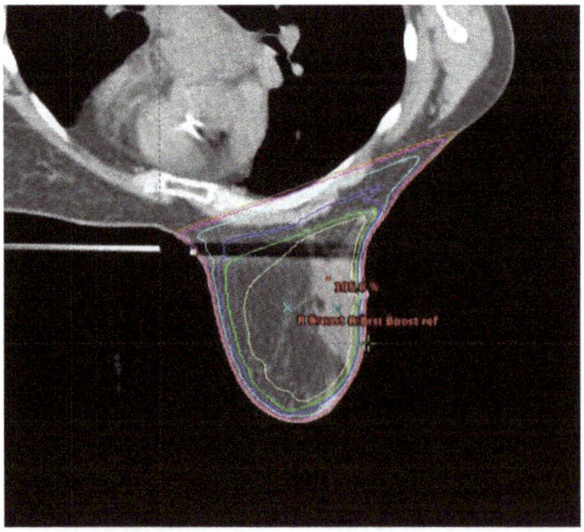

Figure 17.6. Right breast treatment with 48 Gy in 15 fractions using field within field IMRT. The maximum point dose is 105.6%. Courtesy of Carmen Perez, M.D., New York University School of Medicine.

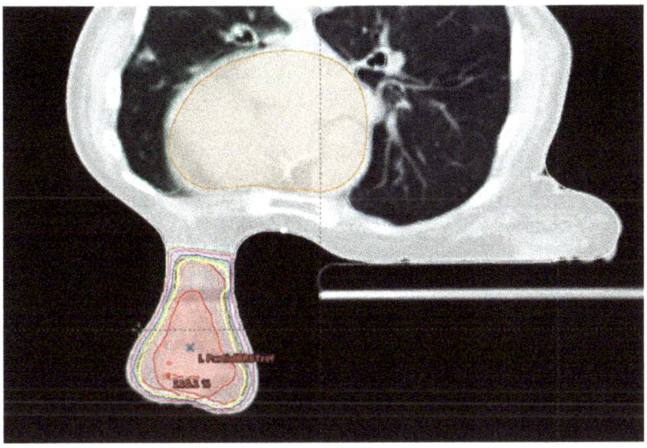

Figure 17.7. Accelerated partial breast irradiation using IMRT in the prone position. A dose of 30 Gy in five fractions was delivered with maximum point dose of 110.1%. Courtesy of Naamit Gerber, M.D., New York University School of Medicine.

grade 2 or higher ($p = 0.0001$). Other reports, however, have shown conflicting results. A multi-institutional study of 2135 women compared WBI (42.5 Gy in 16 or 50 Gy in 25 daily fractions ± boost irradiation) with APBI (38.5 Gy in ten fractions given twice daily over one week) in patients with tumors less than 3 cm after breast conserving surgery and found increased toxicity and inferior cosmetic outcome in patients who received APBI [42]. 3D techniques were used in this study, but inferior outcomes have also been observed in similar studies of APBI with IMRT. For example, investigators from the University of Michigan prospectively enrolled 34 women with stage 0-I breast cancer onto a study where they received APBI with IMRT [43]. Patients received 38.5 Gy in 3.85-Gy fractions given twice daily over five consecutive days with the planning target volume defined as the lumpectomy cavity with a 1.5 cm margin. Deep inspiration breath hold was used for improved accuracy. The trial was terminated early because fair or poor cosmesis developed in seven of 32 women (22%) at a median follow-up of 2.5 years. At a median follow-up of five years, further decline in the cosmetic outcome was observed in five women. Cosmetic outcome was 43.3% excellent, 30% good, 20% fair, and 6.7% poor. Given these conflicting data, the use of APBI after breast conserving surgery remains controversial and patients are encouraged to enter clinical trials so that factors relating to patient selection, radiation dose, and technique may be more clearly defined.

Another potential advantage of IMRT in terms of long-term toxicity is the reduction of heart dose so as to reduce late cardiac effects which were described earlier in this chapter. Investigators from The Hague examined cardiac dose in 20 patients with left sided tumors using IMRT versus 3DCRT [44]. Specifically four plans were compared: 3DCRT with free breathing, IMRT with free breathing, 3DCRT with breath holding, and IMRT with breath holding. The study showed that for heart and left anterior descending atery (LAD), a significant dose reduction was found using breath hold ($p < 0.01$) and for both breath hold and free breathing,

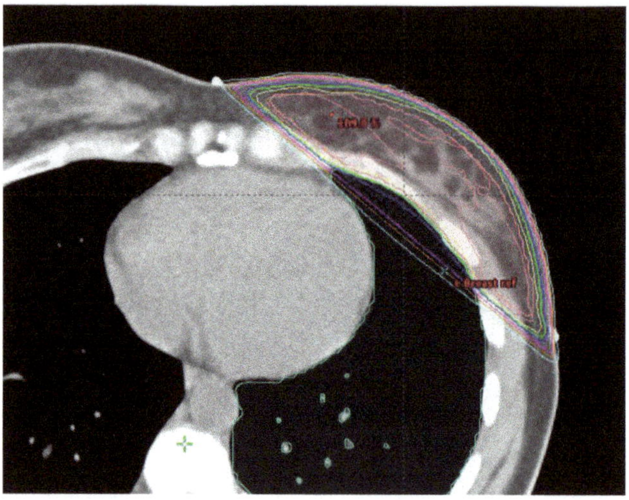

Figure 17.8. IMRT for left sided breast cancer using deep inspiratory breath holding. Note minimal cardiac dose and homogeneous breast dose with maximum point dose of 109%. Patient received 40.05 Gy in 15 fractions. Courtesy of Carmen Perez, M.D., New York University School of Medicine.

a significant dose reduction was found using IMRT ($p < 0.01$). For some metrics the differences were dramatic: mean dose the LAD-region using 3DCRT and free breathing was 18.6 Gy while for IMRT with breath holding it was 6.7 Gy. IMRT resulted in an average reduction of 5% in the LAD-region for the volume receiving 20 Gy. In 5 cases, the LAD-region remained situated in the vicinity of the radiation portals even when breath holding and IMRT still resulted in reduced dose to the LAD-region. An example of deep inspiratory breath holding with IMRT is shown in figure 17.8.

Others have examined prone treatment as a method for reducing cardiac dose. Lymberis reported on 100 patients treated prospectively using IMRT in the prone position and ran dose plans for the same treatment when supine. All patients received 40.5 Gy to the entire breast in 15 fractions of 2.7 Gy^{-1} fraction with a simultaneous boost to the tumor bed of 0.5 Gy^{-1} fraction. RT was delivered Monday to Friday for three weeks to a total dose of 40.50 Gy to the breast and 48 Gy to the tumor bed. The intent was to deliver 95% of the prescribed dose to 95% of the breast volume and planning tumor volume (PTV) tumor bed volume, using concomitant boost inversely planned IMRT (10). Normal tissue constraints required that <10% of the heart and lung volumes received >18 Gy and >20 Gy, respectively. In all patients, the prone position was superior for sparing lung volume compared to the supine setup (mean lung volume reduction was 93.5 c.c. for right and 103.6 c.c. for left breast cancer patients). In 46/53 (87%) left breast cancer patients best treated prone, in-field heart volume was reduced by a mean of 12 c.c. and by 1.8 c.c. for the other 7/53 (13%) patients best treated supine. Thus, there are different methods to optimize dose when using IMRT for breast cancer treatment and there is no broad consensus on any single best technique. Furthermore, while these studies illustrate improved dose distribution with sparing of myocardium, lung, and coronary vessels, only further follow-up will determine if this translates into a reduction in clinical events such as myocardial infarction or congestive heart failure.

References

[1] http://cancer.org/acs/groups/content/@research/documents/document/acspc-046381.pdf

[2] Kushi L H, Doyle C, McCullough M, Rock C L, Demark-Wahnefried W, Bandera E V, Gapstur S, Patel A V, Andrews K and Gansler T 2012 American Cancer Society 2010 Nutrition and Physical Activity Guidelines Advisory Committee. American Cancer Society Guidelines on nutrition and physical activity for cancer prevention: reducing the risk of cancer with healthy food choices and physical activity *CA Cancer J. Clin.* **62** 30–67

[3] Anderson K N, Schwab R B and Martinez M E 2014 Reproductive risk factors and breast cancer subtypes: a review of the literature *Breast Cancer Res. Treat.* **144** 1–10

[4] Collaborative Group on Hormonal Factors in Breast Cancer 2002 Breast cancer and breastfeeding: collaborative reanalysis of individual data from 47 epidemiological studies in 30 countries, including 50302 women with breast cancer and 96973 women without the disease *Lancet* **360** 187–95

[5] Bassuk S S and Manson J E 2015 Oral contraceptives and menopausal hormone therapy: relative and attributable risks of cardiovascular disease, cancer, and other health outcomes *Ann. Epidemiol.* **25** 193–200

[6] Beral V, Reeves G, Bull D and Green J 2011 Million Women Study Collaborators. Breast cancer risk in relation to the interval between menopause and starting hormone therapy *J. Natl Cancer Inst.* **103** 296–305

[7] Preston D L, Mattsson A, Holmberg E, Shore R, Hildreth N G and Boice J D Jr. 2002 Radiation effects on breast cancer risk: a pooled analysis of eight cohorts *Radiat. Res.* **158** 220–35

[8] Clemons M, Loijens L and Goss P 2000 Breast cancer risk following irradiation for Hodgkin's disease *Cancer Treat. Rev.* **26** 291–302

[9] Travis L B *et al* 2003 Breast cancer following radiotherapy and chemotherapy among young women with Hodgkin disease *JAMA* **290** 465–75

[10] Roth J G and Elmore J P *et al* 2011 Self-detection remains a key method of breast cancer detection for U.S. women *J. Womens Health (Larchmt)* **20** 1135–9

[11] Gøtzsche P C and Jørgensen K J 2013 Screening for breast cancer with mammography *Cochrane Database Syst. Rev.* CD001877

[12] Nelson H D, Tyne K, Naik A, Bougatsos C, Chan B, Nygren P and Humphrey L 2009 Screening for Breast Cancer: Systematic Evidence Review Update for the US Preventive Services Task Force [Internet] (Rockville, MD: Agency for Healthcare Research and Quality (US))

[13] Oeffinger K C *et al* 2015 American Cancer Society. Breast Cancer Screening for Women at Average Risk: 2015 guideline update from the American Cancer Society *JAMA* **314** 1599–614

[14] Lu Q, Hua J, Kassir M M, Delproposto Z, Dai Y, Sun J, Haacke M and Hu J 2013 Imaging lymphatic system in breast cancer patients with magnetic resonance lymphangiography *PLoS One* **8** e69701

[15] Yu Y H, Liang C and Yuan X Z 2010 Diagnostic value of vacuum-assisted breast biopsy for breast carcinoma: a meta-analysis and systematic review *Breast Cancer Res. Treat.* **120** 469–79

[16] https://nccn.org/professionals/physician_gls/pdf/breast.pdf

[17] Houssami N, Ciatto S, Macaskill P, Lord S J, Warren R M, Dixon J M and Irwig L 2008 Accuracy and surgical impact of magnetic resonance imaging in breast cancer staging:

systematic review and meta-analysis in detection of multifocal and multicentric cancer *J. Clin. Oncol.* **26** 3248–58

[18] Houssami N and Hayes D F 2009 Review of preoperative magnetic resonance imaging (MRI) in breast cancer: should MRI be performed on all women with newly diagnosed, early stage breast cancer? *CA Cancer J. Clin.* **59** 290–302

[19] Veronesi U, Saccozzi R and Del Vecchio M *et al* 1981 Comparing radical mastectomy with quadrantectomy, axillary dissection, and radiotherapy in patients with small cancers of the breast *N. Engl. J. Med.* 6–11

[20] Sarrazin D, Le M G and Arriagada R *et al* 1989 Ten-year results of a randomized trial comparing a conservative treatment to mastectomy in early breast cancer *Radiother. Oncol.* 177–84

[21] van Dongen J A, Voogd A C and Fentiman I S *et al* 2000 Long-term results of a randomized trial comparing breast-conserving therapy with mastectomy: European Organization for Research and Treatment of Cancer 10801 trial *J. Natl Cancer Inst.* 1143–50

[22] Jacobson J A, Danforth D N and Cowan K H *et al* 1995 Ten-year results of a comparison of conservation with mastectomy in the treatment of stage I and II breast cancer *N. Engl. J. Med.* 907–11

[23] American College of Radiology 2007 Practice guideline for the breast conservation therapy in the management of invasive breast carcinoma *J. Am. Coll. Surg.* **205** 362–76

[24] Wang Y-S, Qiu P-F and Cong B-B 2017 Internal mammary sentinel lymph lode biopsy *Breast Cancer—From Biology to Medicine* ed P Van Pham (Rijeka: IntechOpen)

[25] Veronesi U *et al* 1997 Sentinel-node biopsy to avoid axillary dissection in breast cancer with clinically negative lymph-nodes *Lancet* **349** 1864–7

[26] Fisher B, Anderson S, Bryant J, Margolese R G, Deutsch M, Fisher E R, Jeong J H and Wolmark N 2002 Twenty-year follow-up of a randomized trial comparing total mastectomy, lumpectomy, and lumpectomy plus irradiation for the treatment of invasive breast cancer *N. Engl. J. Med.* **347** 1233–41

[27] Specht J and Gralow J R 2009 Neoadjuvant chemotherapy for locally advanced breast cancer *Semin. Radiat. Oncol.* **19** 222–8

[28] Overgaard M *et al* 1999 Postoperative radiotherapy in high-risk postmenopausal breast-cancer patients given adjuvant tamoxifen: Danish Breast Cancer Cooperative Group DBCG 82c randomised trial *Lancet* **353** 1641–8

[29] Dosani M *et al* 2017 Severe late toxicity after adjuvant breast radiotherapy in a patient with a germline ataxia telangiectasia mutated gene: future treatment decisions *Cureus* **9** e1458

[30] Al-Ghazal S K, Fallowfield L and Blamey R W 1999 Does cosmetic outcome from treatment of primary breast cancer influence psychosocial morbidity? *Eur. J. Surg. Oncol.* **25** 571–3

[31] Bouillon K *et al* 2011 Long-term cardiovascular mortality after radiotherapy for breast cancer *J. Am. Coll. Cardiol.* **57** 445–52

[32] Hooning M J, Botma A, Aleman B M, Baaijens M H, Bartelink H, Klijn J G, Taylor C W and van Leeuwen F E 2007 Long-term risk of cardiovascular disease in 10-year survivors of breast cancer *J. Natl Cancer Inst.* **99** 365–75

[33] Darby S C, McGale P, Taylor C W and Peto R 2005 Long-term mortality from heart disease and lung cancer after radiotherapy for early breast cancer: prospective cohort study of about 300,000 women in US SEER cancer registries *Lancet Oncol.* **6** 557–65

[34] Perez C A 2003 Conservation therapy in T1-T2 breast cancer: past, current issues, and future challenges and opportunities *Cancer J.* **9** 442–53

[35] Kestin L L, Sharpe M B, Frazier R C, Vicini F A, Yan D, Matter R C, Martinez A A and Wong J W 2000 Intensity modulation to improve dose uniformity with tangential breast radiotherapy: initial clinical experience *Int. J. Radiat. Oncol. Biol. Phys.* **48** 1559–68

[36] Vicini F A, Sharpe M, Kestin L, Martinez A, Mitchell C K, Wallace M F, Matter R and Wong J 2002 Optimizing breast cancer treatment efficacy with intensity-modulated radiotherapy *Int. J. Radiat. Oncol. Biol. Phys.* **54** 1336–44

[37] Mukesh M B *et al* 2013 Randomized controlled trial of intensity-modulated radiotherapy for early breast cancer: 5-year results confirm superior overall cosmesis *J. Clin. Oncol.* **31** 4488–95

[38] Pignol J P, Truong P, Rakovitch E, Sattler M G, Whelan T J and Olivotto I A 2016 Ten years results of the Canadian breast intensity modulated radiation therapy (IMRT) randomized controlled trial *Radiother. Oncol.* **121** 414–9

[39] James M L, Lehman M, Hider P N, Jeffery M, Francis D P and Hickey B E 2008 Fraction size in radiation treatment for breast conservation in early breast cancer *Cochrane Database Syst. Rev.* **18** CD003860

[40] Ishihara T, Yoden E, Konishi K, Nagase N, Yoshida K, Kurebayashi J, Sonoo H, Murashima N, Sasaki R and Hiratsuka J 2014 Long-term outcome of hypofractionated radiotherapy to the whole breast of Japanese women after breast-conserving surgery *Breast Cancer* **21** 40–6

[41] Meattini I *et al* 2015 Accelerated partial breast irradiation using intensity-modulated radiotherapy technique compared to whole breast irradiation for patients aged 70 years or older: subgroup analysis from a randomized phase 3 trial *Breast Cancer Res. Treat.* **153** 539–47

[42] Olivotto I A *et al* 2013 Interim cosmetic and toxicity results from RAPID: a randomized trial of accelerated partial breast irradiation using three-dimensional conformal external beam radiation therapy *J. Clin. Oncol.* **31** 4038–45

[43] Liss A L, Ben-David M A, Jagsi R, Hayman J A, Griffith K A, Moran J M, Marsh R B and Pierce L J 2014 Decline of cosmetic outcomes following accelerated partial breast irradiation using intensity modulated radiation therapy: results of a single-institution prospective clinical trial *Int. J. Radiat. Oncol. Biol. Phys.* **89** 96–102

[44] Mast M E, van Kempen-Harteveld L, Heijenbrok M W, Kalidien Y, Rozema H, Jansen W P, Petoukhova A L and Struikmans H 2013 Left-sided breast cancer radiotherapy with and without breath-hold: does IMRT reduce the cardiac dose even further? *Radiother. Oncol.* **108** 248–53

IOP Publishing

Intensity Modulated Radiation Therapy

A clinical overview
Indra J Das, Nicholas J Sanfilippo, Antonella Fogliata and Luca Cozzi

Chapter 18

Prostate cancer

18.1 Epidemiology

Prostate cancer is second only to skin cancer as the most common cancer in men in the United States with approximately 180 890 new cases and 26 120 deaths per year according to the American Cancer Society [1]. This corresponds to a lifetime risk of about 1 in 7 American men developing the disease over their lifetime. Risk of death from the disease, however, is approximately 1 in 39, and there are an estimated 2.9 million men alive with prostate cancer in the United States [1]. The etiology of prostate cancer is largely unknown. Established risk factors include advancing age, race of African or Caribbean ancestry, and family history of the disease [2]. There are certain genetic changes such as BRCA1 and BRCA2, which may increase risk for prostate cancer [3]. Men with Lynch Syndrome, which is caused by inherited genetic changes, increases risk for several cancers including prostate cancer [3]. Diet and obesity are somewhat controversial as risk factors. Some have suggested that high intake of vegetables and lower fat intake may reduce prostate cancer risk [4]. A population based study of obesity, as defined by body mass index, found it was associated with a more aggressive from of prostate cancer, but only in Caucasians and not in African-Americans [5]. Other factors such as chronic prostate inflammation, sexually transmitted diseases, and vasectomy, are even more controversial with conflicting data on their role in the development of prostate cancer [3].

18.2 Anatomy

The prostate gland is a walnut sized structure located in the pelvis under the urinary bladder and in front of the rectum [6]. Its normal role is to secrete fluid that nourishes and protects the sperm. These secretory cells represent the major cell type in the gland and are androgen dependent for growth [7]. Early anatomists described the prostate in terms of lobes even though in adult males these are not readily discernible. In the late 1980s, McNeal and colleagues described the concept of anatomic zones rather than lobes, which is more widely recognized to describe prostate cancer development [8].

doi:10.1088/978-0-7503-1335-3ch18

There are four major zones within the normal prostate a shown in figure 18.1: the peripheral zone (70% of glandular tissue), the central zone (20% of glandular tissue), the transition zone (75% of glandular tissue), and the anterior fibromuscular stroma. The peripheral zone is the most common site for prostate cancer to develop and extends postero-laterally around the gland from the apex to the base. The transition zone, which is centrally located and makes up the majority of the base of the gland, often represents the location of benign prostatic hypertrophy. Some have suggested that transition zone tumors are less aggressive but others suggest no difference when accounting for stage of disease [9, 10].

Prostate lymphatic drainage consists of a periprostatic subcapsular network, from which three groups of ducts originate: (1) the ascending ducts from the cranial prostate draining into the external iliac lymph nodes; (2) the lateral ducts running to the hypo-gastric lymph nodes and (3) the posterior ducts draining from the caudal prostate to the sub-aortic sacral lymph nodes of the promontory [11]. Internal, external iliac and obturator lymph nodes are the most frequently involved by prostate carcinoma while metastases to pre-sacral and common iliac lymph nodes are rare.

18.3 Prostate cancer: general considerations

Management of prostate cancer, as in other tumors, depends on a number of factors. These include patient factors such as age and co-morbid conditions as well as tumor related factors such as PSA level, Gleason score, and clinical stage. Clinicians will generally assign patients to one of three risk categories (low, intermediate, or high) based on risk of recurrence after definitive local therapy. The National Comprehensive Cancer Network (NCCN), for example, utilizes a

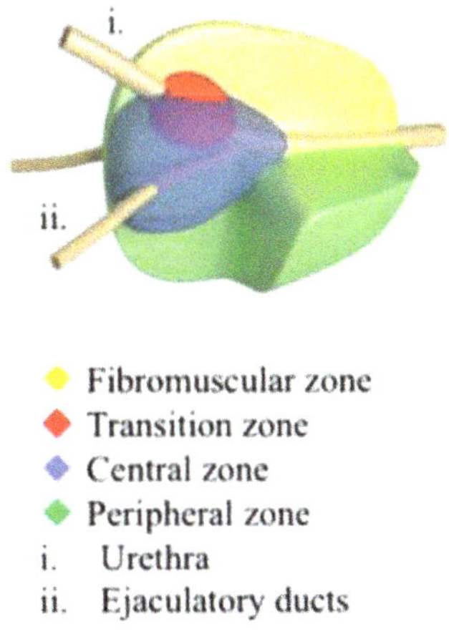

Figure 18.1. Prostate gland zonal anatomy. Reproduced from [12]. Open access CC BY 4.0.

system that incorporates PSA level, Gleason score, and clinical stage [13]. Risk group stratification may differ slightly from institution to institution, but generally allows for more refined treatment options than if using stage alone [14]. By NCCN criteria, low risk patients have a PSA < 10 ng/dL; Gleason sum or $\leqslant$ 6; and clinical stage of T1c–T2a which indicates small volume disease. Intermediate risk patients have PSA 10–20 or Gleason sum = 7 or clinical stage T2b–T2c, which is organ confined but of high volume. High risk patients have PSA > 20 or clinical T3 disease or Gleason sum $\geqslant$8. There is heterogeneity within groups, particularly the intermediate risk group, which may result in unexpected treatment outcomes. For example, Reese and colleagues evaluated over 12 000 men with prostate cancer and found that for men deemed intermediate risk, the ten year biochemical disease free survival was significantly greater for men assigned to the this group due to clinical stage (88.8%) than for those assigned by Gleason score (73.6%) or prostate-specific antigen (PSA) level (79.5%; $p = 0.01$). The authors advised that within-group heterogeneity must be taken into account when considering treatment options for individual patients.

The diagnostic evaluation of newly diagnosed prostate cancer includes a digital rectal examination, pathologic evaluation of Gleason score, PSA level, and assessment of life expectancy. In patients with low risk disease and limited life expectancy, for example, definitive treatment need not be undertaken in all cases, and often no further diagnostic evaluation is done. However, in cases where life expectancy is greater than ten years, an evaluation of local and/or systemic disease is performed. NCCN guidelines suggest and pelvic CT or MRI scan in cases where there is clinical suspicion on DRE and extra-prostatic disease is present or in cases of Gleason score 8–10 or Gleason sum of seven with PSA greater than 15 [15]. Recent advances in MRI have improved diagnostic accuracy not only for evaluating features such as extra-capsular disease, but also to facilitate and improve the accuracy of biopsy [16]. For these reasons, MRI is commonly used in the diagnostic evaluation of patients with prostate cancer. An example of prostate MRI is shown in figure 18.2.

For evaluation of systemic disease, bone scan is the most common test due to the proclivity of this disease to develop osseous metastases. However, the routine use of this study is controversial: The American Urological Association (AUA) and European Urologic Association (EUA) recommend bone scan in patients with localized disease only if PSA is >20 ng dL^{-1} [17, 18]. The NCCN, by contrast, recommends bone scan be obtained if PSA > 20 but also if PSA >10 with T2 disease or any case with Gleason sum $\geqslant$8 or T3/T4 disease. In a study comparing these methods, Chong found that the AUA/EUA criteria were superior for detecting bone metastases [19]. Still, there is no broad consensus and clinicians make these decisions on a case by case basis with all of these criteria in mind. After staging, patients with localized disease have a number of management options, which include surveillance, radical prostatectomy, external beam radiation therapy, brachytherapy, and emerging strategies with focal ablation.

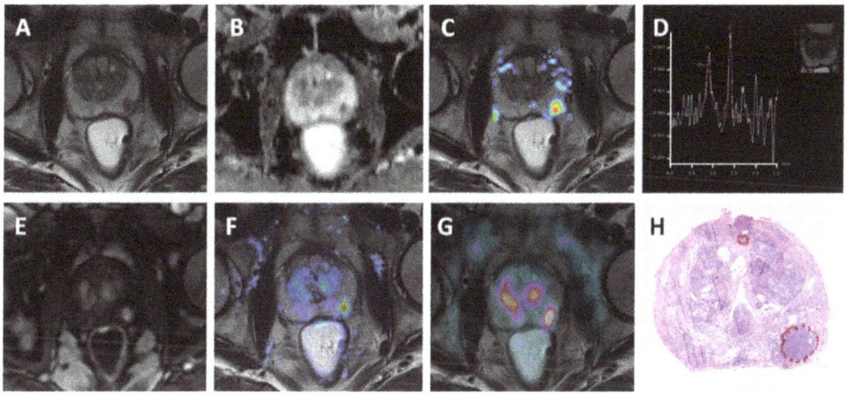

Figure 18.2. MP [11C]Acetate PET-MRI performed in a 68-year-old patient with an elevated prostate-specific antigen (PSA) level (5.3 ng ml^{-1}) at the time of imaging. (a) Axial 3 mm thick T2w image (TR/TE/TI 4000/101/230 ms) of the middle third of the prostate. The observers described a focal hypointense lesion in the left peripheral zone (T2w-positive). (b) On the ADC map, the lesion presents as a focal area with low signal intensity, with corresponding high signal intensity on b800s/mm2 images (DWI-positive). (c) and (d) 1H-MRSI shows an elevated choline/citrate ratio in the suspicious region (1H-MRSI-positive). (e) and (f) The DCE-MRI shows a focal contrast enhancement for the suspicious area (e—T1w image 80 s post contrast, f—Ktrans map overlaid on T2w image) (DCE-positive). (g) [11C]Acetate PET-MRI shows a focal tracer hotspot in this area with a maximal SUV 6.5 (PET positive). Multiparametric [11C]Acetate PET-MRI was rated true-positive in this patient. (h) Histopathological work-up after RPE confirmed a high-grade PCa Gleason 9 (5+4) tumor. Reproduced from [20]. Open access CC BY 4.0.

It is beyond the scope of this text to examine all of these approaches in detail. Briefly, cases that are more favorable and indolent on the disease spectrum are more suitable for surveillance strategies as it offers the patient the chance to avoid side effects until the disease is more clinically concerning. In men with advanced age or significant medical problems, treatment may be avoided indefinitely since these other medical problems may have greater impact on survival than their prostate cancer and patients can avoid treatment related side effects completely. Conservative management also requires some level of patient compliance for follow-up visits and psychological commitment since they are living with their cancer as opposed to having definitive treatment. This approach appears to be safe in large studies: Bul and colleagues examined the outcome of 221 patients with low or intermediate risk prostate cancer who initially deferred radical treatment [21]. The ten year disease specific survival rates were 99% and 96% for low and intermediate risk cases, respectively. Radical prostatectomy is also a highly effective treatment in well selected patients. In a meta-analysis of patients who underwent robotic assisted laparoscopic prostatectomy (RALP) with five year minimum follow up, Wang observed that the five year biochemical relapse free survival rate and cause specific survival rate were 80% and 97%, respectively [22]. Thus, with appropriate patient selection, extremely different management options, namely surveillance or radical surgery, can both yield excellent results.

18.4 Prostate cancer IMRT

As with most solid tumors, the interest in more focused radiation for prostate cancer comes from a desire to escalate dose to the tumor while avoiding side effects from excessive exposure to adjacent organs. Indeed, the most notable difference in the radiotherapeutic management of prostate cancer over the last several decades has been dose escalation. In a historic study by Bagshaw, results of 1119 patients treated between 1956 and 1990 by medium energy linear accelerators at Stanford University were reported [23]. The authors reported that doses of 70 Gy in seven weeks appeared to be safe and effective, with 15 year survival rates of 50% to those with localized disease to 18% in cases with extensive disease. These results obviously cannot be compared to modern series since most were diagnosed before PSA screening and advanced imaging for staging. In all likelihood, these patients had much more advanced disease than was detectable at the time. Still, the authors concluded that more desirable outcomes could be achieved with higher radiation dose and suggested integrated external beam RT with interstitial RT or hyperthermia. Multiple studies using a variety of techniques have shown that biochemical outcome can be improved with dose escalation. Zeitman and collegaues conducted a prosepective randomized trial of 393 men where dose was escalated from 70.2 Gy to 79.2 Gy equivalents (patients received a combination of x-ray therapy and proton beam therapy) [24]. Biochemical failure, as defined by the American Society of Therapeutic Radiology and Oncology was reduced from 32.4% to 16.7% with the higher dose. Kuban and associates from the MD Anderson Cancer Center similarly found improved outcome with dose escalation [25]. In this study, 301 patients with T1b-T3a prostate cancer were randomly assigned to 70 Gy versus 78 Gy with the initial pelvis volume of 46 Gy done with 4-field box arrangement and the boost done with 6-field conformal technique. With median follow up of 7.8 years, the overall failure free rate was 78% for the 78 Gy arm and 50% for the 70 Gy arm ($p = 0.04$). Gastrointestinal toxicity, however, was greater in the high-dose arm (26% versus 13%). As these large data sets demonstrated improved outcome with radiation doses of 78–80 Gy, efforts to reduce toxicity became increasingly important, and thus paved the way for IMRT for prostate cancer.

Several studies in medical dosimetry have demonstrated improved dose distribution of IMRT over 3DCRT: De Meerleer and colleagues examined CT data on 32 consecutive patients planned with 3DCRT and IMRT to determine which technique allowed for superior dose escalation while keeping the anterior rectal wall to 72 Gy and found that a lower volume of rectum received doses in the 40–65 Gy range with IMRT and the V65 was 37.9% for IMRT and 47% for 3DCRT [26]. Figure 18.3 illustrates dosimetry plans for 3DCRT versus IMRT.

The difference is perhaps more dramatic when clinicians are treating pelvis lymph nodes. Nutting and associates examined ten CT plans in patients with prostate cancer with elective pelvic nodal irradiation to a dose of 50 Gy [27]. The small bowel and colon dose was 18.3 for 3DCRT and for 9-field IMRT it was 5.3 ($p < 0.001$ compared to 3DCRT). The authors also investigated different IMRT plans and found that for seven, five, and three IMRT fields, bowel dose was 6.4%, 7.2%, and

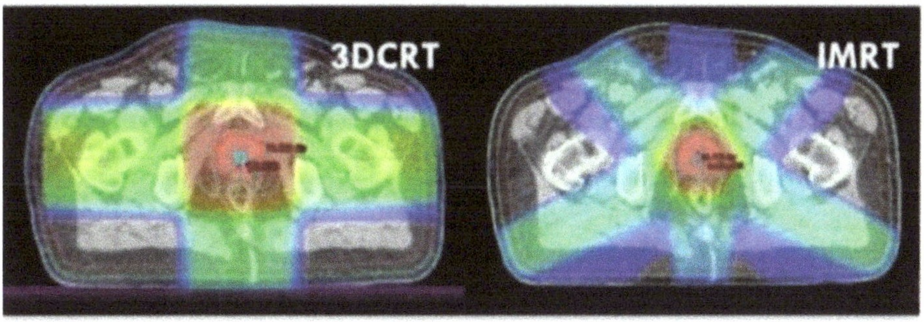

Figure 18.3. Left: Treatment plan for 3DCRT (2 cm PTV margin). Right: Treatment plan for fixed-angle IMRT (5–7 mm PTV margin). Reproduced from [28]. Copyright 2014 Sveistrup *et al.* Open access CC BY 2.0.

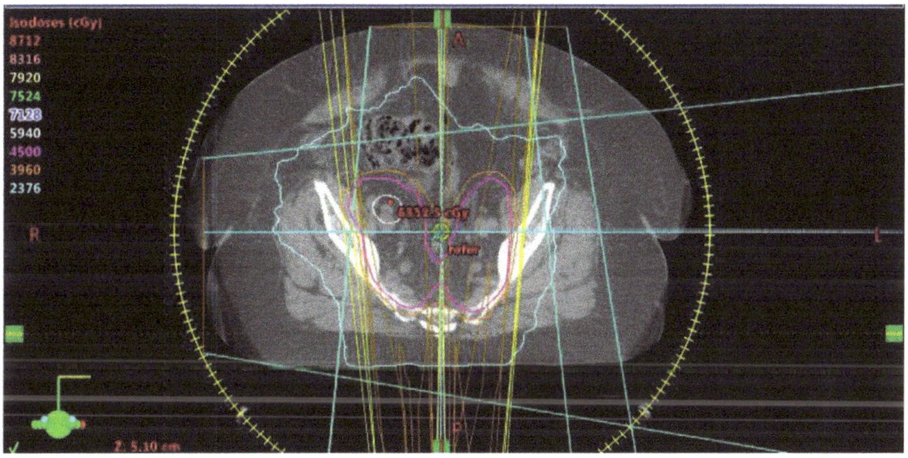

Figure 18.4. Axial image of prostate cancer patient with enlarged pelvic lymph nodes receiving IMRT (VMAT). The bilateral internal and external iliac nodes are receiving 45 Gy (magenta isodose line) while the pathologically enlarged node is receiving greater than 59.4 Gy (white isodose line). The bowel located anteriorly is receiving between 23.7 Gy and 39.6 Gy as noted by the orange and blue isodose lines, respectively. Courtesy of Nicholas J Sanfilippo, M.D., New York University School of Medicine.

8.4%, respectively,which were significantly better than 3DCRT plans ($p < 0.01$). The rectal V45 was reduced from 50.5% for 3DCRT to 5.8 by 9-field IMRT ($p < 0.\ 001$) and bladder from 52.2% to 7% ($p < 0.001$). Indications for elective pelvic irradiation, which is defined as irradiation of nodal stations without any visible disease on imaging, have been controversial and randomized studies do not support its routine use [29]. However, in cases where there are pathologically enlarged nodes on imaging, studies have shown a benefit to radiation therapy in addition to hormonal therapy [30] and IMRT may better allow clinicians to deliver adequate doses while limiting risk of complications, namely related to small and large bowel. Figure 18.4

illustrates a plan for a patient with enlarged pelvic lymph nodes being treated with definitive IMRT. The dose to the enlarged nodes in these cases can typically be escalated to 59–65 Gy while keeping bowel doses to acceptable limits while the prostate can be treated to total dose of 75–80 Gy.

Investigations of IMRT have also shown reduction in bladder dose. DePalma and colleagues conducted an investigation of 10 patients planned for 3DCRT, IMRT, or volumetric modulated arc therapy with either constant dose rate (cdr-VMAT) or variable dose rate (vdr-VMAT) to a total dose (prostate only) to 74 Gy [31]. The bladder 40 was 55% for 3DCRT, 27% for IMRT, 29% for cdr-VMAT, and 26% for vdr-VMAT. The vdr-VMAT resulted in generally more favorable dose plans than IMRT or cdr-VMAT with fewer monitor units required. The dose directive used at NYULMC for prostate cancer patients for IMRT planning is shown in table 18.1, which reflects accepted tolerances for normal structures.

While these dosimteric studies have shown the capacity of IMRT to reduce dose to normal organs, it is still important to examine if these benefits 'on paper' actually translate into reduced side effects for patients. Fortunately, there are clinical data available to shed light on this issue. In a prospective trial from The Netherlands, Al-Mamgani reported on patients randomly assigned to 68 Gy or 78 Gy and treated with either 3DCRT or IMRT [32]. The randomization was for radiation dose (68 Gy versus 78 Gy) and not technique (3DCRT versus IMRT). Thus, this study represented a subset analysis of 78 patients treated in the high-dose arm (37 with 3DCRT, and 41 with IMRT). Patients treated with IMRT experienced significantly less acute grade 2 or greater GI toxicity than 3DCRT (20% versus 61%, $p = 0.001$). IMRT also appeared to reduce late grade 2 or greater GI toxicity (21% vs 37% at 5 years) although this was not statistically significant, likely due to small sample size. A large retrospective study by Zelefsky reported similar clinical benefits with IMRT [33]. This study compared outcomes of 1571 patients treated with 3DCRT to doses of 66–81 Gy to those treated to 81 Gy with IMRT. Despite being treated to a higher dose, patients treated with IMRT experienced less grade 2 or greater GI side effects (13% versus 5%, $p < 0.01$). Genitourinary toxicity, however, was higher in the IMRT group (37% versus 22%, $p < 0.01$). This may be due to the higher total dose and that fact that the bladder neck and prostatic urethra, which are often responsible for these complications, must receive the entire dose regardless of technique.

From a practical standpoint, IMRT has supplanted 3DCRT in the clinical management of prostate cancer with RT [34]. However, other modalities such as proton beam therapy and variations of IMRT with stereotactic body radiation therapy have become more widely available, and considerable controversy exists as to which method is superior. Proton beam therapy, with its Bragg Peak, has the potential for further reduction in toxicity and/or dose escalation, as shown in figure 18.5.

However, claims based studies have cast doubt on this assumption. Sheets and colleagues from the University of North Carolina examined data from the Surveillance, Epidemiology, and End Results (SEER) program of Medicare from 2000 to 2009 on patients with prostate cancer treated with 3d-RT, IMRT, or proton therapy [34]. In a propensity score-matched comparison between IMRT and proton

Table 18.1. NYULMC IMRT/VMAT planning directive for prostate cancer treatment. Courtesy of Nicholas J Sanfilippo, M.D., New York University School of Medicine.

Treatment planning directive: prostate IMRT & VMAT			
Structure	Parameter	Constraint	Comments
	Targets		
PTV (total Rx)	$V_{100\%\ of\ Rx}$	⩾ 95% of PTV	Ideally, 98% covered by prescription dose
	$V_{98\%\ of\ Rx}$	⩾ 98% of PTV	
	D_{min}	⩾ 93% of Rx	
	D_{max}	< 110% of Rx	
PTV (initial phase)	$V_{100\%\ of\ Rx\ (initial\ phase\ Rx)}$	⩾ 95% of PTV	
CTV	$D_{98\%\ of\ CTV}$	⩾ 100% of Rx	
	Normal structures		
Bladder	$D_{15\%}$	< 8000 cGy	
	$D_{25\%}$	< 7500 cGy	
	$D_{35\%}$	< 7000 cGy	
	$D_{50\%}$	< 6500 cGy	
	D_{max}	< 105% of Rx	
Rectum	$D_{15\%}$	< 7500 cGy	
	$D_{25\%}$	< 7000 cGy	
	$D_{35\%}$	< 6500 cGy	
	$D_{50\%}$	< 6000 cGy	
	D_{max}	< 105% of Rx	
Femoral head/neck	$V_{4500cGy}$	< 25% of each	
	D_{max}	< 5400 cGy	
Penile bulb	Dmean	< 5250 cGy	
Small/large bowel	$V_{4000cGy}$	< 70%	
	D_{max}	⩽4500 cGy	
Body	D_{max}	⩽110%	

Guide to Abbreviations: D_{min} = minimum dose received by a structure, D_{max} = maximum dose received by a structure, $D_{x\%}$ = Dose received by x% of volume [cGy or as a % of prescription], Rx = prescription dose, Vx = Volume of structure receiving greater than or equal to x dose [% or c.c.].

therapy (n = 1368), IMRT patients had a lower rate of gastrointestinal morbidity (absolute risk, 12.2 versus 17.8 per 100 person-years). There were no significant differences in rates of other morbidities or additional therapies between IMRT and proton therapy. Yu and associates performed a similar study looking only at IMRT and proton beam therapy in patients treated in 2008 and 2009 [35]. The investigators

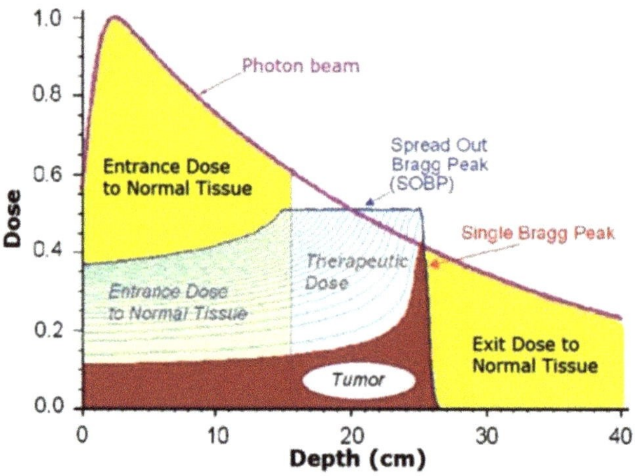

Figure 18.5. Radiation dose profiles: photons versus protons. Photon radiation enters the body and deposits dose along the entirety of the beam path. Dose delivery is maximal just below the skin surface and continues until exiting the body. Proton radiation delivers the majority of its dose at the end of its range, a phenomenon termed a Bragg peak. Passively scattered proton radiation requires a spread out Bragg peak to cover the entire target volume, increasing dose at the skin surface. Notable in this figure is the relative decrease in entry dose compared to photons and the lack of any dose distal to the tumor with proton treatment. Dose as a ratio of maximum dose in represented on the y-axis. Depth of penetration into the patient is represented in centimeters on the x-axis. A tumor is depicted from 17 to 24 centimeters. Reproduced from [36]. Open access CC BY-NC 3.0.

found proton therapy resulted in less genitourinary side effects at 6 months (5.9% versus 9.5%, $p = 0.03$) but no difference at 12 months. They also found no difference in any other toxicity at 6 or 12 months. The authors concluded proton beam therapy added substantial cost to the treatment program but no significant benefit to the toxicity profile.

Hypo-fractionation for prostate cancer has become more popular for prostate cancer out of an interest to reduce the overall treatment from more than 40 sessions with conventionally fractionated IMRT to schedules of 20 sessions or even as short as five treatment sessions with SBRT. The rationale for hypo-fractionation is based on radio-biologic theory that prostate cancer cells may respond greater to higher doses fraction while adjacent normal tissues do not [37]. In a prospective randomized study from the United Kingdom, Dearnaley and colleagues reported non-inferiority of using 60 Gy in 20 fractions compared with 74 Gy in 37 fractions [38]. Comparable levels of biochemical control were observed in the two groups as were overall long term complications. However, short term gastrointestinal morbidity was increased in the hypo-fractionation arm (figure 18.6).

Still, the investigators have recommended 60 Gy in 20 fractions as a new standard of care for prostate cancer as these differences resolved at longer follow-up. In an effort to further exploit any potential radio-biologic advantage, investigators have tested 5-fraction treatments with doses in excess of 7 Gy per fraction. King reported

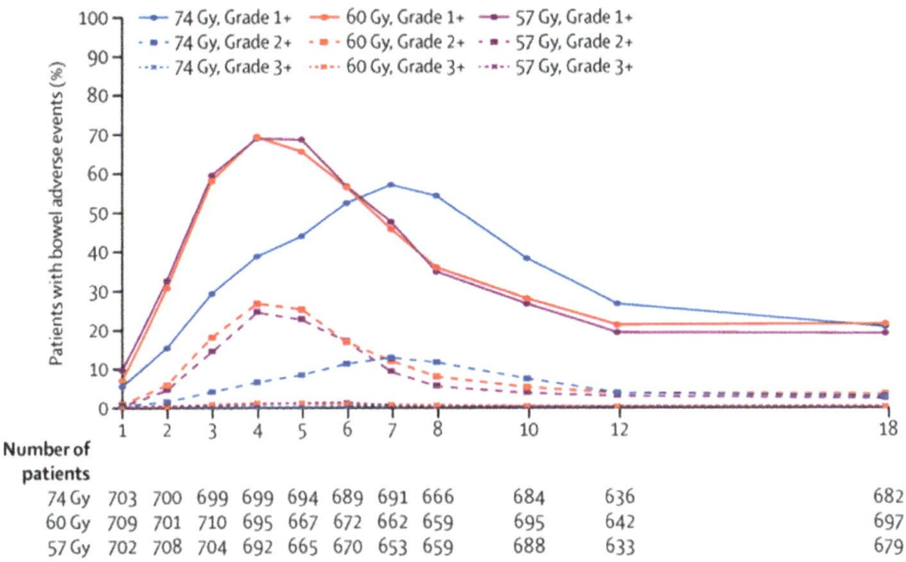

Figure 18.6. Acute bowel effects (radiation therapy oncology group toxicity grade) by time point (weeks). Reproduced from [38]. Copyright 2016 the authors. Open access CC BY 4.0.

on 1100 patients treated in eight institutions between 2003 and 2011 [39]. Most patients had either low (58%) or intermediate (30%) risk disease and were treated with 36.25 Gy in 4–5 fractions using the CyberKnife system. With a relatively short median follow up of 36 months, the five year biochemical relapse free survival rate was 93% for all patients and 95%, 84% and 81% for low-, intermediate- and high-risk patients, respectively ($p < 0.001$). Quality of life data were reported separately, but illustrated generally that patients returned to baseline function after an initial period.

However, as seen in the proton beam literature, claims based studies have suggested that when comparing SBRT to conventionally fractionated IMRT, some disadvantages to SBRT may exist. Yu and associates examined data from Medicare beneficiaries who received IMRT ($n = 2670$) or SBRT ($n = 1335$) between 2008 and 2011 [40]. They found that while SBRT was associated with lower cost, genitourinary toxicity at 24 months was significantly higher in the SBRT group (44% versus 36%, $p = 0.01$) and the increase in genitourinary toxicity was due to claims of urethritis, incontinence, and/or obstruction. Thus, as in other clinical situations, prospective randomized trials are needed to further examine these treatment strategies.

References

[1] http://cancer.org/cancer/prostatecancer/detailedguide/prostate-cancer-key-statistics

[2] Hsing A W and Chokkalingam A P 2006 Prostate cancer epidemiology *Front Biosci.* **1** 1388–413

[3] http://cancer.org/cancer/prostatecancer/detailedguide/prostate-cancer-risk-factors

[4] Cohen J H, Kristal A R and Stanford J L 2000 Fruit and vegetable intakes and prostate cancer risk *J. Natl Cancer Inst.* **92** 61–8

[5] Khan S, Cai J, Nielsen M E, Troester M A, Mohler J L, Fontham E T, Hendrix L H, Farnan L, Olshan A F and Bensen J T 2016 The association of diabetes and obesity with prostate cancer aggressiveness among Black Americans and White Americans in a population-based study *Cancer Causes Control* **27** 1475–85

[6] Oh W K, Hurwitz M and D'Amico A V *et al* 2003 Biology of prostate cancer *Holland-Frei Cancer Medicine* 6th edn ed D W Kufe, R E Pollock and R R Weichselbaum *et al* (Hamilton, ON: BC Decker)

[7] Isaacs J T 1983 Prostatic structure and function in relation to the etiology of prostatic cancer *Prostate* **4** 351–66

[8] McNeal J E, Redwine E A, Freiha F S and Stamey T A 1988 Zonal distribution of prostatic adenocarcinoma: Correlation with histologic pattern and direction of spread *Am. J. Surg. Pathol.* **12** 897–906

[9] Reissigl A, Pointner J and Strasser H *et al* 1997 Frequency and clinical significance of transition zone cancer in prostate cancer screening *Prostate* **30** 130–5

[10] Greene D R, Wheeler T M and Egawa S *et al* 1991 Relationship between clinical stage and histological zone of origin in early prostate cancer: morphometric analysis *Br. J. Urol.* **68** 499–509

[11] Cellini N, Luzi S, Mantini G, Mattiucci G C, Morganti A G, Digesù C, Bavasso A, Deodato F, Smaniotto D and Valentini V 2003 Lymphatic drainage and CTV in carcinoma of the prostate *Rays* **28** 337–41

[12] Theophilou G, Lima K M G, Briggs M, Martin-Hirsch P L, Stringfellow H F and Martin F L 2015 A biospectroscopic analysis of human prostate tissue obtained from different time periods points to a trans-generational alteration in spectral phenotype *Sci. Rep.* **13** 465

[13] https://nccn.org/professionals/physician_gls/pdf/prostate.pdf

[14] D'Amico A V *et al* 2002 15 Biochemical outcome after radical prostatectomy or external beam radiation therapy for patients with clinically localized prostate carcinoma in the prostate specific antigen era *Cancer* **95** 281–6

[15] https://nccn.org/professionals/physician_gls/pdf/prostate.pdf

[16] Shaish H, Taneja S S and Rosenkrantz A B 2017 Prostate MR imaging: an update *Radiol. Clin. North Am.* **55** 303–20

[17] Heidenreich A *et al* 2011 EAU guidelines on prostate cancer. Part 1: screening, diagnosis, and treatment of clinically localised disease *Eur Urol.* **59** 61–71

[18] Greene K L *et al* 2009 Prostate specific antigen best practice statement: 2009 update *J Urol.* **182** 2232–41

[19] Chong A *et al* 2014 Application of bone scans for prostate cancer staging: which guideline shows better result? *Can. Urol. Assoc. J.* **8** E515–9

[20] Polanec S H *et al* 2017 Multiparametric [11C] Acetate positron emission tomography-magnetic resonance imaging in the assessment and staging of prostate cancer *PLoS One* **12** e0180790

[21] Bul M, van den Bergh R C, Zhu X, Rannikko A, Vasarainen H, Bangma C H, Schröder F H and Roobol M J 2012 Outcomes of initially expectantly managed patients with low or intermediate risk screen-detected localized prostate cancer *BJU Int.* **110** 1672–77

[22] Wang L, Wang B, Ai Q, Zhang Y, Lv X, Li H, Ma X and Zhang X 2017 Long-term cancer control outcomes of robot-assisted radical prostatectomy for prostate cancer treatment: a meta-analysis *Int. Urol. Nephrol.* **49** 995–1005

[23] Bagshaw M A, Kaplan I D and Cox R C 1993 Prostate cancer. Radiation therapy for localized disease *Cancer* **71** 939–52

[24] Zietman A L *et al* 2010 Randomized trial comparing conventional-dose with high-dose conformal radiation therapy in early-stage adenocarcinoma of the prostate: long-term results from proton radiation oncology group/american college of radiology 95-09 *J. Clin. Oncol.* **28** 1106–111

[25] Kuban D A, Tucker S L, Dong L, Starkschall G, Huang E H, Cheung M R, Lee A K and Pollack A 2008 Long-term results of the M. D. Anderson randomized dose-escalation trial for prostate cancer *Int. J. Radiat. Oncol. Biol. Phys.* **70** 67–74

[26] De Meerleer G O, Vakaet L A, De Gersem W R, De Wagter C, De Naeyer B, De and Neve W 2000 Radiotherapy of prostate cancer with or without intensity modulated beams: a planning comparison *Int. J. Radiat. Oncol. Biol. Phys.* **47** 639–48

[27] Nutting C M, Convery D J, Cosgrove V P, Rowbottom C, Padhani A R, Webb S and Dearnaley D P 2000 Reduction of small and large bowel irradiation using an optimized intensity-modulated pelvic radiotherapy technique in patients with prostate cancer *Int. J. Radiat. Oncol. Biol. Phys.* **48** 649–56

[28] Sveistrup J *et al* 2014 Improvement in toxicity in high risk prostate cancer patients treated with image-guided intensity-modulated radiotherapy compared to 3D conformal radiotherapy without daily image guidance *Radiat. Oncol.* **2014** 44

[29] Asbell S O, Krall J M, Pilepich M V, Baerwald H, Sause W T, Hanks G E and Perez C A 1988 Elective pelvic irradiation in stage A2, B carcinoma of the prostate: analysis of RTOG 77-06 *Int. J. Radiat. Oncol. Biol. Phys.* **15** 1307–16

[30] Lin C C, Gray P J, Jemal A and Efstathiou J A 2015 Androgen deprivation with or without radiation therapy for clinically node-positive prostate cancer *J. Natl. Cancer Inst.* **107** djv119

[31] Palma D, Vollans E, James K, Nakano S, Moiseenko V, Shaffer R, McKenzie M, Morris J and Otto K 2008 Volumetric modulated arc therapy for delivery of prostate radiotherapy: comparison with intensity-modulated radiotherapy and three-dimensional conformal radiotherapy *Int. J. Radiat. Oncol. Biol. Phys.* **72** 996–1001

[32] Al-Mamgani A, Heemsbergen W D, Peeters S T and Lebesque J V 2009 Role of intensity-modulated radiotherapy in reducing toxicity in dose escalation for localized prostate cancer *Int. J. Radiat. Oncol. Biol. Phys.* **73** 685–91

[33] Zelefsky M J, Levin E J, Hunt M, Yamada Y, Shippy A M, Jackson A and Amols H I 2008 Incidence of late rectal and urinary toxicities after three-dimensional conformal radiotherapy and intensity-modulated radiotherapy for localized prostate cancer *Int. J. Radiat. Oncol. Biol. Phys.* **70** 1124–29

[34] Sheets N C *et al* 2012 Intensity-modulated radiation therapy, proton therapy, or conformal radiation therapy and morbidity and disease control in localized prostate cancer *JAMA* **307** 1611–620

[35] Yu J B, Soulos P R, Herrin J, Cramer L D, Potosky A L, Roberts K B and Gross C P 2013 Proton versus intensity-modulated radiotherapy for prostate cancer: patterns of care and early toxicity *J. Natl. Cancer Inst.* **105** 25–32

[36] Cotter S E, McBride S M and Yock T I 2012 Proton radiotherapy for solid tumors of childhood *Technol. Cancer Res. Treat.* **11** 267–78

[37] Thames H D, Bentzen S M, Turesson I, Overgaard M and Van den Bogaert W 1990 Time-dose factors in radiotherapy: a review of the human data *Radiother. Oncol.* **19** 219–35

[38] Dearnaley D *et al* 2016 Conventional versus hypofractionated high-dose intensity-modulated radiotherapy for prostate cancer: 5 year outcomes of the randomized, non-inferiority, phase 3 CHHiP trial *Lancet Oncol.* **17** 1047–60

[39] King C R *et al* 2013 Stereotactic body radiotherapy for localized prostate cancer: pooled analysis from a multi-institutional consortium of prospective phase II trials *Radiother. Oncol.* **109** 217–21

[40] Yu J B, Cramer L D, Herrin J, Soulos P R, Potosky A L and Gross C P 2014 Stereotactic body radiation therapy versus intensity-modulated radiation therapy for prostate cancer: comparison of toxicity *J. Clin. Oncol.* **32** 1195–201

IOP Publishing

Intensity Modulated Radiation Therapy
A clinical overview
Indra J Das, Nicholas J Sanfilippo, Antonella Fogliata and Luca Cozzi

Chapter 19

Cervical cancer

19.1 Epidemiology

Cancer of the uterine cervix is the fourth most common female cancer and fourth most common cause of death from cancer in women worldwide with approximately 528 000 cases and 266 000 deaths worldwide in 2012 [1]. Infection with human papilloma virus (HPV) is the primary risk factor with types 16 and 18 accounting for approximately 75% of cases and types 31 and 45 for an additional 10% globally [2]. Smoking is the second leading risk factor, primarily through the development of cervical intraepithelial neoplasia type 3 (CIN 3), even in women who are not affected by HPV [3]. In addition, heavy smokers who are infected with HPV have a greater likelihood of contracting cervical cancer than non-smokers [4]. Thus it appears smoking can directly and indirectly increase risk for development of cervical cancer. Oral contraceptive use is associated with increased risk of cervical cancer development in a time dependent fashion: women who have used oral contraception for 5–9 years have an approximately three-fold higher incidence of the disease, and those with greater than ten years of oral contraceptive use have a four-fold higher incidence [5]. Multiple pregnancies are also associated with higher risk of cervical cancer development. Among HPV positive women, those with greater than or equal to seven full term pregnancies have a four-fold risk of being diagnosed with cervical cancer compared to women with no pregnancy history and two to three times the risk of women who have one or two pregnancies [5].

19.2 Cervical cancer: general considerations

Cervical cancer can present with a variety of signs and symptoms. Since the majority are caused by infection with HPV, vaccination against the high risk strains of the virus can prevent the vast majority of cases [6]. Vaccination is typically done at a young age (9–26 years) since it is important to vaccinate prior to infection. The duration of activity of the vaccine is not entirely clear, but is believed to be effective for 5–10 years [7]. The cost of the vaccine is an area of concern, particularly in less developed countries. Early pre-cancerous lesions may have no symptoms at all and can be discovered as part of routine screening with the Papanicoloau test, or PAP smear. It is generally recommended that women undergo PAP test every 3 to 5 years with adequate follow-up and that up to 80% of invasive cervical cancer cases can be prevented in this way [8]. As with vaccination, screening with PAP tests is also challenging in developing countries. According the World Health Organization, this is due to under-developed health care infrastructure with a paucity of workers trained to execute and interpret these tests in a timely fashion [9].

In patients with cervical cancer at presentation, the most common presenting symptom is bleeding after sexual intercourse. Other symptoms may include pain with intercourse, pelvic pain, or symptoms related to metastases, such as bone pain when osseous metastases are present. Confirmation of a diagnosis of cervical cancer, like other solid tumors, is through biopsy. Several methods can be used to obtain tissue for diagnosis including punch forceps, brushing, or electrocautery. Following tissue diagnosis, the extent of disease is then determined through physical examination and imaging. Cervical cancer staging system is done in accordance with rules of the International Federation of Obstetrics and Gynecology (FIGO) and only certain tests are allowed for determination of stage: palpation, inspection, colposcopy, endocervical curettage, hysteroscopy, proctoscopy, intravenous urography, cervical conization, and plain x-ray examination of the lungs and cytoskeleton. This does not mean more advanced imaging studies, such as CT, MRI, or PET-CT scan are not done in cervical cancer to guide treatment. An example of PET-CT for cervical cancer is shown in figure 19.1.

However, these advanced tests, do not influence the FIGO stage. For example, if a patient based on FIGO criteria had small tumor disease localized to the cervix and a negative chest x-ray, a FIGO stage of IB could be assigned. However, if the same patient underwent a PET scan which showed small lung nodules too small to see on x-ray, she would still have IB disease per FIGO rules. However, she would not be managed with definitive local therapy such as surgery or radiation since lung metastases were present. Thus, the FIGO stage does not always guide treatment due to its limitations.

Treatment of cervical cancer varies based on a variety of factors including access to surgeons with skill in radical pelvic surgery, access to radiation therapy treatment facilities, and even institutional, clinician, or patient preferences. Generally, tumors limited to the cervix or proximal vagina that are less than 4 cm (FIGO stages IA, IB1 or IIA) may be managed with surgery. In these cases, adjuvant radiation or chemoradiation may be recommended for adverse pathologic features such as involved lymph nodes, parametrial involvement, or positive surgical margins. More advanced cases, such as those with clinical parametrial, pelvic sidewall or bladder or rectal involvement are typically managed with radiation and concurrent cisplatin based chemotherapy.

Radiation has had a curative role in the curative management of cervical cancer for many decades. A key technical method for successful disease control is the integration of external beam therapy and intracavitary brachytherapy. These two techniques work in a complimentary fashion since brachytherapy cannot adequately

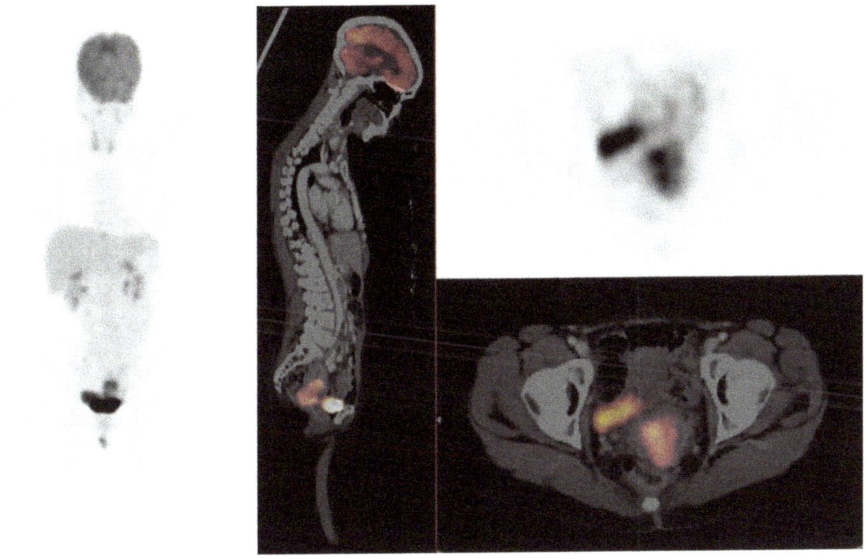

Figure 19.1. FDG-PET/CT images of a 46-year-old HIV-infected female referred for imaging with stage IIB squamous cell carcinoma of the cervix (SUVmax = 13.06, SUVmean = 4.22, MTV = 186.66, and TLG = 787.77). (a) Coronal PET, (b) sagittal fused PET/CT, (c) axial PET and (d) axial fused PET/CT images show disease localized to the cervix with no distant metastasis. Reproduced from [10]. Open access CC BY 4.0.

treat disease in lymph nodes or at the pelvic sidewall while external RT is unlikely to provide sufficient dose to eradicate the primary tumor in many cases. Therefore, treatment usually commences with external RT to the whole pelvis with the intent of eradicating micro-metastatic disease throughout the pelvis and simultaneously shrinking the primary tumor so that an effective intracavitary implant can be performed. Although specific dose schedules vary from institution to institution, patients are usually treated with external RT to doses of 40–45 Gy prior to brachytherapy. This will reduce the size of the primary tumor so that effective implant geometry can be accomplished. Patients then undergo a series of intracavitary brachytherapy treatments, often four or five, so as to provide a curative dose to the primary tumor. Brachytherapy can be done with low dose rate (LDR) or high dose rate (HDR) systems, but most centers in the United States utilize high dose rate brachytherapy (figure 19.2). Both methods are effective but HDR allows for outpatient delivery, reduction of exposure to staff, and temporary maneuvers such as rectal retraction which can be done easily for treatment that last 15–30 min but would be difficult for LDR treatments that may last for a few days.

19.3 IMRT for cervical cancer

Radiotherapeutic management of cervical cancer, while effective, carries both acute and long term side effects. IMRT is therefore being tested and, as in other tumors, early studies focused on dosimetric advantages for both tumor coverage and dose to normal structures: Chan and colleageus examined dosimetry plans of 12 patients

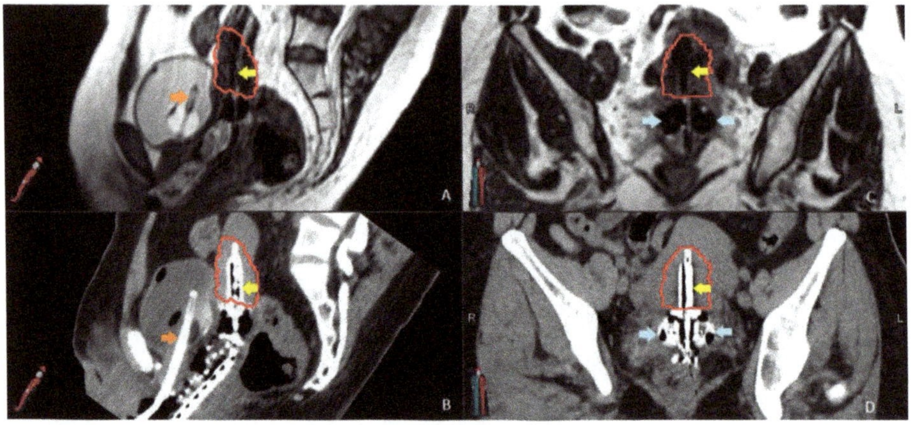

Figure 19.2. HDR brachytherapy for cervical cancer. Reproduced from [11]. Open access CC BY 3.0.

with gynecologic tumors (eight cervical, two endometrial, and two vaginal) [12]. Dose conformity was significantly improved with IMRT versus conformal technique. Specifically, the volume of rectum in the high dose volume (>66% of the prescription) was reduced by 22% ($p < 0.001$) with IMRT relative to conformal RT and bladder volume was reduced by 19% ($p < 0.001$). This was at the expense of an increase in the volume of these organs receiving low doses (<33% of prescription dose). Whether or not this difference in dose distribution provides the clinical benefit of reduced toxicity is a subject of debate. However, a recent randomized trial has shed some light on the issue. Naik and colleagues performed a randomized trial where 40 patients with intact-uterus cervical cancer were randomly assigned to IMRT or 3DCRT [13]. All patients received external RT with concurrent cisplatin which was followed by three brachytherapy treatments of 7 Gy each. Conformal and IMRT plans were done for all patients and all were followed for acute toxicity. Results showed that both techniques achieved planning target volume coverage, but mean conformity index was significantly better in IMRT plans ($p = 0.001$). Dose to 35% volume (D35) and D50 for bladder was reduced by 14.62% and 32.57% and for rectum by 23.82% and 43.68% with IMRT. In addition, V45 (volume receiving 45 Gy) of bowel was significantly lower ($p = 0.0001$), non-tumor integral dose was significantly higher ($p = 0.0240$) and V20 of bone marrow was found significantly reduced (p-value = 0.019) in IMRT cases compared to 3DCRT. More importanty, clinical outcomes were also improved. There was significant reduction of grade 2 or higher (20% versus 45%; $p = 0.058$) and grade ⩾3 (5% versus 15%, $p = 0.004$) acute genitourinary toxicity and grade 2 or more (20% versus 45%, $p = 0.003$) and grade ⩾3 (5% versus 20%, $p = 0.004$) acute gastrointestinal toxicity. No significant difference for grade 2 and 3 or more hematological toxicity was observed in patients treated with IMRT compared to 3D conformal radiotherapy. In recent years, the routine use of IMRT for intact-uterus cervical cancer has been controversial. However, data such as these which demonstrate clinical benefit will likely support

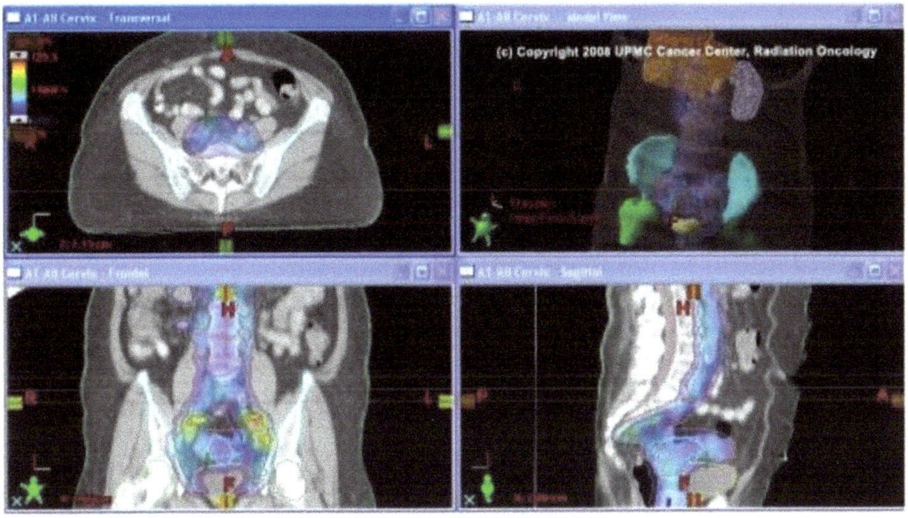

Figure 19.3. Extended-Field IMRT plan for Cervical Cancer. Note color wash radiation distribution and integrated boost treating the pathologically positive pelvic lymph nodes. Reproduced from [14]. Open access CC BY-SA 3.0.

greater utilization of this technology. An example of IMRT dose distribution is shown in figure 19.3.

Consensus is building on the use of IMRT in the post-operative setting and in cases where there is bulky pelvic sidewall disease or if para-aortic nodes are being treated [15]. Internal organ motion and associated target delineation are areas of concern that are being investigated. The routine use of IMRT for intact-uterus cervical cancer should be used cautiously and ideally in the setting of a clinical trial.

References

[1] World Cancer Report 2014 (World Health Organization)

[2] Dillman R 2009 *Principles of Cancer Biotherapy* 5th edn ed R K Oldham (Dordrecht: Springer)

[3] Agorastos T, Miliaras D, Lambropoulos A F, Chrisafi S, Kotsis A, Manthos A and Bontis J 2005 Detection and typing of human papillomavirus DNA in uterine cervices with coexistent grade I and grade III intraepithelial neoplasia: biologic progression or independent lesions? *Eur. J. Obstet. Gynecol. Reprod. Biol* **121** 99–103

[4] Jensen K E, Schmiedel S, Frederiksen K, Norrild B, Iftner T and Kjær S 2005 Risk for cervical intraepithelial neoplasia grade 3 or worse in relation to smoking among women with persistent human papillomavirus infection *Cancer Epidemiol. Biomark. Prevent.* **21** 1949–55

[5] National Institutes of Health 12/17/2015 *National Cancer Institute: PDQ® Cervical Cancer Prevention* (Bethesda, MD: National Cancer Institute)

[6] Tran N P, Hung C F, Roden R and Wu T C 2014 Control of HPV infection and related cancer through vaccination *Recent Results Cancer Res.* **193** 149–71

[7] Harper D, Gall S, Naud P, Quint W, Dubin G and Jenkins D *et al* 2008 Sustained immunogenicity and high efficacy against HPV 16/18 related cervical neoplasia: Long-term follow up through 6.4 years in women vaccinated with Cervarix (GSK's HPV-16/18 AS04 candidate vaccine) *Gynecol. Oncol.* 158–9

[8] Arbyn M, Anttila A, Jordan J, Ronco G, Schenck U, Segnan N, Wiener H, Herbert A and von Karsa L 2010 European guidelines for quality assurance in cervical cancer screening. Second Edition—Summary Document *Ann. Oncol.* **21** 448–58

[9] World Health Organization 2014 *Comprehensive Cervical Cancer Control. A Guide to Essential Practice* 2nd edn (Geneva: World Health Organization)

[10] Lawal I O *et al* 2019 Fluorodeoxyglucose Positron Emission Tomography integrated with computed tomography in carcinoma of the cervix: its impact on accurate staging and the predictive role of its metabolic parameters *PLoS One* **14** e0215412

[11] Asher D *et al* 2018 Magnetic resonance-guided external beam radiation and brachytherapy for a patient with intact cervical cancer *Cureus* **10** e2577

[12] Chan P, Yeo I, Perkins G, Fyles A and Milosevic M 2006 Dosimetric comparison of intensity-modulated, conformal, and four-field pelvic radiotherapy boost plans for gynecologic cancer: a retrospective planning study *Radiat Oncol.* **1** 13

[13] Naik A, Gurjar O P, Gupta K L, Singh K, Nag P and Bhandari V 2016 Comparison of dosimetric parameters and acute toxicity of intensity-modulated and three-dimensional radiotherapy in patients with cervix carcinoma: A randomized prospective study *Cancer Radiother.* **20** 370–6

[14] Heron D E, Shogan J E and Mucenski J W 2008 Innovations in chemotherapy and radiation therapy: Implications and opportunities for the Asia-Pacific Rim *Biomed. Imag. Interv. J.* **4** e40

[15] Loiselle C and Koh W J 2010 The emerging use of IMRT for treatment of cervical cancer *J. Natl Compr. Canc. Netw.* **8** 1425–34

Chapter 20

Summary and outlook

This book has provided the nuts and bolts of the IMRT process from the beginning of its evolution to its current state. Now, nearly 60%–80% curative cases of radiation therapy use this technology. In very complex cases and cases of retreatment where OAR dose could be detrimental to the patient, IMRT is a solution. In general, one can paint the dose as desired like an artist who has medical knowledge. A lot is happening in the industry, as every vendor is now providing automated plans based on *a priori* knowledge of the class and types of patients planned. These plans have various names such as smart plans, rapid plans, knowledge based plans, etc. Still, the complexities of the IMRT process require human efforts in planning and plan verification. However, there is a lot more to be achieved in future.

The success of IMRT has to be evaluated in terms of better survival and reduced toxicity. Over the last 30 years, IMRT has gained a place in radiation oncology in fulfilling the outcome goals as shown in various disease sites. IMRT outcomes in prostate cancer [1, 2], nasopharynx [3, 4], oropharynx [5], lung cancer [6, 7], rectum [8] and breast cancer [9–11] are shown to be superior to 3DCRT and are now accepted in most complex cases.

20.1 Plan automation, adaptive therapy and artificial intelligence: A glance into the crystal ball

The entire process of 'radiotherapy' has become significantly more challenging over the past few years than in the early days of 3DCRT that was developed in the 1990s. The advances in the delivery devices with all the flavors of intensity modulation techniques and the increased complexity of the input data (from multi-modality imaging to the choice of optimization strategies) require an advanced level of management and sophisticated skills. The process of automating the treatment planning in radiotherapy aims, among its most important objectives, for harmonization (i.e. the reduction of the inter-patient variance) and improved quality (i.e. the search for the optimal solution of the inverse planning problem).

doi:10.1088/978-0-7503-1335-3ch20

At the same time, the increase in the patient's burden and the often-limited resources in clinics are in conflict with the quest for individualized treatments. The increase of productivity and the alignment of the planning outcome, irrespective of the resources or the skills of the operators, are relevant drivers for automation as IMRT is generally time consuming [12].

All of these elements coincide with the aim of providing top-class treatments under all types of conditions related to patients/treatments and workload/resources available in clinics.

The practical solutions to the problem of automation might be grouped into two major categories: (i) use of artificial intelligence (AI) to perform the task of plan optimization and (ii) the implementation of (semi)-automated class solutions for specific treatment techniques/cases. Both of the main groups can be further divided into several sub-branches.

The research conducted by several groups led to the commercial and research-based implementation of planning automation engines widely used in the practice. Knowledge-based planning, protocol-based automatic iterative optimization, and multi-criteria optimization are the main 'names' associated with the different automated planning algorithms [13–17].

The core of the knowledge-based methods (KBP) consists of the development of mathematical models capable of predicting achievable dose-volumes and objective function constraints for new patients. The predictive models should be developed with training and validation out of libraries of good and representative cases from historical databases. The extraction of relevant features descriptive of the problem and valuable for prediction is the 'knowledge' component and is based on AI methods of learning. The models, once trained, can be applied to any new patient (of the same 'type') without any need to access the original data, making them portable and sharable. Some earlier attempts applied to cases were atlas-based algorithms, which optimize new cases by matching them to prior cases from atlases (requiring similarity criteria to be implemented) and transfer the planning rules inferred from the library to the current cases. The AI implementation of KBP planning included studies aiming to predict the entire curve of dose-volume histograms or more detailed dose-volume metrics. Some efforts were put also in the prediction of the dose maps at the voxel level [18].

An alternative approach consists in automatically exploring/navigating multiple alternative solutions with the addition of eventual sequential optimization (i.e. sequential achievement of planning objectives according to predefined priorities or wish-lists). A typical workflow could be realized by the means of a navigation system through a Pareto optimal front (identified through a large number of alternative plans, eventually in the hundreds, obtained by varying clinical goals and/or techniques of treatment). Human planners (or further AI-based robots) would then finally select the ideal plan by a critical assessment of the various trade-offs.

Another typical workflow consists of adding a pre-optimization phase based on lexicographic multi-criterial plan generation. For each individual patient, the automatic plan generation can be based on a fixed wish-list with hard and soft constraints with assigned priorities. The objectives would be sequentially optimized, generating at the end a Pareto-optimal solution without any need of further interaction. This method could allow for site-specific wish-lists adaptable to physicians' intentions on a case-by-case base.

The development of AI-based optimization will guide the automation of treatment planning in the near future. With our current computational power, it is possible that in the timescale of seconds, highly accurate, complex dose distributions can be 'determined' in a completely unsupervised manner. Similarly, the process is ongoing for the segmentation of the patient's anatomy. This is the actual basis for a huge 'dematerialization' of the treatment planning process with all the positive and negative aspects of it. On the positive side, we might just mention the possibility to effectively and routinely implement the old dream of adaptive treatments. From the negatives, there is the risk to delegate too much 'brain' to the machines. Our future will not be in opposing this but to ensure that enough 'knowledge' is modeled into the AI tools. This will also require adequate quality assurance and the preservation of some 'manual' instruments to continue the search for the unexplored and to teach the machines how to better serve the patients of tomorrow.

20.2 Decision-making artificial intelligence (AI) guided radiotherapy

Adaptive radiotherapy (ART) is the natural evolution of radiotherapy. It will encompass all the technological advancements of intensity modulation and automated planning with the ultimate goal of truly personalizing the treatment of each patient at each fraction [16].

ART will involve the possibility to alter an initial treatment plan (intent) according to the tumor or anatomical evolution/changes over the course of therapy in a cost/effective, time efficient, and safe manner.

The ultimate goal is to enable a simple and effective adaptive therapy workflow for both initial and daily re-planning. The key points of the process will require the identification of the best plan (based on geometry and dosimetry) in the initial planning and, on each treatment day, the possibility to re-optimize (adapt) a new plan from the initial set of target and OAR goals, given the daily anatomy.

The AI will guide this technology by offering (i) a decision tree throughout the entire adaptive process; (ii) a treatment planning and management ecosystem that is tightly coupled and context-aware; (iii) a plan engineered for high quality, high speed/throughput, and extreme safety.

In the future, the challenges that AI-guided technology will have to solve are:

i. The challenge of enabling the complete treatment planning optimization during the treatment fraction while the patient is on the treatment couch;
ii. The challenge of performing automated segmentation of the daily anatomy (on high quality images) and to identify the structures mostly influencing the plan adaptation workflow;
iii. The challenge of generating high quality adaptive plans with full inverse planning methods in a very amount of short time;
iv. The challenge of monitoring the delivered doses (i.e. dose accumulation) over the entire course of treatment.

References

[1] Sheets N C, Goldin G H and Meyer A-M *et al* 2012 Intensity-modulated radiation therapy, proton therapy, or conformal radiation therapy and morbidity and disease control in localized prostate cancer *JAMA* **307** 1611–20

[2] Pan H Y, Jiang J and Hoffman K E *et al* 2018 Comparative toxicities and cost of intensity-modulated radiotherapy, proton radiation, and stereotactic body radiotherapy among younger men with prostate cancer *J. Clin. Oncol.* **36** 1823–30

[3] Lee A W, Ng W T and Chan L L *et al* 2014 Evolution of treatment for nasopharyngeal cancer - Success and setback in the intensity-modulated radiotherapy era *Radiother. Oncol.* **110** 377–84

[4] Wu P, Zhao Y and Xiang L *et al* 2020 Management of chemotherapy for stage II nasopharyngeal carcinoma in the intensity-modulated radiotherapy era: a review *Cancer Manag. Res.* **12** 957–63

[5] Clavel S, Nguyen D H A and Fortin B *et al* 2012 Simultaneous integrated boost using intensity-modulated radiotherapy compared with conventional radiotherapy in patients treated With concurrent carboplatin and 5-fluorouracil for locally advanced oropharyngeal carcinoma *Int. J. Radiat. Oncol. Biol. Phys.* **82** 582–9

[6] Appel S, Bar J and Ben-Nun A *et al* 2019 Comparative effectiveness of intensity modulated radiation therapy to 3-dimensional conformal radiation in locally advanced lung cancer: pathological and clinical outcomes *Br. J. Radiol.* **92** 20180960

[7] Shirvani S M, Juloori A and Allen P K *et al* 2013 Comparison of 2 common radiation therapy techniques for definitive treatment of small cell lung cancer *Int. J. Radiat. Oncol. Biol. Phys.* **87** 139–47

[8] Ng S Y, Colborn K L and Cambridge L *et al* 2016 Acute toxicity with intensity modulated radiotherapy versus 3-dimensional conformal radiotherapy during preoperative chemo-radiation for locally advanced rectal cancer *Radiother. Oncol.* **121** 252–7

[9] Freedman G M, Anderson P R and Li J *et al* 2006 Intensity modulated radiation therapy (IMRT) decreases acute skin toxicity for women receiving radiation for breast cancer *Am. J. Clin. Oncol.* **29** 66–70

[10] Pignol J P, Olivotto I and Rakovitch E *et al* 2008 A multicenter randomized trial of breast intensity-modulated radiation therapy to reduce acute radiation dermatitis *J. Clin. Oncol.* **26** 2085–92

[11] Harsolia A, Kestin L and Grills I *et al* 2007 Intensity-modulated radiotherapy results in significant decrease in clinical toxicities compared with conventional wedge-based breast radiotherapy *Int. J. Radiat. Oncol. Biol. Phys.* **68** 1375–80

[12] Das I J, Moskvin V and Johnstone P A 2009 Analysis of treatment planning time among systems and planners for intensity-modulated radiation therapy *J. Am. Coll. Radiol.* **6** 514–7

[13] Zhang X, Wang X and Dong L *et al* 2006 A sensitivity-guided algorithm for automated determination of IMRT objective function parameters *Med. Phys.* **33** 2935–44

[14] Yan H, Yin F F and Guan H Q *et al* 2003 AI-guided parameter optimization in inverse treatment planning *Phys. Med. Biol.* **48** 3565–80

[15] Ge Y and Wu Q J 2019 Knowledge-based planning for intensity-modulated radiation therapy: A review of data-driven approaches *Med. Phys.* **46** 2760–75

[16] Archambault Y, Boylan C and Bullock D *et al* 2020 Making on-line adaptive radiotherapy possible using artificial intelligence and machine learning for efficient daily re-planning *Med. Phys. Int.* **8** 77–86
[17] Cozzi L, Heimen B J M and Muren L P 2019 Advanced treatment planning strategies to enhance quality and efficiency of radiotherapy *Phys. Imag. Radiat. Oncol.* **11** 69–70
[18] Shen C, Nguyen D and Chen L *et al* 2020 Operating a treatment planning system using a deep-reinforcement learning-based virtual treatment planner for prostate cancer intensity-modulated radiation therapy treatment planning *Med. Phys.* **47** 2329–36

www.ingramcontent.com/pod-product-compliance
Ingram Content Group UK Ltd.
Pitfield, Milton Keynes, MK11 3LW, UK
UKHW051905100926
8556IPUK00005B/765

9 780750 313360